HELPING BEREAVED CHILDREN
A Handbook for Practitioners

THIRD EDITION

Edited by
Nancy Boyd Webb

Foreword by Kenneth J. Doka

THE GUILFORD PRESS
New York   London

© 2010 The Guilford Press
A Division of Guilford Publications, Inc.
72 Spring Street, New York, NY 10012
www.guilford.com

Printed in the United States of America

This book is printed on acid-free paper.

Last digit is print number: 9 8 7 6 5 4 3 2 1

Library of Congress Cataloging-in-Publication Data is available
from the publisher.

ISBN: 978-1-60623-597-3

HELPING BEREAVED CHILDREN

*To my husband, children, and grandchildren
for their love, support, and promise for the future*

About the Editor

Nancy Boyd Webb, DSW, BCD, RPT-S, a board-certified diplomate in clinical social work and a registered play therapy supervisor, is a leading authority on play therapy with children who have experienced loss and traumatic bereavement. Her bestselling books are considered essential references for clinical courses and for agencies that work with children. These include *Play Therapy with Children in Crisis* (3rd edition): *Individual, Group, and Family Treatment, Culturally Diverse Parent–Child and Family Relationships: A Guide for Social Workers and Other Practitioners, Working with Traumatized Youth in Child Welfare, Mass Trauma and Violence: Helping Families and Children Cope, Social Work Practice with Children* (2nd edition), and *Helping Children and Adolescents with Chronic and Serious Medical Conditions: A Strengths-Based Approach.* In addition, she has published widely in professional journals and produced a video, *Techniques of Play Therapy: A Clinical Demonstration,* which won a bronze medal at the New York Film Festival's International Non-Broadcast Media Competition. Dr. Webb is the editor of The Guilford Press book series Social Work Practice with Children and Families; serves as a consulting editor for the *Journal of Child and Adolescent Trauma;* is on the editorial advisory board for the journal *Trauma and Loss: Research Interventions;* and is a past board member of the New York Association for Play Therapy.

Dr. Webb was a professor on the faculty of the Fordham University Graduate School of Social Service from 1979 until 2008, where she held the endowed James R. Dumpson Chair in Child Welfare Studies and was named University Distinguished Professor of Social Work in 1997. In 1985, she founded Fordham's Post-Master's Certificate Program in Child and Adolescent Therapy to meet the need in the New York metropolitan area for training in play therapy. In April 2000, she appeared as a panelist in a satellite teleconference, *Living with Grief: Children,*

Adolescents, and Loss, sponsored by the Hospice Foundation of America. Hosted by Cokie Roberts, the conference was beamed to more than 2,100 sites.

In addition to teaching, writing, and consulting, Dr. Webb supervises practitioners, trains child welfare workers, and consults with schools and agencies. She has given keynote presentations and conducted workshops throughout the United States, Canada, Australia, Europe, Hong Kong, and Taiwan on play therapy, social work, trauma, and bereavement.

Contributors

Patti Homan Anewalt, PhD, LPC, FT, is Director of the PATHways Center for Grief & Loss at Hospice of Lancaster County. Her clinical training, practice, writing, and teaching are focused on issues related to end of life, compassion fatigue, crisis, trauma, and loss, about which she presents regularly at the national, state, and local level. Dr. Anewalt is certified as a Fellow in Thanatology with the Association for Death Education and Counseling and chairs the Body of Knowledge Committee. She is active with the National Council of Hospice and Palliative Professionals and served two 3-year terms as section leader for the Bereavement Professionals Section. A disaster mental health specialist for the American Red Cross, Dr. Anewalt serves on several community crisis teams, providing training, debriefings, and support when local tragedies occur.

Jennifer Baggerly, PhD, LMHC-S, RPT-S, is Associate Professor in the Counselor Education Program at the University of South Florida and Director of the Graduate Certificate in Play Therapy. A board member of the Association for Play Therapy, Dr. Baggerly is a licensed mental health counselor supervisor, a registered play therapist supervisor, and a field traumatologist. Her research projects and publications focus on the effectiveness of play therapy with children who are homeless and counseling interventions for traumatized children, and she has given national and international presentations on these topics. Dr. Baggerly provided trauma interventions for children after the 2004 Florida hurricanes, the tsunami in Sri Lanka, and Hurricane Katrina.

Derek Brown, MSW, is an adjunct faculty member and doctoral student at Fordham University's Graduate School of Social Service. He has 10 years of social work experience, including direct and administrative services to homeless and formerly homeless women and people infected with HIV. Mr. Brown also served as a public servant for the city of Philadelphia, where he performed public health planning and research. His research interests include health disparities, oppression, and complementary and alternative medicines, including yoga therapy.

Roxia Bullock, PhD, LCSW, has taught master's-level courses on social work and served as Assistant Director of the Post-Master's Certificate Program in Child and Adolescent Therapy at Fordham University. She served many years as a counselor at the Department of Education in New York City. It was in this capacity, in an urban school setting and in her private practice, that she dealt with children experiencing the death of family members, including children. Dr. Bullock presently has a private practice in Ossining, New York.

Lois Carey, LCSW, RPT-S, is in private practice and offers Sandplay training and supervision through the Center for Sandplay Studies in Nyack, New York. Ms. Carey has presented Sandplay in many sites in the United States, Canada, England, Ireland, Switzerland, and South Africa. She has also authored and/or edited four books, as well as numerous articles and chapters in other books. She is an approved provider for the Association for Play Therapy.

David A. Crenshaw, PhD, ABPP, RPT-S, is founder of the Rhinebeck Child and Family Center, LLC, in Rhinebeck, New York. He is board certified in clinical psychology by the American Board of Professional Psychology and is a registered play therapist supervisor for the Association for Play Therapy. Dr. Crenshaw is the author of *Bereavement: Counseling the Grieving throughout the Life Cycle* and numerous book chapters and journal articles related to grief and trauma in children. He is also past president of the New York Association for Play Therapy (2004–2008).

Betty Davies, RN, CT, PhD, FAAN, is Professor and Senior Scholar, School of Nursing, University of Victoria, Canada, and Professor Emerita, Department of Family Health Care Nursing, University of California, San Francisco. She has conducted extensive research on sibling bereavement and has worked with bereaved siblings in group settings. Dr. Davies was one of the founders of Canuck Place, North America's first free-standing hospice in Vancouver, Canada, and developed its bereavement program. Her research resulted in numerous publications, including *Shadows in the Sun: Experiences of Sibling Bereavement in Childhood.* Her current research focuses on pediatric palliative care, including the needs of siblings. Past chair of the International Work Group on Death, Dying and Bereavement, she received the 2008 Distinguished Career Achievement Award from the Hospice and Palliative Nurses Association and the Canadian Nurses Association Centennial Award.

Kenneth J. Doka, PhD, is Professor of Gerontology at the Graduate School of The College of New Rochelle and Senior Consultant to the Hospice Foundation of America. A prolific author, Dr. Doka's 24 books include *Grief: Children and Adolescents*; *Children Mourning, Mourning Children*; and *Living with Grief: Children, Adolescents, and Loss.* He has also published over 100 articles and book chapters. Dr. Doka is editor of both *Omega: The Journal of Death and Dying* and *Journeys: A Newsletter to Help in Bereavement.* He was elected President of the Association for Death Education and Counseling in 1993 and served as chair of the International Work Group on Death, Dying and Bereavement from 1997 to 1999. Dr. Doka is an ordained Lutheran minister and a licensed mental health counselor.

Jennifer Lee, PhD, is a clinical psychologist in private practice specializing in the treatment of adolescents and families. She also serves as Adjunct Instructor at Marist College in Poughkeepsie, New York, where she teaches graduate students in mental health counseling. Her research focuses on mindfulness-based interventions, ethnic-minority identity development, and adolescent mental health. She has published scientific articles and book chapters on these topics.

Rana Limbo, PhD, RN, PMHCNS-BC, is Director of Bereavement and Advance Care Planning Services for Gundersen Lutheran Medical Foundation, Inc., in La Crosse, Wisconsin. She is one of the founders of the perinatal bereavement program Resolve Through Sharing.

Tina Maschi, PhD, LCSW, is Assistant Professor in the Graduate School of Social Service at Fordham University. She is also a licensed clinical social worker with extensive practice experience working with traumatized and bereaved youth and adults in correctional, school, and community mental health settings. She incorporates the use of creative arts in clinical practice as a tool to process grief and loss and facilitate empowerment. Dr. Maschi's community-based research projects include research on trauma and resilience among juvenile and criminal justice populations and the use of creative arts as a therapeutic intervention strategy.

Cynthia McCormack, LMSW, is a primary therapist at Rochester Mental Health Center, where she provides psychotherapy for adults. She also worked for 6 months in a community mental health center in Ridgewood, New Jersey, providing psychotherapy. Ms. McCormack has participated in the American Foundation for Suicide Prevention's Out of the Darkness Overnight Walk, and is a member of the National Association of Social Workers and the Association for Death Education and Counseling.

Sharon M. McMahon, RN, EdD, is Associate Professor on the Faculty of Nursing at the University of Windsor, Windsor, Ontario, Canada, where she is the Undergraduate Coordinator for the Faculty of Nursing. Dr. McMahon was the cofounder of the Companion Animal Visitation Programme and Pet Bereavement Support Services of Essex County, the first service agency of its kind funded by the United Way/Centraide in Canada beginning in the late 1980s. Her bereavement support of children began during her pediatric nursing practice over 40 years ago. Dr. McMahon's work has been published and presented to many peer-reviewed conferences and world gatherings on topics associated with the human–companion animal bond.

Kathleen Nader, DSW, is former Director of Evaluations for the Trauma, Violence, and Sudden Bereavement Program at the University of California, Los Angeles, and is currently Director of Two Suns, dedicated to assisting traumatized children and adolescents. Her work has included the provision of consultation, training, and specialized interventions following catastrophic events. In the United States, Europe, Australia, and the Middle East, she has trained psychologists, psychiatrists, social workers, and counselors in methods of screening and treating traumatized youth. She has written and coauthored a variety of publications, screening instruments, and videotapes on the assessment and treatment of trauma in youth and school interventions. Her publications include *Honoring Differences: Cultural Issues in the Treatment of Trauma and Loss* and *Understanding and Assessing Trauma in Children and Adolescents: Measures, Methods, and Youth in Context*, which addresses the many issues important to the assessment and treatment of children, especially after trauma.

Donna O'Toole, MA, is a counselor, author, trainer, and storyteller. She is Founding Director of Compassion Books, Inc., an international resource center distributing a variety of written and electronic materials related to loss and grief. She is a working member of the International Work Group on Death, Dying and Bereavement, and the winner of state and national awards for her written and training work in bereavement.

Priscilla A. Ruffin, RN, MS, NPP, is founding President and CEO of East End Hospice, a free-standing community-based interdisciplinary program for end-of-life care located in Westhampton Beach, New York. She is licensed as a nurse practitioner in psychiatry, specializing in emotional trauma, grief, and bereavement. Dr. Ruffin has established innovative programs for the treatment of grief in children and adults, and is cofounder, with Sarah A. Zimmerman, of Camp Good Grief, a day camp in Long Island, New York, for grieving children, now in its 14th year. She is also coauthor, with Sarah A. Zimmerman, of *Jeremy Goes to Camp Good Grief*, a book for grieving children, and *A Parent's Guide to Children's Grief*, a work in progress. She lectures extensively on topics of grief, bereavement, and end-of-life care in professional, academic, and community settings.

Alison Salloum, PhD, is Assistant Professor in the School of Social Work at the University of South Florida. She has extensive clinical experience working with children, adolescents, and families after violence and death. She is the author of *Group Work with Adolescents after Violent Death: A Manual for Practitioners* and *Reactions: A Workbook for Children Experiencing Grief and Trauma*. Based on her work in New Orleans and in partnership with the Children's Bureau of New Orleans, Dr. Salloum developed a grief and trauma intervention for children. Her research continues to focus on effective ways to help traumatized children and adolescents and their families.

Diane L. Scott, PhD, is Associate Professor in the School of Justice Studies and Social Work at the University of West Florida. Her research interests include program evaluation, service learning, domestic violence, and veteran issues. Dr. Scott's publications appear in the *Journal of Offender Rehabilitation, Journal of Social Welfare and Family Law, Journal of Policy Practice, Journal of Social Policy*, and the *American Journal of Criminal Justice*. Her practice experience primarily included work as a social worker for Department of Defense programs serving military personnel and their family members. She is also a military spouse and grew up in a military family.

Janine Shelby, PhD, is Assistant Professor in the Geffen School of Medicine at the University of California, Los Angeles, and Director of Child Psychology Training as well as the Child Trauma Clinic at Harbor–UCLA Medical Center. She has devoted her career to the study and treatment of young trauma survivors, having provided humanitarian relief work and consultation in more than a dozen countries. As a frequent presenter across North America and in numerous countries abroad, Dr. Shelby integrates empirical with clinical findings to provide research-based, practical suggestions for the treatment of young trauma survivors. She is the recipient of service awards from the American Red Cross and the Association for Play Therapy, and has served as the Association's Foundation President, consulting to both the National Child Traumatic Stress Network and Operation USA.

Patricia Van Horn, JD, PhD, is Associate Clinical Professor of Psychiatry at the University of California, San Francisco, and Associate Director of its Child Trauma Research Program. She is coauthor of *Losing a Parent to Death in the Early Years: Guidelines for the Treatment of Traumatic Bereavement in Infancy and Early Childhood*; *Don't Hit My Mommy!: A Manual of Child–Parent Psychotherapy with Young Witnesses of Family Violence*; and *Psychotherapy with Infants and Young Children: Repairing the Effects of Stress and Trauma on Early Attachment*.

Nancy Boyd Webb, DSW, BCD, RPT-S. See "About the Editor."

Sarah A. Zimmerman, LCSW-R, is Bereavement Coordinator at East End Hospice in Westhampton Beach, New York, where she developed the children's bereavement program. Ms. Zimmerman is cofounder, with Priscilla A. Ruffin, of Camp Good Grief, a bereavement day camp for children who have suffered a loss, and coauthor, with Priscilla A. Ruffin, of *Jeremy Goes to Camp Good Grief* as well as *A Parent's Guide to Children's Grief*. She has also developed a holiday coping program, now in its 14th year, and lectures to educators and civic groups on various aspects of trauma, grief, bereavement, and hospice care.

Foreword

When I was about 9 years old, an elder of my Lutheran church was waked in the church. I remember a few of us more adventuresome boys snuck in to see the body. Alone, without adult supervision, we dared each other to touch the corpse. We commented on the coldness and unnatural feel of the skin. I do not think any of us shared the experience with our parents, or, for that matter, any other adult. It was part of the code of silence that we all followed. This was not my first experience with death, however. My aunt had died 5 years earlier, and I had experienced the loss of some pets. But it was the first time I had ever seen or touched a dead body. Some years later, in the middle of adolescence, a group of us restrained one of our friends, heartbroken about a breakup with her boyfriend, from drowning herself in a dangerous river. Again, that event remained a secret unshared with the adults around us.

Adults like to think of childhood as a kingdom where nobody dies. But in our attempt to protect children from death, we are in fact only protecting ourselves. Children detect this discomfort about death in adults, and they then join in and perpetuate the code of silence about death.

As my opening remembrances remind us, children are no strangers to loss and death. They may experience the deaths of grandparents, neighbors, and pets. They may even experience the deaths of friends, parents, and siblings. In the graduate course on Children, Adolescents, Death, and Loss that I teach at The College of New Rochelle, I ask each student to recount his or her first death experience. Most experiences occur prior to the students' being 6 years old. Rarely has a student had a first encounter when he or she was older than 12. Even if children have never suffered a death, they are not strangers to loss. Many of them have had loss experiences, such as divorce, separation, or family relocation.

Children, then, do grieve. But their grief is often unrecognized and disenfranchised by others around them. They may be denied the opportunity to publicly mourn and to express their grief. With limited opportunities to understand their reactions to death or to receive support, their grief becomes manifest in indirect ways—sleep disturbances, physical complaints, acting-out behaviors, and regressive behaviors.

We need to find effective ways to help children deal with their grief. Yet helping grieving children is not easy. It is both difficult and different from helping adults cope with grief for a number of reasons. First, children do not usually have the opportunity to choose counseling. Their parents and guardians make that choice. This violation of the counseling contract—the assumption that the individual has reached out for assistance—is further complicated by the triangulated approaches to confidentiality that need to be negotiated between the child, counselor, and guardian.

Methods and approaches to helping grieving children have to be different as well. No phrase strikes more terror into the heart of many children than when an adult, especially an unknown adult, sits them in a room and says, "Let's talk." Children speak in their own language—a language of play, art, and story. This is why expressive methods are far better approaches for working with children. Yet these methods also have to be intentional and prescriptive. Different children will each have their own special modality. Counselors, therefore, need to be "eclectically expressive" when working with these children.

Children, too, are at different developmental levels. As they get older, they are developing cognitively, gaining a more mature and richer conception of the meanings of loss and death. Children develop in other ways as well. They grow in affect. Very young children may find it difficult to identify the emotions that they are experiencing. They may have a "short feeling span," unable to sustain strong emotions for long periods of time. Their sense of empathy develops as well. Young children tend to see loss only from their perspective, only responding to personal implications, while older children can see how the loss affects others, offering support even within the family system.

Children also grow spiritually. From the earliest ages, children explore questions of meaning ("Why did he have to die?"). At very young ages, children still may be exploring their beliefs, trying to figure out answers to their questions, attempting to make sense of the world. As they get older, they may develop spiritual constructs, beliefs that can be applied to various crises that they face.

So children are in a paradoxical situation. They do face death and loss. Yet it is not always easy to approach and assist them as they encounter loss.

That is one reason why the third edition of *Helping Bereaved Children* is so welcome. Nancy Boyd Webb brings four great gifts to the task. Two are personal. She is a superb and sensitive therapist who is a pioneer in play therapy. The third gift is that once again she has assembled a wonderful group of colleagues who contribute their own special expertise. The fourth gift is the very timeliness of this book. Dr. Webb is always willing to periodically revisit and to re-examine her work. While the earlier editions were contributions to the field, this new edition continues to add to our understanding of the experiences of the contemporary child. She has added chapters that deal with war-related deaths and the impact of terrorism and school violence on children. She expands on the modalities available to children, including groups and camps and innovative therapeutic approaches to help grieving children. She has also added a section that focuses on empowering children's natural support system—their parents and teachers. And therapists will especially find beneficial the updated and enriched appendix of resources.

In my reading, the book offers five contributions to the task of helping grieving children. First, it offers solid theory and concepts. This work is on the cutting edge of grief theory, incorporating insights such as the importance of retaining continuing bonds with the deceased, the value of narrative approaches, and the possibility of growth in loss. Dr. Webb continues to develop here one of her significant conceptual contributions, disabling grief. To Dr. Webb, one of the critical factors in assessing grief reactions is the degree to which these reactions are disabling—that is, how much they impair the individual's ability to function. This idea is a welcome alternative to fruitless debates about pathological grief.

A second contribution is the book's sensitivity to the world of the child. Children live in families and go to schools. The sensitivity of the school and the ability of the family to support the grieving child will be critical factors in the eventual outcome—the implication of the loss in the child's ongoing life. A third contribution is Dr. Webb's sensitivity to the needs of therapists, as noted in particular in the strengthened section on self-care and the prevention of secondary trauma.

A fourth contribution lies in the grounded methodologies and diverse modalities offered. As stated earlier, children are all different, and they will respond differently to varied methodologies: Some will prosper with art therapy; others will respond well to play; still others will benefit from the use of storytelling. There is no "one size fits all." Ultimately, readers will find an eclectic array of methodologies so that they may be intentional in prescribing the most effective approach for their young clients.

There is a final contribution: In her early remarks, Dr. Webb notes that students often want formulas—what to do in each situation and circumstance. She wisely notes that this is an impossible, and in fact dangerous, approach. There is no formula that can substitute for sensitivity and skill. But in the place of one standard formula she and the book's contributors offer much else—tools, case vignettes, and clear methodological approaches. This will do much to assisting those who wish to help bereaved children. Most important, though, the frequent use of methodological examples should spur the reader's creativity. And that is the book's greatest gift.

KENNETH J. DOKA, PhD
Professor of Gerontology, The College of New Rochelle
Senior Consultant, Hospice Foundation of America

Preface

At the end of the first decade of the 21st century, death continues to be a topic that adults avoid discussing with children. As if agreeing with the more than 75-year-old views of the poet Edna St. Vincent Millay that "childhood is the kingdom where nobody that matters dies" (1934/1969, p. 203), many adults try to shield children from the reality that *everyone* does die eventually. The rationale of avoiding the subject of death in order to protect children also keeps adults themselves from having to face this truth. It is ironic that despite the universality of death, few are comfortable talking about it, and the resulting silence shrouds the subject in even greater mystery and fear.

Millay's poetry has particular meaning for me, since she wrote some of her earlier works under the pseudonym Nancy Boyd. Furthermore, her father rented a room in my grandparents' home in Kingman, Maine, long before I was born. Millay, who was the first woman to receive the Pulitzer Prize for Poetry, was very intrigued about the topic of death, and many of her poems struggle to understand the meaning of loss. Although this book addresses practitioners who are working with bereaved children, sometimes the wisdom of creative artists can also offer evocative insights into profound topics such as death.

In the 8 years since the publication of the second edition, there has been an increased occurrence of widely publicized violent deaths in natural disasters, wars, and drug-associated killings. Furthermore, many men and women in the military have died in the wars in Iraq and Afghanistan, and their child relatives require both short- and long-term assistance with their bereavement. Schools and communities are now more aware of the need for specialized services for children following incidents of murder, bombings, natural disasters, and terrorist attacks. The second edition of this book contained several chapters dealing with traumatic death, and this third edition has expanded this focus by including new chapters on child bereavement following deaths in war and terrorist attacks, as well as sudden, violent deaths at schools. New content is also included on cognitive-behavioral therapy, parent–child relationship interventions, and bereavement camps. And all the chapters have all been revised to include updated literature and methods for helping bereaved children.

At the numerous conferences and workshops where I have presented in recent years, I have benefited from listening to questions from participants, learning first-hand from what they ask about how best to help bereaved children. This new edition reflects my enhanced awareness about the needs of clinical practitioners and counselors. It includes nine new chapters with topics not covered in previous editions. A dozen new chapter authors (and five new coauthors) have contributed their knowledge and expertise to this important project. In order to keep them in a unified format, all the chapters follow the same outline: detailed cases with actual recreated dialogue and a section on Discussion Questions and Role-Play Exercises in order to facilitate classroom and workshop interactions.

The book is divided into five major sections. As in previous editions, Part I presents the theoretical framework for understanding the child's views about death and for assessing the bereaved child. Chapter 2, on assessment of the bereaved child, includes several forms that can be used to record significant information about the child's background as well as particulars about the death situation and the family, social, and religious supports. Each death occurs in a context that affects survivors uniquely. Therefore, it is essential to consider this context thoroughly to understand the nature of the child's bereavement and the appropriate helping role of the therapist/counselor.

Part II focuses on deaths occurring in families, including a range of situations from the anticipated, timely death of a grandparent to sudden deaths of parents by suicide and war-related deaths. Included as well are chapters on sibling death and helping children following the death of a pet. Situations of disenfranchised bereavement indicate the complications associated with deaths that family members consider shameful. The treatment modalities in these various chapters reflect a range of interventions, including family therapy, individual play therapy, and groups for bereaved children.

Part III deals with deaths that have occurred in the community and when groups of schoolchildren have been affected by the shared loss of a peer, counselor, or teacher, or by random, violent deaths. The critical role of the media in possibly adding to traumatic aftereffects is discussed in Chapter 11. Several chapters demonstrate the need for multilevel interventions, including individual, small-group, and large-group approaches to helping bereaved children. As always, the age of the children and their unique personal histories affect their responses to death. Often school-based counselors must identify children who require individual follow-up and referral to mental health practitioners.

Part IV presents specific methods of intervention with bereaved children. These include parent–child relationship therapy, individual counseling and therapy, cognitive-behavioral therapy, play therapy, bereavement groups and camps for children, and the use of specialized methods of art therapy and storytelling.

The final section, Part V, focuses specifically on helping counselors, parents, and teachers. Chapter 17 deals with the importance of self-care for bereavement counselors, and Chapter 18 presents guidelines and suggested bibliographic resources for parents and teachers of bereaved children.

The Appendix lists numerous resources, including locations of training programs for play therapy, grief counseling, and trauma/crisis counseling. It also provides a list of references to different religious, cultural, and ethnic practices related to death.

This book serves two major groups of professionals who work and come into contact with bereaved children: those who are trained in the mental health fields of psychology, psychiatry, psychiatric nursing, and clinical social work, and those who are trained in counseling fields such as pastoral counseling and educational counseling. School-based personnel have extensive contact with children. They can provide bereavement counseling in the school and refer at-risk children to mental health specialists when the grief is traumatic or complicated. As discussed in the book, a timely referral places initial focus on the trauma in order to permit subsequent grief work.

The important "unfinished business" at the completion of this book involves the advisability of helping children *before* a death occurs. Preventive psychoeducational approaches are valid and should be offered in schools to help familiarize children with the concept of death and the types of responses that may help survivors. I would be very happy if this book leads to the routine inclusion of death education units at the elementary school level. We must not continue to act as if children should be excluded from experiences with death. More open discussion of the topic would serve as a primary prevention model to educate and prepare children before they have to deal with the pain of a loss. Death touches children's lives in many ways, and we must do everything we can to help them before, during, and after their inevitable death experiences.

NANCY BOYD WEBB

REFERENCE

Millay, E. S. V. (1969). Childhood is the kingdom where nobody dies. In *Edna St. Vincent Millay collected lyrics*. New York: Harper & Row. (Original work published 1934)

Acknowledgments

I knew that this book needed to be written when a former student with many years' post-MSW experience in hospice told me that as a father with young children, he could not bear the pain of working with bereaved children. With the publication of this edition, I hope that he and others who counsel bereaved families will now be more knowledgeable and comfortable when circumstances bring them into contact with a bereaved child.

As in the first and second editions, the evolution of this third edition depended heavily on the 20 chapter authors who contributed their rich practice and research experience in this field. My circle of personal and professional contacts has continued to widen in the course of seeking out and working with the skilled practitioners who have written about their direct interventions with bereaved children. I am grateful to them, as well as their child and adolescent clients, who proudly and eagerly agreed to share their counseling/therapy experiences for the benefit of others.

Jill Krementz was especially open and generous about permitting me to quote excerpts from her wonderful book *How It Feels When a Parent Dies*.

My own child clients and their families have also been open in granting me permission to write about our work together. I value the trust they have accorded me and hope they will take deserved pride in knowing that their experiences of loss can train therapists/counselors to help other bereaved children. Except for the examples noted otherwise, all the clinical cases have been disguised to protect the confidentiality of the children and their families. The situations and the dynamics are based on reality, but the identities of the individuals have been altered.

Time is a serious pressure in producing a book such as this. I especially appreciate the help and support of my husband, who has witnessed the full range of both the satisfactions and the difficulties entailed in such a project. He has helped in numerous ways, both substantive and logistically, always managing to buoy me up and move me ahead.

It has again been a pleasure to work with the editors at The Guilford Press. I would like to recognize both Seymour Weingarten, Editor-in-Chief, and Jim Nageotte, Senior Editor. Over the past 18 years of my association with The Guilford Press, I have been impressed and pleased by the high professional standards of the entire staff. I also thank all the dozens of individuals who have been involved in the production of this book. I hope that they will take pride in participating in this effort to break through the taboo surrounding the topic of children and death. Bereaved children *can* be helped, and this book is dedicated to that helping process.

Contents

PART I

INTRODUCTION

CHAPTER 1

The Child and Death

NANCY BOYD WEBB

A simple child
that lightly draws its breath
And feels its life in every limb
What should it know of death?
—WORDSWORTH
(1798/1928, pp. 74–75)

What, indeed, should any child know about death, and when should he or she know it, and by what means should he or she find out? The notion of childhood innocence as portrayed by the poet Wordsworth conveys the wish that children's knowledge about death could be avoided or postponed. Edna St. Vincent Millay said that "childhood is the kingdom where nobody dies" (1934/1969), and Becker refers to adults' "ever-present fear of death" (1973, p. 17). If adults cannot confront and make peace with their own fears about the end of life, how can they possibly help children understand these realities? Many adults refrain from discussing death with children because of their own anxiety about the subject. In addition, they may want to avoid distressing the child and having to respond to questions for which they have no answers. Many parents and other adults find it easier to talk to children about sex than about death. As in both Wordsworth's and Millay's eras, discussion about death today still represents a powerful taboo.

The above paragraph was written for the first edition of this book in 1991, and repeated in the second edition in 2002. In preparation for the publication of this current, third edition in 2009 we would hope that there would have been progression in the degree of openness in discussions with children about death. There have been numerous books published to help adults help children with this difficult topic, and certainly children's exposure to death has increased through hearing and seeing numerous reports of deaths in natural disasters, in accidents such as plane crashes, and in wars. Some children who live in dangerous, inner-city neighborhood know firsthand about drug-related killings. The contemporary child, through television, views hundreds of deaths, both real and fictionalized, in the daily course of watching cartoons, news, and General Audiences/Parental Guidance Suggested (G/PG-rated) dramatizations and movies. Images of all types of deaths make imprints on the minds and psyches of the watching children, but different children respond differently to what they see and hear. And many adults still prefer to avoid discussing death with children.

Does familiarity bring desensitization about death or easy acceptance of it? Obviously, children must take a huge leap from knowing that death occurs to strangers or fantasy creatures on television to awareness that it occurs to everyone, including their own family members, and that in real life, unlike on television cartoons, the dead person does not return.

CHILDREN'S PROGRESSION TOWARD MATURE UNDERSTANDING ABOUT DEATH

The necessary truth about death that we all eventually come to know is that it is irreversible, inevitable, and universal. Most children achieve this knowledge by approximately 7 or 8 years of age due to their normal cognitive development and life experience. Some may achieve a mature conception at younger ages (Wass & Stillion, 1988) if they have had experience with the death of an animal (Yalom, 1980), or if they have had early experience with the death of a family member (Kane, 1979). For most children, the natural evolution of their ability to think rationally leads gradually to a mature understanding about death.

Cognitive Development: From Immaturity to Conceptual Understanding

Although Jean Piaget's work did not focus on children's understanding about death, I have applied his theories concerning children's cognitive development to this topic. I focus on the three major developmental phases identified by Piaget and connect these with children's ideas about death in each phase.

The Young Child: Ages 2–7; Piaget's Preoperational Stage

According to Piaget, the preschooler tends toward magical thinking and egocentricity. He or she does not differentiate between thoughts and actions, and therefore a young boy of this age may believe, when his sister dies suddenly in an accident, that his anger toward her caused her death (see example in Kaplan & Joslin, 1993). The young child also cannot comprehend the irreversibility of death, and at this age may think that if he screams loudly enough he can awaken his deceased father, who he believes is sleeping (example in Saravay, 1991). Even when the young child has witnessed a burial he or she may not realize that the dead body in the casket no longer feels anything or performs its usual bodily functions. The child may wonder how the dead man can breathe with dirt on him, and how he will go to the bathroom (Fox, 1985). A child in the movie *My Girl* insisted on putting eye glasses on her deceased friend in the casket so that he could see!

These vignettes all relate to Piaget's *preoperational stage* (ages 2–7), during which the child's concrete (literal) thinking may distort reality to conform to his or her idiosyncratic understanding, despite contradictions. Piaget refers to this type of thinking as "egocentric," since the child believes that everyone else sees the world as he or she sees it.

The work of Maria Nagy (1948) continues to be widely quoted with regard to her study and identification of three stages in children's perceptions of death. Nagy's first stage (ages 3–5) corresponds roughly to Piaget's preoperational phase. Nagy found that children at this age deny that death is a final condition; they consider the state of death as temporary and reversible. Therefore, they wonder and may ask when their dead father is coming home, even though they viewed his body in the casket at the wake. In summary, the preschool child (ages 2–6) has the following ideas about death:

- Does not understand that death is final.
- Often believes that death is reversible or temporary.
- Believes in magical thinking and that wishes come true.
- May believe that something he or she did caused the death.
- May ask repeatedly about the whereabouts of the deceased person.
- May not show outward expected signs of grieving, except intermittently (because he or she expects the dead person to return).
- May be afraid that someone else may die (leading to regressive clinging).
- May be angry with the deceased, or with the surviving parent or sibling.

Before proceeding I caution against taking these age references too literally. Development is an individual process that proceeds generally as outlined, but—as with all matters human—individual variations are the rule. Furthermore, the lack of synchrony between ages in Nagy's and Piaget's stages should not cause serious concern. The main point is that development progresses gradually from immature to mature understanding about death, and it is unrealistic to expect a young child to have a mature understanding of death.

The Latency-Age (Elementary-School-Age) Child: Ages 7–11; Piaget's Concrete Operational Stage

Reduced egocentricity and improved capacity for reasoning contribute to the progressive realization among children of elementary school age that death is irreversible. Fox states that "latency youngsters begin to know that dead is dead and that at some time each of us will die. However, their own increasing sense of power and control make it difficult for them to believe such a thing could happen to *them*" (1985, p. 11; emphasis in original). Solnit, referring to this realization, states that "the concept that inevitably each of us has to die becomes a threatening, unpleasant, ineffable quality of the *future*. Most children *are able to lay aside this oppressive sense of inevitability,* denying the feel of it because it is so far off. . . . [The] juices of life and the joy of living help block out the fearful, painful conviction about death" (1983, p. 4; emphasis added). The elementary-school-age child's improved understanding of time permits this conceptualization about the "future" as a remote, distant expectation.

Piaget notes children's increased capacity for reasoning and the ability to organize sequentially and count backwards (subtract) during the period from 6 to 8 years (Piaget, 1955, 1972). The fact that children are learning to read and use language further signals their developing cognitive abilities.

This development not only facilitates mastery of reading, writing, and arithmetic but it also opens the child's thinking to more accurate comprehension of the mysteries of life and death. Whereas the concept of the body and the spirit confuses the preschool child, who cannot understand how the deceased can simultaneously be in heaven and in a grave at the cemetery (Saravay, 1991), children of 9 or 10 are able to dramatize a puppet play that expresses their wish to visit their parents in heaven, despite clearly knowing that they are buried in a cemetery (Bluestone, 1999).

The elementary-school-age child knows that death is final, and that it will happen to everybody "sometime." However, children of this age believe that death happens primarily to the elderly and weak, who cannot run fast enough to escape the pursuing "ghost, angel, or space creature" who will cause their death (Fox, 1985; Nagy, 1948); 6- to 8-year-olds therefore believe that young people their age usually do not die, because they can run fast! According to Lonetto, "death for the child from six to eight years old is personified, externalized, and can be avoided if seen in time. Death is not yet finalized; rather, it assumes various external forms (skeletons, ghosts, the death-man)" (1980, p. 100). The popularity of skeleton costumes at Halloween speaks to young people's fascination with death and their attempts to gain control over their fears about it. When children reach 9 or 10 years of age they may develop a more realistic understanding about death, although they still may have difficulty dealing with it. In summary, some typical responses of school-age children (6–12 years old) about death include the following:

- Inability to deal with death.
- May use denial to cope with the loss and may act like the death did not occur.
- May hide their feelings in an effort not to seem childish, and do their grieving in private (this is especially true for boys).
- May feel guilty and/or different from peers because of the death.
- May express anger or irritability rather than sadness.
- May overcompensate for feelings of grief by becoming overly helpful and caretaking of others (this is especially true for girls).
- May develop somatic symptoms or hypochondria.
- Anxiety may occur due to increased fear of death.

The Prepubertal Child: Ages 9–12;
Bordering on Piaget's Formal Operational Stage

"The mental development of the child appears as a succession of three great periods. Each of these extends the preceding period, reconstructs it on a new level, and later surpasses it to an ever greater degree" (Piaget & Inhelder, 1969, p. 152). Thus, as we consider Piaget's third and "final" stage of cognitive development, that of "formal operations," we note the building on preceding stages, in addition to the ultimate spurt into the complex arena of mature thought and understanding.

Piaget's stage of formal operations usually begins around age 11 or 12, when the youngster's thinking becomes truly logical, able to handle many variables at once, and capable of dealing with abstractions and hypotheses. Many authorities on the topic of children's understanding about death (Anthony, 1971; Grollman, 1967; Kastenbaum, 1967; Lonetto, 1980; Nagy, 1948; Wolfelt, 1983) believe that children acquire a realistic perception of the finality and irreversibility of death by age 9 or 10. Speece and Brent (1996), in an examination of more than 100 studies of children's understanding of death, conclude that by 7 years of age most children have achieved a mature understanding. This is quite a bit earlier than Piaget's designation of the inception of formal thought "around the age of eleven or twelve" (1968, p. 63). Yet perhaps it attests to the complexity of death itself—connecting both "concrete" elements, that is, a body that no longer functions (comprehensible to 7- and 8-year-olds), and the "abstract," that is, a notion of spirituality and life after death (understood by children older than 10). In Lonetto's (1980) study of children's drawings at different ages, an intriguing shift was found in the representation of death in abstract terms among 12-years-olds. They portrayed death with black crayon markings that they described as "darkness." Lonetto states that

> children from nine to twelve years old seem capable not only of perceiving death as biological, universal, and inevitable, but of coming to an appreciation of the abstract nature of death, and of describing the feelings generated by this quality. This complex recognition pattern associated with death is joined by an emerging belief in the mortality of the self, but for these children death is far off in the future and remains in the domain of the aged. (1980, p. 157)

As the prepubescent youth moves into adolescence, greater maturity in thinking can result in more complex responses. The bereaved young person:

- May feel helpless, frightened, or numb.
- May behave in a manner younger than his or her years (regression).
- May feel conflicted between the desire to behave in an adult manner and the wish to be taken care of as a child.
- May experience guilt about teen behaviors, which were a normal part of the individuating process, at the time of the death.
- May use anger to defend against feelings of helplessness.
- May respond in a self-centered or callous way.

CHILDREN'S EMOTIONAL RESPONSES TO DEATH

What is the implication of children's cognitive development on their ability to mourn the death of a loved one? Can children grieve, and, if so, how do they grieve? Is children's grieving different from that of adults? What factors other than the child's age and level of cognitive development impact on the nature of the child's emotional response to death? This chapter (and others in this book) explores these questions in detail after first defining and distinguishing between the concepts of "grief," "mourning," and "bereavement." Obviously, these terms all relate to loss following death, but they are not synonyms, even though the general public and some professionals use them interchangeably.

Bereavement

The term "bereavement" refers to the status of the individual who has suffered a loss and may be experiencing psychological, social, and physical stress because a meaningful person has died; the term does not, however, spell out the precise nature of that stress (Kastenbaum, 2008). Three elements are essential in all bereavement: "1) a relationship with some person or thing that is valued; 2) the loss—ending, termination, separation—of that relationship; and 3) a survivor deprived by the loss" (Corr, Nabe, & Corr, 2000, p. 212).

Grief

Bowlby describes grief as "the sequence of subjective states that follow loss and accompany mourning" (1960, p. 11). Wolfelt (1983) points out that grief is a process, rather than a specific emotion like fear or sadness; it can be expressed by a variety of thoughts, emotions, and behaviors. A simple definition is that "grief is the reaction to loss" (Corr, Nabe, & Corr, 2000, p. 213). These reactions can occur in feelings, in physical sensations, in cognitions, and in behaviors (Worden, 1991).

Mourning

The psychoanalytic definition describes mourning as "the mental work following the loss of a love object through death" (Furman, 1974, p. 34, quoting Freud, 1915/1954). This "mental work," often called "grief work," involves the "painful, gradual process of detaching libido from an internal image" (A. Freud, 1965, p. 67), thereby freeing libidinal energy for new relationships. This theoretical model of grief *requires disengagement from attachment to the deceased* in order for the grief to be resolved. The psychoanalytical definition of mourning, therefore, encompasses not only the initial grief reaction to the loss but also the future resolution of that grief (Grossberg & Crandall, 1978). In order for mourning to be resolved, according to Krueger, the bereaved person must comprehend the "significance, seriousness, permanence, and irreversibility" of his or her loss (1983, p. 590). In other words, in addition to feeling typical grief reactions, such as sadness and anger, the individual must also come to understand that the deceased person will never return, but that life can be meaningful nonetheless. This adaptation or acceptance of the irrevocable loss is referred to by Bowlby as "relinquishing the object" (1960, p. 11).

An alternative, very different model of bereavement (Klass, Silverman, & Nickman, 1996) emphasizes the mourner's *continuing bonds* with the deceased. This approach differs drastically from conceptualizations that posit disengagement and relinquishment as a goal of grief resolution. In contrast, in this view, "it is normative for mourners to maintain a connection with the deceased" (p. 18) and this connection *continues throughout the life of the mourner.* This conceptualization has great implications for bereavement counseling, which, in this view, emphasizes remembering and honoring cherished memories of the deceased.

Can Children Mourn?

This question has been asked and debated in the literature, with responses depending on both the definition of "mourning" and on the specific theoretical framework of the respondent. If one's definition of mourning requires mature awareness regarding the finality of death, as stated earlier by Krueger (1983), a positive response would not be possible until prepuberty. This is the position of Nagera (1970). At the other extreme, Bowlby argues forcefully for the existence of grief and mourning in even very young children when they are separated from their mothers. Quoting Robertson's 10-year study of children ages 18–24 months who experienced maternal separation, Bowlby presents the following position:

> If a child is taken from his mother's care at this age, when he is so possessively and passionately attached to her, it is indeed as if his world has been shattered. His intense need of her is unsatisfied, and the frustration and longing may send him frantic with grief. It takes an exercise of imagination to sense the intensity of this distress. *He is overwhelmed as any adult who has lost a beloved person by death.* To the child of two with his lack of understanding and complete inability to tolerate frustration, it is really as if his mother had died. *He does not know death, but only absence;* and if the only person who can satisfy his imperative need is absent, *she might as well be dead.* (1960, p. 15, quoting Robertson, 1953; emphasis added)

Sigmund Freud, toward the end of his life, in discussing the responses of young children to their mothers' absences, referred to their crying and facial expressions as evidence of both anxiety and pain. Freud stated, with regard to the distressed child, "it cannot as yet distinguish between temporary absence and permanent loss. As soon as it loses sight of its mother, it behaves as if it were never going to see her again" (1926/1959, p. 169). These desperate reactions point to the child's total lack of understanding that the mother continues to exist when she goes away ("object constancy"). They also indicate the child's lack of a "mental representation" (memory) of the mother that can be evoked in her absence. The beginning stage of object constancy usually occurs in the second half of the first year of life, but the child's capacity to recall the mother's image in her absence is ephemeral until completion of M. Mahler's rapprochement stage at around 25 months of age (Furman, 1974; Masur, 1991).

It seems only logical that the child must have a clear idea about the separate, independent existence of a person before being able to grieve the loss of that person after his or her death. Anna Freud (1960) maintained that the child can mourn only when he or she has developed reality testing and object constancy, and Furman (1974) agrees with this position.

While it is indisputable that even very young children react strongly to the absence and loss of a meaningful person, and that they show their reactions in conformity with Bowlby's (1960) stages of protest, despair, and detachment, it seems to me inaccurate to refer to these responses as "mourning" when the young child understands neither the finality of the loss not its significance in his or her life. Thus, feelings of sadness, rage, and longing following the loss of a significant person may qualify as *grief reactions* but, without mature understanding of the finality and meaning of that loss, cannot accurately be termed as "mourning" in my view.

Although this may appear to be semantic hairsplitting, the implications for the grief counselor or therapist point to the necessity of respecting children's feelings without expecting more of the child than is developmentally appropriate. Thus, the question "Can children mourn?" should instead be "Can children grieve?", to which an unqualified affirmative response can be given.

Does the Expression "Relinquishing the Object" Apply to Children—or Is the Concept of "Continuing Bonds" More Relevant?

The idea that mourning can be "resolved" and that this resolution involves "decathecting" or "relinquishing" emotional investment in the deceased seems problematic when applied to children's mourning. Some traditional child therapists (Buchsbaum, 1987; Nagera, 1970; Wolfenstein, 1969) have pointed to children's ongoing psychological need to hold on to their relationship with their parents to successfully complete the tasks of development. Such a fantasized relationship with a deceased parent obviously hinders any "relinquishing" of libido from that fantasy until the adolescent stage has been completed. Nagera states that "the evidence seems to point to the fact that the latency child strongly cathects a fantasy life where the lost object may be seen as alive and at times as ideal" (1970, p. 381). This explains the position of Nagera and Wolfenstein that mourning is not possible until "detachment from parental figures has taken place in adolescence" (Nagera, 1970, p. 362).

A different view about childhood grief (Baker, Sedney, & Gross, 1992) conceptualizes it as a series of psychological tasks that must be accomplished over time. For these authors, decathexis, or detachment, is not essential to the mourning process, because they found that many children maintain an internal attachment to the mental image of the lost person that serves an important function in terms of their child and later their adult development. This is consistent with the views about continuing bonds as discussed previously (Klass et al.,1996).

Therefore, in my opinion, decathexis/detachment and "relinquishing the object" are not appropriate concepts in describing the mourning of children. While a child may certainly grieve the absence of the person who died and long to be with that person, these feelings need not interfere with the child's developmental course. In fact, my own experience as a bereavement counselor supports the convincing reports in the literature that an ongoing attachment relationship after the death of a loved person can help children withstand and overcome many stresses, as illustrated in the following examples.

CASE VIGNETTES

The Grief of a 4-Year-Old

This example of the accidental death of the father of four children comes from the second edition of this book (Webb, 2002) and is used with permission. The youngest child, Lisa, age 4, was unable to understand the reality of her father's death, even though she attended both the funeral and the burial service. Several months after her father's tragic death in a house fire Lisa still became very excited whenever someone would come to the house in the late afternoon at the time that her father used to return from work. When she heard keys in the lock or someone entering the front door, Lisa would shout, "Daddy's home, Daddy's home!" Her two brothers, ages 6 and 9, who knew that their father could *not* return because he was dead, would become angry and respond to Lisa, "Daddy's dead. Why do you think he can come back?" Sometimes in frustration one of the boys would hit Lisa in the hope that this would change her expectations about their dead father's return. It was partly the mother's exasperation about how to deal with episodes such as these among her children that prompted the referral for grief counseling. I comment on aspects of the children's behavior in treatment that demonstrate their developmental issues with regard to their expressions of grief. In my role as a bereavement counselor, I typically employ play therapy as the ideal manner of intervention with young children.

Counseling with Lisa

In the first play therapy session, this little 4-year-old was immediately drawn to the dollhouse, which had movable furniture and numerous family figurines. The therapist told Lisa that she could set up the dollhouse any way she wished and use any of the dolls she wanted. Lisa focused on the kitchen and created a scene there with a mother doll, and four "child" dolls of different sizes. There was no male doll in evidence, and the therapist asked: "Where is the daddy in this family?" Lisa immediately responded: "They can't find him; he is 'lost.' " The child's use of this term made the therapist think about how often people refer to death as a "loss"; she wondered whether Lisa had heard her mother or someone else say that the family members "lost" their husband or father. With this assumption, the therapist replied to Lisa: "Maybe he is dead, and that is why he can't be with the family." Lisa said: "That's what they say; the daddy is dead; but I think he is lost and they should try to find him." The therapist then replied, "When a person is dead, he cannot come back, no matter what." Later, the therapist spoke privately to the mother and suggested that she explain to the boys that Lisa was not yet old enough to understand the reality of death, so that she and others would need to be patient with her and keep repeating that when people are dead, they cannot come back to their families.

Comment

This girl's reactions demonstrate the inability of this preschool child to comprehend the finality of her father's death. She very much wanted him to return and seemed to be in some pain due to his absence. The play therapy sessions occurred only 3 months after the death, and suggest that the child was still actively remembering her father and was very aware of missing him.

The Grief of a 6-Year-Old

This example involves Lisa's 6-year-old brother Brian, who was also seen individually for bereavement counseling. Because of Brian's age, play therapy was also the method of treatment. This boy was very active in the sessions, moving quickly from one activity to another. Sometimes he would draw, and other times he would play with wooden blocks, creating a rectangular building, then destroying it. Typically, after throwing all the blocks into the center of the floor, he would also toss human figures, cars, and animals in the pile, and then he would say, "It's a mess!" The therapist believed that this child was referring symbolically to his life, so she responded with an affirmative reply, "Yes it *is* a mess, and we need to try to help these poor people!" Brian would then say "They are all dead, all dead!!" in a very sad and hopeless voice. The therapist then would comment about how sad this was, and how she wanted to find some way to help.

Brian repeated this play scene for several weeks, showing through his play how very devastated he felt. After about a month had passed, the therapist decided to comment more specifically about the dead people, and she said that the people's families must be very sad because they miss their dead relatives. Brian made eye contact and said, "they need to have a funeral." The remainder of the session consisted of putting one of the male bodies into a toy casket, covering it carefully, and creating a goodbye message from the family.

Comment

This boy, at the age of 6 years, was struggling with his intense feelings of grief over the loss of his father. Initially he could convey only his distraught feelings that his life was now a mess. After playing this out repeatedly and receiving some verbal and emotional support from the grief counselor, he was then able to reconstruct the funeral preparations and prepare a goodbye message for his beloved father. This appeared to be very meaningful to this young child, who, through play, was able to reconstruct what he had witnessed (but probably not understood) at the time of his father's death.

The Grief of a 9-Year-Old

Brian's brother Greg also participated in grief counseling that included both play therapy and verbal discussion of Greg's memories of his father.

Since his father's death, Greg had had some problems hitting other children on the school playground. This behavior was very unusual for him, and the teacher had called Greg's mother to express her concerns. In the initial meeting with Greg, the therapist mentioned that she knew Greg had been getting into some fights at school, and that this behavior was not typical for him. The therapist asked whether Greg might want to draw a picture, and the boy drew a volcano. This stimulated a discussion about how anger can be "stuffed down" and then it explodes like a volcano. The therapist assured Greg that people usually feel angry after someone dies unexpectedly. They then talked about how else he could express his anger without getting in trouble. The remainder of that session, and many others to follow, consisted of playing with toy cars on the floor as Greg reminisced about his father. He had many happy memories. However, he was worried, because other people told him that because he was the oldest male, he was the man of the family now. Greg did not like this idea, because he realized that he was *not* a man, and the therapist agreed with him. She also said that she would speak to his mother to have her reassure the boy about her expectations for him.

Comment

At age 9, this boy fully understood the meaning of death; he knew that his father would not come back, and he welcomed the chance to grieve his father's loss by talking about his many happy memories of his father. The therapist encouraged him to do so, while also helping him understand his feelings of anger about the loss of his father, and about the unrealistic expectations that others were trying to put on his small shoulders.

The Grief of a 12-Year-Old

Mary, the eldest child in this family, at age 12, took on a protective and parenting-type role with her younger siblings. Initially she denied the opportunity to participate in therapy, but a year later she spontaneously asked her mother to arrange an appointment. At that time this preteen girl was preoccupied with her friends and peer relationships, which is a normal focus for a youngster of that age. She worried that some of her friends were nice to her only because they were sorry for her as a result of her father's death. After discussing this issue with the therapist, Mary began to realize that she felt very different since the death, and she thought that her friends must have noticed. The fact that she had had certain friends for many years seemed to suggest that they liked her for herself, not because they felt sorry for her. As the therapist pointed this out, Mary began to feel better during this discussion and said that she was glad she brought it up with the therapist.

Comment

This example exhibits this girl's age-appropriate, preteen development related to concerns about making and keeping friends. Often bereaved children feel very different from their peers, and they are so painfully aware of the death in their family that they believe it will alienate other people. This reflects both the bereaved child's anxiety and the difficulty many children may have in expressing their condolences and sympathy toward their bereaved friend.

IS CHILDREN'S GRIEF DIFFERENT FROM THAT OF ADULTS?

Case vignettes, professional literature, and clinical experience with bereaved children all attest to some marked differences, as well as some similarities, between the grief of children and that of adults. Wolfelt reminds us that "grief does not focus on one's ability to 'understand,' but instead upon one's ability to 'feel.' Therefore any child mature enough to love is mature enough to grieve" (1983, p. 20).

Denial, anger, guilt, sadness, and longing are felt by young and old alike in response to the death of a loved person. Adults, who expect children to have many of the same feelings they themselves experience at a time of bereavement, may be able to help children realize that these feelings are justified. It is even more important, however, for adults to recognize that most children have *limited ability to verbalize their feelings,* as well as very *limited capacity to tolerate the pain* generated by open recognition of their loss. Thus, in these vignettes, we note the children's various attempts to avoid talking about their losses.

We also note in the vignette about Mary the *fear of being "different" from one's peers with regard to having a deceased parent.* Unlike adults, who may obtain solace and comfort from the condolences of their friends, bereaved children *dread* this process, and frequently their peers feel equally uncomfortable at the prospect of having to speak to them. They do not know what to say, and they are afraid that they themselves or their friend will start crying. Children in latency and adolescence are trying hard to gain control over their feelings, so they resist and feel uncomfortable with an invitation to express their emotions openly. Furman (1974) comments that children consider crying babyish, so they may do their crying in private. The child's "short sadness span" (Wolfenstein, 1966) reflects the low capacity to tolerate acute pain for long periods, characteristic of childhood. Rando (1988/1991) explains that a child may manifest grief on an intermittent basis for many years in an approach–avoidance cycle with regard to painful feelings.

Children often use play as an escape from their pain and as a way to gain mastery over their complex and confused feelings about the death. Insofar as play is the language of childhood, children can deal with their feelings through play in a displaced, disguised manner. The trained play therapist understands and knows how to communicate in this symbolic language and, through the use of play therapy, can help the child work through his or her painful feelings. This book contains various examples of play therapy that can help bereaved children with their grief.

In summary, the following considerations serve to differentiate the grief of children from that of adults:

1. Children's immature cognitive development interferes with their understanding about the irreversibility, universality, and inevitability of death.
2. Children have a limited capacity to tolerate emotional pain. I refer to this as a "short sadness span," which means that they cannot spend long periods of time grieving.
3. Children's acute feelings of loss may occur in spurts over many years.
4. Children have limited ability to verbalize their feelings.
5. Children are sensitive about "being different" from their peers. A death in their family makes them feel different and uncomfortable, so they may not wish to acknowledge the death.
6. Children are able to express their feelings in play therapy.

RELIGIOUS/CULTURAL INFLUENCES ON CHILDREN'S CONCEPTIONS OF DEATH

Any analysis of a child's understanding about death must include not only the individual factors related to the child's cognitive and emotional development but also the influences impacting on the child that emanate from the cultural and religious beliefs in the child's home environment.

This is discussed more fully in Chapter 2. A psychosocial assessment of the child examines both internal and external elements contributing to the child's understanding about death. McGoldrick et al. warn that "clinicians should be careful about definitions of 'normality' in assessing families' responses to death, [since] the manner of, as well as the length of time assumed normal for mourning differs greatly from culture to culture" (1991, pp. 176–177). These family therapists/authors further point out that "cultures differ in major ways about public versus private expressions of grief" (p. 178). Because of these differences, it behooves therapists to try to find out from a family member "what its members believe about the nature of death, the rituals that should surround it, and the expectations about afterlife" (p. 178). The child absorbs and interprets these beliefs and customs, questioning what is not clear, and supplying his or her own answers when the responses to his or her questions are vague and incomprehensible.

The Appendix to this book lists resources for information about the different religious practices and mourning observances in different cultures. It is not practical to attempt a comprehensive overview of various religions and cultures. However, grief counselors and therapists working with bereaved children must learn about the typical practices in the cultural and religious group of the bereaved child's family. It is especially important to know whether the children are expected to participate in the formal and informal rituals of grieving, or whether they are excluded from these rituals due to the belief that involving the children would be upsetting to them. Most Western thanatologists believe that it assists the child's grieving when he or she is included in the funeral and other rituals associated with the death of a loved one (Rando, 1988/1991; Wolfelt, 1983; Kastenbaum, 2008). When children are told in advance about what to expect and are given the opportunity to decide whether or not to participate, many elect to do so. Rando points out that rituals are well suited to children, who are fascinated by these types of behaviors (1988/1991, p. 216). Of course, if there is an open casket at the funeral, the child must be prepared for this in advance and assured that the family will have some private time to say their farewells to the deceased. James Agee's Pulitzer Prize–winning novel *A Death in the Family* contains a moving, detailed account of a 5-year-old viewing his dead father at the wake, during which time the child came to synthesize his observations about his father's appearance in the casket with his first true understanding of the meaning of the word "dead" (1938/1969, pp. 288–298).

Children's accounts about attending wakes and funerals often project their ambivalence about the death. They prefer to remember their loved one when alive, but they also want to be included in the services. A 15-year-old boy, whose mother died when he was 9, reflects as follows:

> "The night before the funeral we all went to the funeral parlor, and I spent a lot of time right next to her coffin. She was wearing a white dress, but that's all I remember. I remember her more when she was alive because *I think my mind wants to remember her alive rather then dead.* I'm glad, though, that I got a chance to get a last look at her. I drew a picture for her and wrote a little note on it, asking her to wait in heaven for all of us. I gave it to Daddy to put in her coffin with her, and even though she was dead, I like to think that she got that last message from me." (in Krementz, 1981/1991, p. 54; emphasis added)

Children differ in their feelings about how they want to remember their deceased relative, but the idea of avoidance of the cemetery is a repeated theme for many children. A 16-year-old Puerto Rican girl whose mother died when she was 11 stated:

> "I'm not sold on going to the cemetery. That's the worst place to remember her because I associate it with putting her into the ground. Why would I want to remember that part? My aunt is very religious and she's really into going to the cemetery and lighting candles in church and all that stuff. I don't think anybody should have to go the cemetery. I can't see it. I think the most vivid thing in a person's mind should be the happy moments, and when you visit the grave, you're left with the sad parts. . . . I *cannot* relate to my mother by looking at her tombstone. It's hard to imagine there's a body underneath the ground even if I know it's there. The body's not that important to me. It's the soul that counts, and once that's gone, forget it. I wish my mother had been cremated." (in Krementz, 1981/1991, pp. 48–49; emphasis in original)

This child clearly has attained a mature understanding of death, and she appears to have accepted the finality of her loss while being able to appreciate and remember "the happy moments" of her mother's life.

REFERENCES

Agee, J. (1969). *A death in the family.* New York: Bantam. (Original work published 1938)

Anthony, S. (1971). *The discovery of death in childhood and after.* London: Penguin.

Baker, J. E., Sedney, M. A., & Gross, E. (1992). Psychological tasks for bereaved children. *American Journal of Orthopsychiatry, 62*(1), 105–116.

Becker, E. (1973). *The denial of death.* New York: Free Press.

Bluestone, J. (1999). School-based peer therapy to facilitate mourning in latency-age children following sudden parental death: Cases of Joan, age 10½, and Roberta age 9½, with follow-up 8 years later. In N. B. Webb (Ed.), *Play therapy with children in crisis: Individual, group, and family treatment* (2nd ed., pp. 225–251). New York: Guilford Press.

Bowlby, J. (1960). Grief and mourning in infancy and early childhood. *Psychoanalytic Study of the Child, 15,* 9–52.

Buchsbaum, B. C. (1987). Remembering a parent who has died: A developmental perspective. *Annual of Psychoanalysis, 15,* 99–112.

Corr, C. A., Nabe, C. M., & Corr, D. M. (2000). *Death and dying, life and living.* Belmont, CA: Wadsworth.

Fox, S. S. (1985). *Good grief: Helping groups of children when a friend dies.* Boston: New England Association for the Education of Young Children.

Freud, A. (1960). Discussion of Dr. John Bowlby's paper. *Psychoanalytic Study of the Child, 15,* 53–62.

20 INTRODUCTION

Freud, A. (1965). *Normality and pathology in childhood.* New York: International Universities Press.

Freud, S. (1954). Mourning and melancholia. In *Standard Edition* (Vol. 14, pp. 237–258). London: Hogarth Press. (Original work published 1915)

Freud, S. (1959). Inhibitions, symptoms and anxiety. In *Standard Edition* (Vol. 20, pp. 77– 175). London: Hogarth Press. (Original work published 1926)

Furman, E. (1974). *A child's parent dies.* New Haven, CT: Yale University Press.

Grollman, E. (Ed.). (1967). *Explaining death to children.* Boston: Beacon Press.

Grossberg, S. H., & Crandall, L. (1978). Father loss and father absence in preschool children. *Clinical Social Work Journal, 6*(2), 123–134.

Kane, B. (1979). Children's concepts of death. *Journal of Genetic Psychology, 134,* 141– 153.

Kaplan, C. P., & Joslin, H. (1993). Accidental sibling death: Case of Peter, age 6. In N. B. Webb (Ed.), *Helping bereaved children: A handbook for practitioners* (pp. 118–136). New York: Guilford Press.

Kastenbaum, R. J. (1967). The child's understanding of death: How does it develop? In E. Grollman (Ed.), *Explaining death to children* (pp. 89–109). Boston: Beacon Press.

Kastenbaum, R. J. (2008). *Death, society, and human experience* (10th ed.). New York: Merrill.

Klass, D., Silverman, P. R., & Nickman, S. L. (1996). *Continuing bonds: New understandings of grief.* Washington, DC: Taylor & Francis.

Krementz, J. (1991). *How it feels when a parent dies.* New York: Knopf. (Original work published 1981)

Krueger, D. W. (1983). Childhood parent loss: Developmental impact and adult psychopathology. *American Journal of Psychotherapy, 37*(4), 582–592.

Lonetto, R. (1980). *Children's conceptions of death.* New York: Springer.

Masur, C. (1991). The crisis of early maternal loss: Unresolved grief of 6-year-old Chris in foster care. In N. B. Webb (Ed.), *Play therapy with children in crisis: A casebook for practitioners* (pp. 164–176). New York: Guilford Press.

McGoldrick, M., Almeida, R., Hines, P. M., Garcia-Preto, N., Rosen, E., & Lee, E. (1991). Mourning in different cultures. In F. Walsh & M. McGoldrick (Eds.), *Living beyond loss: Death in the family* (pp. 176–206). New York: Norton.

Millay, E. St. V. (1969). Childhood is the kingdom where nobody dies. In *Edna St. Vincent Millay collected lyrics* (p. 203). New York: Harper & Row. (Original work published 1934)

Nagera, H. (1970). Children's reactions to the death of important objects: A developmental approach. *Psychoanalytic Study of the Child, 25,* 360–400.

Nagy, M. (1948). The child's theories concerning death. *Journal of Genetic Psychology, 73,* 3–27.

Piaget, J. (1955). *The child's construction of reality.* New York: Basic Books.

Piaget, J. (1968). *Six psychological studies.* New York: Vintage Books.

Piaget, J. (1972). Intellectual evolution from adolescent to childhood. *Human Development, 15,* 1–12.

Piaget, J., & Inhelder, B. (1969). *The psychology of the child.* New York: Basic Books.

Rando, T. A. (1991). *How to go on living when someone you love dies.* New York: Bantam. (Original work published 1988)

Robertson, J. (1953). Some responses of young children to the loss of maternal care. *Nursing Times, 49,* 382–389.

Saravay, B. (1991). Short-term play therapy with two preschool brothers following sudden paternal death. In N.B. Webb (Ed.), *Play therapy with children in crisis: A casebook for practitioners* (pp. 177–201). New York: Guilford Press.

Solnit, A. J. (1983). Changing perspectives: Preparing for life or death. In J. E. Schowalter, P. R. Patterson, M. Tallmer, A. H. Kutscher, S. V. Gullo, & D. Peretz (Eds.), *The child and death* (pp. 4–18). New York: Columbia University Press.

Speece, M. W., & Brent, S. B. (1996). The development of children's understanding of death. In C. A. Corr & D. M. Corr (Eds.), *Handbook of childhood death and bereavement* (pp. 29–49). New York: Springer.

Wass, H., & Stillion, J. (1988). Dying in the lives of children. In H. Wass, F. Berardo, & R. Neimeyer (Eds.), *Dying: Facing the facts* (pp. 201–228). Washington, DC: Hemisphere.

Webb, N. B. (Ed.). (2002). *Helping bereaved children: A handbook for practitioners.* New York: Guilford Press.

Wolfelt, A. (1983). *Helping children cope with grief.* Muncie, IN: Accelerated Development.

Wolfenstein, M. (1966). How is mourning possible? *Psychoanalytic Study of the Child, 21,* 93–126.

Wolfenstein, M. (1969). Loss, rage and repetition. *Psychoanalytic Study of the Child, 24,* 432–460.

Worden, J. W. (1991). *Grief counseling and grief therapy: A handbook for the mental health practitioner* (2nd ed.). New York: Springer.

Wordsworth, W. (1928). Now we are seven. In *The complete poetical works of William Wordsworth.* London: Macmillan. (Original work published 1798)

Yalom, I. D. (1980). *Existential psychotherapy.* New York: Basic Books.

CHAPTER 2

Assessment of the Bereaved Child

NANCY BOYD WEBB

Thanatologists agree that expressions of grief take many forms and that its duration varies (Wolfelt, 1983; Fox, 1985; Rando, 1988/1991) depending on individual, cultural, religious, and circumstantial factors. How, then, do we determine when a bereaved child's grief response is progressing on a "normal" course, and when the child's reaction suggests the need for referral and assessment by a trained mental health professional? This question begs for a precise formula, yet its answer depends on the complex interplay among factors related to the child, the circumstances of the death, and the ability of the concerned adult to weigh these variables and arrive at a decision.

This chapter tackles the thorny question about "normal", "disabling," and "complicated" grief as it applies to children, and offers some guidelines about when a professional assessment would be appropriate. Various helpful therapeutic approaches for bereaved children are outlined in Part IV of this book, as are the qualifications and training of the therapist or grief counselor who works with bereaved children.

DISTINGUISHING AMONG "NORMAL," "DISABLING," AND COMPLICATED GRIEF

Granted the generous leeway for individual variability in both the nature and duration of grieving, how can we determine when the boundaries of "normal" grief have trespassed into the dangerous territory of "disabling" or complicated grief that seriously interferes with the person's life? Furthermore, given the distinctions between adult's and children's grief, as outlined in Chapter 1, this volume, how relevant is the literature on adult grieving to the assessment of children's grief as normal, disabling, or complicated? Is it helpful or pejorative to use the term "disabling" when referring to responses to a death that appear to greatly exceed the range, duration, or intensity of expression considered appropriate in a given situation? I begin with the latter question.

Terminology

Lindemann's landmark article on the symptomatology and management of acute grief spelled out in great detail the "normal" grief reactions following traumatic experiences, such as war or disastrous fire, and contrasted these with delayed or distorted responses considered "morbid" or "pathological" (1944; reprinted in Parad, 1965, pp. 8–16). In studying 101 relatives and survivors of the Coconut Grove fire in Boston, and members of the armed forces, Lindemann concluded:

1. Acute grief is a definite syndrome, with psychological and somatic symptomatology.
2. This syndrome may appear immediately after a crisis; it may be delayed; it may be exaggerated or apparently absent.
3. In place of the typical syndrome, there may appear distorted pictures, each of which represents one special aspect of the grief syndrome.
4. By use of appropriate techniques, these distorted pictures can be successfully transformed into a normal grief reaction with resolution (1944; reprinted in Parad, 1965, p. 7).

I do not review Lindemann's work in detail here since it did not focus specifically on *children's* grief nor did it distinguish between various forms of "acute" grief, and the term "traumatic grief" was not in use at that time. However, Lindemann's designation of delayed or distorted grief reactions does seem applicable to children's grief despite his unfortunate labeling of these responses as "morbid." Lindemann emphasized that "not only over-reactions, but under-reactions of the bereaved, must be given attention because delayed responses may occur at unpredictable moments and the dangerous distortions of the grief reaction, not conspicuous at first, may be quite destructive later" (1944; reprinted in Parad, 1965, p. 18). Rando refers to a category of grief she terms "unresolved grief," and within this group of responses she includes absent grief, inhibited grief, delayed grief, distorted grief, chronic grief, and unanticipated grief (1988/1991, pp. 81–84). Several cases in this book describe children who manifest various forms of unresolved grief. Indeed, one might propose that "absent," "inhibited," and "delayed" grief may be the *norm* for children because of their age-appropriate inability to bear the pain of extended grief.

Bowlby, in contrast to both Lindemann and Rando, focused on the impact of *loss* in childhood. He believed that separation or death of a parent during the years of early childhood may predispose the individual to "unfavorable personality development" that leads to future psychiatric illness (1963, p. 500). Bowlby's views about the impact of loss on subsequent grief presented a rationale about terminology that continues to be applicable in the 21st century:

> If the experience of loss is likened to the experience of being wounded or being burned, the processes of mourning that follow loss can be similar to the processes of healing that follow a wound or burn. Such healing processes, we know, may take a course which in time leads to full, or nearly full, function being restored; or they may on the contrary, take one of many courses each of which has as its outcome an impairment of function of greater or less degree. In the same way, processes of mourning may take a favorable course that leads in time to restoration of function, namely to a renewal of the capacity to make and maintain love relationships, or they may take a course that leaves this function impaired in greater or less degree. *Just as the terms* healthy *and* pathological *are applicable to the different course taken by healing processes, so may they be applied to the different courses run by mourning processes.* (p. 501; emphasis added)

With due respect to Bowlby's concern about the possible devastating effects of separation and loss in early childhood, it is reassuring to note his opinion that "not every child who experiences either permanent or temporary loss grows up to be a disturbed person" (1963, p. 527). This book is dedicated to the process of helping bereaved children, so that their development can proceed despite their loss.

What, then, would be an accurate term to describe harmful grief when referring to a child? Any judgment about the appropriateness of a grief response always considers temporal factors related to the relative recency of the death. Since many, if not most, children avoid facing their upsetting feelings and can tolerate discomfort in only small doses, the terms "unresolved," "absent," or "delayed" grief do not seem apt for describing children's grief. One must expect children's grief to require the passage of time before expression and eventual resolution. Therefore, timeliness is not a useful consideration in evaluating children's grief.

Rather than the length of time of a child's grief reaction, it is *the degree of intrusiveness into the child's life* created by the grieving that must be evaluated. Specifically, we must determine the extent to which a child can carry out his or her usual activities and proceed with developmental tasks despite the presence of grief reactions. When a child's social, emotional, or physical development show signs of blocking, his or her grief process can justifiably be considered "disabling," and our deliberate use of the term indicates that something is wrong.

The grief has become all-encompassing and detrimental, instead of permitting the child to move on with the activities of his or her life. The child is "stuck" and needs help that family members may be unable to provide. It is important to recognize and help such a struggling and blocked child so that, in Lindemann's words, "these distorted pictures *can be successfully transformed into a normal grief reaction with resolution*" (1944; reprinted in Parad, 1965, p. 7; emphasis added).

In the first and second editions of this book I coined the phrase "disabling grief" to describe a cluster of grief reactions that interfere with the youngster's normal developmental course. The intent was to avoid terms, such as "unresolved" or "delayed" grief, that might lead the counselor to join the child's helplessness and hopelessness and to wait for the child to "work it out" according to his or her individual timetable. The term "disabling grief" was welcomed by therapists who wanted to assist the bereaved child who was floundering and even drowning in the throes of bereavement crosscurrents. However, in recent years a new term "complicated grief" has come into use to describe individuals who have difficulty resolving a bereavement loss. This term encompasses, and goes beyond, the expression "disabling grief," in that it includes bereavements associated with traumatic loss.

Traumatic Grief and Posttraumatic Stress Disorder in Children

An argument could be made that all deaths are traumatic for the child insofar as they may generate feelings of "intense fear, helplessness, or horror" (American Psychiatric Association, 2000) stemming from the youth's belief that he or she cannot survive without the person who died. This fear can contribute to some or many of the resulting symptoms of posttraumatic stress disorder (PTSD). However, "although youth demonstrate the re-experiencing, numbing/avoidance, arousal symptoms, and impaired functioning found in PTSD, it has become clear that there are variations by age, and other variables in the manifestations of the disorder" (Nader, 2007, p. 25) and we know that "PTSD fails to sufficiently capture the unique experiences of those who suffer from chronic grief as a result of violent loss of an important attachment figure" (Gray, Prigerson, & Litz, 2004, p. 71).

Complicated Grief

The term "complicated grief" (CG) refers to the individual's inability to return to his or her preloss level of functioning following a bereavement experience (Prigerson et al., 1995). This new diagnosis, which was originally studied in adults, is receiving increased attention as applicable for children and adolescents as well. It has been proposed as a separate diagnosis for the forthcoming DSM-V. It describes grief that is accompanied by symptoms of separation distress and trauma (Prigerson, Shear, & Jacobs, 1999; Prigerson et al., 1997). CG is distinct from major depression, anxiety, and PTSD (Melhem, Moritz, Walker, Shear, & Brent, 2007) although traumatic after effects and preoccupation with the lost relationship are distressing components of CG (Mitchell, Prigerson, & Martimer-Stephens, 2004; Prigerson et al., 1995). Researchers have recently developed a promising assessment tool used to identify CG in children and adolescents, the Inventory of Complicated Grief— Revised (ICG-R; Melhem et al., 2007). Chapter 6 discusses the topic of complicated grief with reference to suicide survivors.

Disabling, delayed, and complicated grief all refer to a person's poor adjustment to a bereavement loss that may signal a need to refer the distressed individual for help. What, then, are the indicators for referral for an evaluation by a mental health professional, and what components does such an assessment include?

Indications for Professional Assessment

Many years before the designation of the concept of complicated bereavement, Grollman (1967) pointed out that the line of demarcation between "normal psychological aspects of bereavement" and "distorted mourning reactions" was thin indeed. He said that

> the difference is not in symptom but in intensity. It is a *continued* denial of reality even many months after the funeral, or a *prolonged* bodily distress, or a *persistent* panic, or an *extended* guilt, or an *unceasing* idealization, or an *enduring* apathy and anxiety, or an *unceasing* hostile reaction to the deceased and to others. Each manifestation does not in itself determine a distorted grief reaction; it is only as it is viewed *by the professional* in the composition of the *total* formulation. (p. 21; emphasis added).

This certainly sounds a lot like many of the characteristics of complicated bereavement. What should be the professional response to youth with such painful reactions?

Some clinicians believe that "professional mental health services are indicated if there are questions about suicidal risk or if a child has been involved in some way in the death of another person" (Fox, 1985, p. 17). Other children who may need professional assistance include the following:

1. Children who themselves have a life-threatening or terminal illness.
2. Children who have already been identified as emotionally disturbed.
3. Children who are developmentally disabled and who may have difficulty understanding what has happened.
4. Children who remain "frozen" and in shock long after most grievers have returned to their usual daily activities. (Fox, 1985, pp. 39–40)

In addition to identifying these groups of potentially vulnerable children, Fox enumerated some symptoms that she considered "red flags," suggesting the need for careful assessment of the grieving child. These "red flag" symptoms include the following:

- Suicidal hints
- Psychosomatic problems
- Difficulties with schoolwork
- Nightmares or sleep disorders
- Changes in eating patterns
- Temporary regressions

Although "none of these presentations suggests a formal diagnosis of emotional problems, each is a possible indicator that the child's grief work may not be proceeding smoothly. Therefore, *each deserves the attention of someone who has been trained in the broad field of mental health so, if intervention is indicated, it can begin promptly*" (Fox, 1985, p. 42; emphasis added). Rando (1988/1991) wisely admonished us that when there is a question, it is better to err on the side of going for professional help.

Symptoms of Depression

Many of the "red flag" behaviors noted by Fox (1985) and the distorted reactions listed by Grollman (1967) duplicate the clinical syndrome of depression as listed in the text revision of the fourth edition of the *Diagnostic and Statistical Manual of Mental Disorders* (DSM-IV-TR; American Psychiatric Association, 2000). Rapoport and Ismond (1990) state that depression has been underdiagnosed in children. As indicated in DSM-IV-TR criteria, there must be at least five of nine symptoms present during the same 2-week period (see Table 2.1), and this must represent a change from previous functioning.

**TABLE 2.1. DSM-IV-TR Symptoms
of Major Depression**

5 of 9 Symptoms for Two Weeks

1. Depressed mood most of the day
2. Diminished pleasure
3. Weight loss
4. Insomnia or hypersomnia
5. Agitation or retardation
6. Fatigue or low energy
7. Feelings of worthlessness or guilt
8. Reduced ability to concentrate
9. Recurrent thoughts of death or suicide

An important and possibly confusing consideration in identifying a child with "disabling" grief is the requirement in DSM-IV-TR that "the symptoms are not better accounted for by Bereavement, i.e., after the death of a loved one" (American Psychiatric Association, 2000, p. 356). The caveat implies that although some bereavement responses might duplicate many of the same symptoms as those for a major depressive episode, if a loss has occurred, the symptoms are considered "secondary" to that; Rapoport and Ismond state that diagnostically "it is crucial . . . that the mood disturbance be primary and not secondary to some other disorder" (1990, p. 101). This argues for a careful history that includes information about the child's prebereavement adjustment.

As previously indicated, there is as yet no DSM diagnostic category for "complicated" or "disabling/ pathological" grief. However, it is clear that extensive overlapping exists between the term "depressed states" as used there and the term "disabling grief" as used by me. The designation of "bereavement" in DSM-IV-TR clarifies that "some grieving individuals present with symptoms characteristic of a Major Depressive Episode (e.g., feelings of sadness and associated symptoms such as insomnia, poor appetite, and weight loss)" (American Psychiatric Association, 2000, p. 740). In the event that the next DSM includes the diagnosis of CG, this will afford greater clarity about these overlapping conditions.

As a child and family therapist, I am familiar with DSM and use it regularly in the assessment of clients who consult with me regarding a variety of problems, some of which include bereavement. Several of my child clients have become bereaved unexpectedly during the course of my contact with them. I believe that all counselors who work with bereaved children would find it helpful to become knowledgeable about DSM criteria for depression, since they describe in detail many of the behaviors and responses that occur in grieving children, especially those whose grief has become "disabling" or complicated. In my own practice, I have treated several children whose life experience combined depression, trauma, and bereavement in different ways.

Preexisting Depression

Sometimes a child exhibits signs of depression prior to and independent of any experience with loss. Many of these children are "undiagnosed," since their form of depression permits minimal or passing school performance, without extreme behaviors that draw attention to them. This category includes the quiet child who seems "withdrawn" but who "gets by." The child may have few or no friends, and sometimes he or she may be scapegoated or bullied because peers consider him or her "different."

These children are at extreme risk when they become bereaved, since their survival was precarious even before the loss. An example of such a child (Webb, 2002) involves a boy with poor self-esteem (related to learning disabilities) who suffered the deaths of two grandparents in 1 year. Without the loving familial support and the preexisting supportive relationship with his therapist, this child's grief might have become disabling.

Depressive Symptoms Following Loss

Sometimes symptoms of depression occur in a child with no previous psychiatric diagnosis. This speaks to the importance of the therapist obtaining a careful history to arrive at the correct diagnosis. The case of Susan (Webb, 2002) illustrates an example of a child who was functioning normally until the sudden violent death of her friend precipitated a grief reaction with some accompanying symptoms of depression. When Susan's grief reaction was treated through play therapy, her depressive symptoms abated.

Suicidal Risk

Fox emphatically states that "each bereaved child must be considered potentially at risk for suicide" (1985, p. 16). While this advice may appear to be extreme, practice wisdom dictates caution. We know that many young children do not comprehend the irreversibility of death. Therefore, their wish to "go to heaven" to be with their deceased mother or father represents a literal interpretation of their experience and their remedy for their loss, rather than a wish for death per se.

Even elementary-school-age children who understand the finality of death may express suicidal thoughts with reference to wanting a reunion with a deceased parent. Bluestone describes her skillful use of puppet play to assist two bereaved latency-age children who therapeutically "play out" their painful losses and longing for reunion with their deceased parents (1999, pp. 225–251). It is noteworthy that the therapist not only helped these children with their grief through play therapy but also conducted a suicide evaluation to determine the degree of suicidal risk of the girl, who had been most upset during the play. When I presented this case at the annual meeting of the Association of Death Education and Counseling in 1992, one member of the audience was surprised that the therapist had taken the child's suicidal ideation "so seriously," since "it is common for bereaved children to fantasize about reunions with their parents."

We never know when a child might try to carry out his or her reunion fantasy. I agree with Bluestone that we must take all such fantasies seriously, especially when they include the desire to escape the pain of the loss. Evaluation of degree of risk for suicide provides information about the individual's degree of intent and, in addition, gives the therapist the opportunity to discuss with the child his or her wish and longing for reunion, while simultaneously emphasizing the vast difference between the wish and the irrevocable action that would implement it.

Counselors who are not familiar with the assessment of degree of suicide risk should consult Table 2.2 and the references at the end of this chapter (especially Goldman, 2001; Pfeffer, 1986; Peck, Farberow, & Litman, 1985). In situations where the counselor or therapist has any lingering doubts about the child's intent, it is wise to seek another opinion, and to tell the child and family that you are doing so because you are so concerned that you want to be certain that the child will not do anything to harm him- or herself. It is better to overreact than to underreact in these circumstances.

TABLE 2.2. Assessment of Suicidal Risk: Five Questions to Ask (Webb)

1. Are you so upset that you are thinking about killing yourself? [Tell me more.]
2. Have you thought about a plan? A method [degree of lethality]? When?
3. Have you made any previous attempts?
4. How much do you drink [alcohol]? Do you use recreational drugs? Are you taking medications?
5. What would keep you from acting on your wish?

I have used this five-question assessment for many years to train Master's of Social Work students in my Death and Dying class, in which we role-play asking these questions with children of different ages. Of course younger children may not be able to fantasize about elaborate plans, and their thinking may be dominated primarily by their longing for reunion with a deceased parent. Therefore this assessment is more relevant for use with older elementary-school-age to adolescent youth. In the first and second editions of this book, I included a lengthy suicide assessment that I now consider too extensive for practical use with the average young person (Pfeffer, 1986, pp. 187–188). Nonetheless that does include some very pertinent questions that readers might like to pursue. One topic from Pfeffer that might lead to a very rich discussion in an adolescent group includes the following questions:

> What happens when people die? Can they come back again? Do they go to a better place? Do they go to a pleasant place? Do you often think about people dying? Do you often think about your own death? Do you often dream about people or yourself dying? Do you know anyone who has died? What was the cause of this person's death? When did this person die? When do you think you will die? What will happen when you die? (1986, pp. 187–188)

Of course, these questions will have meaning only to a child who has a mature understanding of death (as discussed in Chapter 1, this volume).

When the Child's Bereavement Is Due to the Suicidal Death of a Family Member

Hurley (1991) points out that children bereaved by the suicide of a family member require urgent intervention, since there is evidence that such children are at greater risk than children in the general population for suicide and depression. In particular, response to the grief of children bereaved by the suicide of a parent requires great professional skill and sensitivity, since the meaning of such a death "often becomes distorted in the mind of the child, who usually cannot face the 'voluntary' nature of the suicidal death" (Hurley, 1991, p. 238). Also, the family is usually emotionally devastated in this situation and may be incapable of offering the child essential information and support. When the family feels shame associated with the suicide, they may want to disguise or distort the truth about the death. This further confuses the child, who needs and wants accurate information about how his or her loved one died. The shame associated with stigmatized death such as suicide complicates the grief process for all involved and leaves the child bereft and angry. Doka (1989) refers to this as "disenfranchised grief," referring to grief that cannot be openly acknowledged, socially sanctioned, or publicly mourned. Children in this situation should be referred to a mental health professional for evaluation and treatment. (See Hurley, 1991, for an example of play therapy with a 4-year-old whose father committed suicide.)

THE TRIPARTITE ASSESSMENT OF THE BEREAVED CHILD

Mental health practitioners, teachers, religious leaders, nurses, school bus drivers, and scout leaders all on occasion may have counseled a bereaved child. They may or may not have had training in grief counseling or in child development, but nonetheless most respond effectively out of their own compassion and instinctive respect for the child's feelings. Many bereaved children are not referred to mental health professionals, and many can go through their grieving without assistance from specialists.

Since the 1970s, however, there has been growing awareness in the general public about issues related to death and dying, sparked by the work of Kübler-Ross (1969) and reflected in the growth of the interdisciplinary field of death education. Interest in knowing more about how to help children has increased enormously. Furthermore, since the events of 9/11 there has been burgeoning interest in the topic of traumatic death and its impact across the life cycle.

Because of my firm belief in the necessity and value of a thorough assessment prior to counseling or treatment, I now focus on the elements of such an assessment. I developed the tripartite assessment of the bereaved child as an adaptation of the tripartite crisis assessment originally designed to facilitate evaluation of the child in a variety of crisis situations (Webb, 1991, 1993, 1999, 2004, 2007).

Assessment of a bereaved child involves consideration of three groups of factors:

1. Individual factors
2. Factors related to the death
3. Family, social, and religious–cultural factors

All of these interact and must be evaluated in order to appreciate fully the bereavement experience of a given individual. Figure 2.1 illustrates the components and interaction among the three sets of variables.

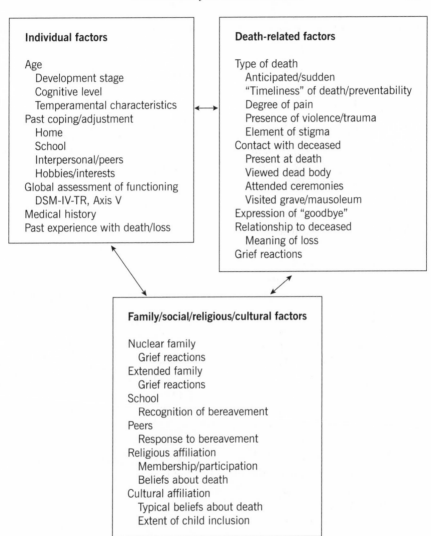

FIGURE 2.1. Tripartite assessment of the bereaved child: Webb.

Individual Factors in Childhood Bereavement

The assessment of a bereaved child begins with study of the background and current status of the individual who is bereaved. Many of the elements in the assessment of the individual focus on the reality of the child's life prior to the death, for example, his or her level of cognitive understanding and overall adjustment. I have developed a form (see Figure 2.2) on which this information can be recorded to assist the bereavement counselor in organizing and summarizing the relevant personal information about the child. The five subcategories in this assessment consist of the following:

- Age/development/cognitive/temperamental factors
- Past coping/adjustment
- Global assessment of functioning: DSM-IV-TR, Axis V
- Medical history
- Past experience with death/loss

Age/Developmental/Cognitive/Temperamental Factors

Chapter 1, this volume, contains a detailed review of age/developmental/ cognitive factors with reference to how these impact upon the child's understanding about death. The temperamental components refer to Chess and Thomas's (1986) profiles of general temperamental style, which reflect a child's typical approach to routine and to stressful life experiences. Chess and Thomas identify three distinct profiles describing children's level of responsiveness: the difficult child, the easy child, and the slow-to-warm child. Although these categories might seem overly simplistic, they are potentially useful to the bereavement counselor. It is valid to expect that a child who has always approached new situations with difficulty would have a more difficult time when faced with a death than would a youngster whose usual adaptation to new and stressful experiences is generally adaptive.

Past Coping/Adjustment

While it may not be entirely true that the past determines the future (and most of us resist this idea strongly), it is only logical that someone who has been successful managing life stresses in the past will benefit from this track record and confront new challenges with a sense of confidence and resolve. Conversely, an individual who has barely managed to "get by" will probably have a more difficult time when he or she is confronted with a death experience. A rather harsh biblical teaching

1. Age _____ years _____ months   Date of birth _____
                                         Date of assessment _____

   a. Developmental stage   b. Cognitive level
      Freud _____   Piaget _____
      Erickson _____   c. Tempermental characteristics
                                            Chess and Thomas _____

2. Past coping/adjustment
   a. Home (as reported by parents) Good _____ Fair _____ Poor _____
   b. School (as reported by parents and teachers) Good _____ Fair ___ Poor _____
   c. Interpersonal/peers Good _____ Fair _____ Poor _____
   d. Hobbies/interests (list) _____
      _____
      _____

3. Global assessment of functioning: DSM-IV-TR, Axis V
   Current _____   Past year _____

4. Medical history (as reported by parents and pediatrician)—describe serious
   illnesses, operations, and injuries since birth, with dates and outcome _____
   _____
   _____
   _____
   _____

5. Past experience with death/loss—give details with dates and outcome *or* complete
   Wolfelt's Loss Inventory. _____
   _____
   _____
   _____
   _____

FIGURE 2.2. Individual factors in childhood bereavement: Webb. This form is one component of a three-part assessment of the bereaved child, which also includes an assessment of death-related factors (Figure 2.3) and family/social/religious/cultural factors (Figure 2.5).

From *Helping Bereaved Children: A Handbook for Practitioners* (3rd ed.), edited by Nancy Boyd Webb. Copyright 2010 by The Guilford Press. Permission to photocopy this figure is granted to purchasers of this book for personal use only (see copyright page for details). Purchasers may download a larger version of this figure from the book's page on The Guilford Press website.

(Matthew 13:12, 25:29) maintains that the person who has much will be given more, whereas the person with less becomes further deprived. The concept of ego strength explains why a child who is well adjusted will be more capable of dealing with the stress of a death than will a child who already is exhibiting difficulties in coping with routine daily stresses.

Global Assessment of Functioning: DSM-IV-TR, Axis V

This scale is of use to mental health practitioners who wish to rate the child's overall psychological, social, and school functioning at the time of the evaluation and during the previous year (see DSM-IV-TR [American Psychiatric Association, 2000, p. 34] for a description of the scale and how to use it). A useful function is that the scale provides ratings for two time periods—the current and the past year—so that the comparison may point to the need for treatment and the prognosis for future functioning, based on the scoring of the previous level of adjustment. The Global Assessment of Functioning constitutes a formalized, validated method of assessing past coping/adjustment.

Medical History

Sickness, injury, and hospitalization all constitute loss experiences in which the child has had to cope with his or her reality as an ill or injured person. None of us likes to be sick or hospitalized, least of all a child, who wants more than anything to view him- or herself as strong and competent. The child who has had extensive past experience in which he or she has felt medically vulnerable or disabled may feel less than confident when confronting a death experience. Children who themselves are terminally or seriously ill may have very diminished reserves with which to undergo grieving for someone who has died.

Past Experience with Death/Loss

In addition to personal experiences of physical vulnerability, it is essential to obtain a history of the child's past experiences with death and loss, no matter how insignificant these may seem. Wolfelt (1983) has devised a detailed Loss Inventory that documents a whole range of losses, from the death of a parent to a change in the child's living situation as a minor having to share a room. Wolfelt scores each loss in terms of degree of impact and also with regard to elapsed time since the loss, ranging from 0–6 months to 1–4 years. The Loss Inventory can help the grieving child understand that losses and attendant grief responses occur not only in response to death experiences but also the myriad seemingly petty problems of everyday life (Wolfelt, 1983, pp. 83–85). It also provides a literal summary of losses that contributes to documenting the possible effects of one individual's cumulative losses.

Death-Related Factors in Childhood Bereavement

Death is simple, and it is complex. A person stops breathing, and that single event can produce a sense of relief or of horror in the survivors. Family members who know that their loved one is in a coma with no hope of recovery may anticipate the death and feel relief when it occurs. In contrast, the cessation of breathing can create feelings of terror in a child who views his or her brother lying lifeless by the side of the road following a fatal car collision.

In evaluating the impact of a death on a child, we must consider the interaction of factors related to his or her personal background and experience, plus factors related to the death itself, and how these interact with influences of family/religion/culture/community to mediate the expression of grief. Death related factors include the following:

- Type of death
- Contact with deceased
- Expression of "goodbye"
- Relationship to deceased
- Grief reactions

Figure 2.3 provides a form for recording these factors.

Type of Death

Children listen and try to understand the many comments made by family and friends about the circumstances associated with a death. Rando refers to "the death surround" to describe all the details of a death; these include the location, type of death, reason for the death, and the degree of preparation of the survivors (1988/1991, p. 52). Factors that I consider especially important with regard to children's understanding include whether the death was anticipated or sudden; whether family members consider it was "timely"; the extent to which it might have been prevented; whether pain, violence, and trauma accompanied the death; and whether the death occurred due to circumstances associated with a sense of "stigma."

A sudden death contributes to a tendency toward denial among survivors. If a classmate who was not sick yesterday drowns today in his family pool, anxious feelings of personal vulnerability are stimulated

1. Type of death
   Anticipated? Yes _____ No _____ If yes, how long? _____ or sudden _____
   "Timeliness" of death: Age of the deceased _____
   Perception of preventability
     Definitely preventable _____ Maybe _____ Not _____
   Degree of pain associated with death
     None _____ Some _____ Much _____
   Presence of violence/trauma   Yes _____ No _____
     If yes, describe, indicating whether the child witnessed, heard about, or was present
     and experienced the trauma personally. _____
     _____
     _____

   Element of stigma   Yes _____ No _____
     If yes, describe, indicating nature of death, and degree of openness of family
     in discussing. _____
     _____
     _____

2. Contact with deceased
   Present at moment of death?   Yes _____ No _____
     If yes, describe circumstances, including who else was present and whether the deceased
     said anything specifically to the child. _____
     _____
     _____

   Did the child view the dead body?   Yes _____ No _____
     If yes, describe circumstances, including reactions of the child and others who
     were present. _____
     _____
     _____

   Did the child attend funeral/memorial service/graveside service?
     Yes _____ No _____ Which? _____
     Child's reactions _____
     _____
     _____

   Has the child visited grave/mausoleum since the death?   Yes _____ No _____
     If yes, describe circumstances. _____
     _____
     _____

3. Did the child make any expression of "goodbye" to the deceased, either spontaneous or
   suggested?   Yes _____ No _____
     If yes, describe. _____
     _____
     _____

FIGURE 2.3. Death-related factors in childhood bereavement: Webb. This form is one component of a three-part assessment of the bereaved child, which also includes an assessment of individual factors (Figure 2.2) and family/social/religious/cultural factors (Figure 2.5).

among all his peers, who probably would not experience the same level of anxiety if the death had been that of a different classmate known to be very sick with cancer. The degree of perceived preventability of the death is important both to adults and to children. Bugen (1983) discusses the interaction between the perception of preventability and the closeness of the relationship with the bereaved as predictors of the grief response.

Children are very sensitive about pain. They fear it with reference to themselves, and hearing details about a very painful death may arouse their anxiety, depending on the extent to which they can empathize. Elements of violence and trauma associated with a death also raise anxiety levels and may interfere with the grief process. Eth and Pynoos warn that "children are particularly vulnerable to the additive demands of trauma mastery and grief work. The obligatory efforts at relieving traumatic anxiety *can complicate the mourning process, and greatly increase the likelihood of a pathological grief response*" (1985, p. 179; emphasis added). Some children exposed to traumatic death may develop posttraumatic stress reactions that require special treatment (Pynoos & Nader, 1993; Nader, 1997). Many authors in this book discuss cases involving treatment of traumatic grief.

Another important consideration with regard to the type of death is the degree to which the death may be associated with stigma. Some examples of stigmatized deaths are those occurring because of suicide, AIDS, drug overdose, or murder/homicide. Doka's (1989) term "disenfranchised grief" applies to the feelings of shame that complicate the grief process and compound reactions of guilt and anger in all of the survivors.

Contact with the Deceased

As I have previously indicated, children are very literal, and they are also curious. Family members may argue about the degree to which they believe that children should be included with the family in various rituals associated with a death. I consider four pivotal points in time at which the child may be permitted to have personal contact with the deceased. These include the following:

- Being present at the death
- Viewing the body
- Attending ceremonies
- Visiting the grave or mausoleum

Rando (1988/1991) is adamant about the appropriateness of including children with the family in all rituals and observances surrounding a death. According to Rando, when children are separated from the family and not given accurate information, they have more difficulty resolving their loss. However, some children may prefer not to attend a funeral when they understand that many people will be crying. Most mental health professionals and thanatologists believe that the child should be given the choice after having been told about the circumstances that may occur at each event.

Expression of "Goodbye"

Some form of farewell to the deceased can help a child comprehend the reality of the death. The wake and/or funeral ritual may serve this purpose for adults, who "pay their last respects" as a final goodbye. Situations of sudden death, in which the body may be lost (as in a drowning at sea) or when families do not engage in any formalized funeral or memorial, deprive all family members of the personal contact with their loved one's body that can help them confirm the reality and finality of the death.

Children, who may be unable to comprehend the abstraction "death," may benefit from doing something tangible for the dead person. Some of the children described by Krementz (1981/1991) expressed their satisfaction about placing a rose on the casket or putting a note with a poem inside the casket. Bowen (1976) relates a moving example of his work with a family in which a young mother died very suddenly of a heart attack, leaving her husband and three young children. The children benefited from the private viewing of their mother's body, during which time each child spontaneously said or did something special or meaningful in the spirit of goodbye. Perhaps the value of these gestures is that they give some measure of personal control in a situation that is beyond everyone's control.

Relationship to the Deceased

The closer the relationship, the more profound will be the impact on the survivor. Wolfelt's Loss Inventory (1983) ranks the death of a parent or sibling as having the highest impact, the death of a close relative next, and the death of a friend several points lower in terms of impact on the child. Unfortunately, there is no ranking for the death of a pet, which constitutes the first experience of death for many and can be quite devastating to a child.

It is very important to consider the personal meaning of each loss in terms of the unique aspects of that relationship to the surviving child. The grief counselor can obtain details about this by asking the child to talk about the dead person and, especially, about what they used to enjoy doing together.

Grief Reactions

In the assessment of the bereaved child, the therapist notes the grief reactions that the child currently demonstrates, including in this review the child's feelings and both self-reported behaviors and those observed by the family and by the counselor. Figure 2.4 provides a means of recording the details about the nature of the child's grief.

Family/Social/Religious/Cultural Factors in Childhood Bereavement

The growing child becomes socialized into the belief systems of the adults in his or her family, school, and community. Those adults, in turn, maintain beliefs about life and death based in large part on their own childhood experiences. A book about childhood bereavement would have to be enormous to include the practices and beliefs of all cultures and religions. This is not my intent here, as I indicated in Chapter 1 of this volume. I believe, however, that the therapist or counselor must take into account the particular belief system (cultural–religious) of any bereaved child with whom he or she is working.

The significance of the following general spheres of influence on the bereaved child are included as part of the assessment, and may be recorded on the form in Figure 2.5:

- Family influences (nuclear and extended)
- School/peer influences
- Religious/cultural influences

Family Influences

Bowen (1976) pointed out that "family systems theory provides a broader perspective of death than is possible with conventional psychiatric theory, which focuses on death as a process within the individual" (quoted in Walsh & McGoldrick, 1991, p. 92). My position is that *both* individual and family systems factors must be assessed. Certainly it is essential to know how the family perceives the death and to what extent the child is included in the mourning rituals of the family. A family that believes it is appropriately shielding a young child from pain by arranging an outing with a favorite babysitter at the time of a grandmother's funeral cannot be criticized for being cruel. Families differ greatly in

Age of child _____ years _____ months   Date of birth _____

                                          Date of assessment _____

See the form "Individual Factors in Childhood Bereavement" (Figure 2.2) for recording of personal history factors.

Date of death _____

Relationship to deceased _____

_____

    Favorite activities shared with deceased _____

_____

    What the child will miss the most _____

_____

    If the child could see the deceased again for 1 hour, what would he or she like to do or say? _____

_____

_____

_____

_____

Nature of grief reactions (describe) _____

_____

_____

_____

    Signs of the following feelings?   Y = Yes; N = No

    Sadness _____   Anger _____   Confusion _____   Guilt _____   Relief _____

    Other _____

    Source of information on which this form has been completed:

        Parent _____   Observation _____   Other _____

FIGURE 2.4. Recording form for childhood grief reactions: Webb. This form is an extension of "Death-Related Factors in Childhood Bereavement" (Figure 2.3), focusing specifically on the nature of the child's grief.

1. Family influencets

   Nuclear family: How responding to death? Describe in terms of relative degree of openness of response.

   Very expressive _____ Moderately expressive _____ Very guarded _____

   To what extent is the child included in family discussions/rituals related to the deceased?

   Some _____ A great deal _____ Not at all _____

   Extended family: How responding to death? Describe, as above, in terms of relative degree of openness of response.

   Very expressive _____ Moderately expressive _____ Very guarded _____

   To what extent do the views of the extended family differ or agree with those of the nuclear family with regard to the planning of rituals and inclusions of the child?

   Very different _____ Very similar _____

   If different, describe the nature of the disagreement. _____

   _____

2. School/peer influences

   The child's grade in school _____

   Did any of the child's friends/peers attend the funeral/memorial services?

   Yes _____ No _____

   Was the teacher informed of death? Yes _____ No _____

   Did the child receive condolence messages from friends/peers? Yes _____ No _____

   Does the child know anyone his or her age who has been bereaved?

   Yes _____ No _____

   If yes, has the child spoken to this person since the death? Yes _____ No _____

   Does the child express feelings about wanting or not wanting peers/friends to know about the death? Yes _____ No _____

   If yes, what has the child said? _____

   _____

3. Religious/cultural influences

   What is the child's religion? _____

   Has he or she been observant? Yes _____ No _____

   What are the beliefs of the child's religion regarding death? _____

   _____

   What about life after death? _____

   _____

   Has the child expressed any thoughts/feelings about this? _____

   _____

FIGURE 2.5. Family/social/religious/cultural factors in childhood bereavement: Webb. This form is one component of a three-part assessment of the bereaved child, which also includes an assessment of individual factors (Figure 2.2) and death-related factors (Figure 2.3).

their degree of comfort about open expression of feelings, and the child might indeed become upset upon witnessing adults in the throes of grief.

Family members may hold differing views about the rightful role of children as participants in significant life passages such as death, and their beliefs will be determined by their cultural backgrounds. Some parents, at a time of diminished emotional reserves, do not have the resolve to argue their position with a member of the older generation, who may appear weak and vulnerable but hold more "traditional" views about "protecting innocent children" from exposure to the pain of death. In the ideal situation, young and old family members cry together and obtain strength and comfort from the unity of their mutual support. Thus, in the years to come, I hope there will be increasing inclusion of children in all of the family's rituals and personal expressions following death.

School/Peer Influences

The preschool child who attends day care may have growing awareness of the wider world outside the family. Nonetheless, young children continue to be influenced mainly by the attachment figures in their close family network. Once a child enters elementary school, however, he or she is much more alert to the opinions of teachers and classmates. When a child experiences the death of a loved one, the reactions of friends and school personnel are important to him or her. As I have already discussed, children have a strong need to "fit in" and feel accepted by their peers. Frequently they interpret this to mean conformity. When someone close to them dies, this event makes them "different" from their peers, and many children feel uncomfortable about the difference. Children may need reassurance that they will still be respected and admired for their own qualities, even though they may no longer have a father or mother. Similar to the need to reassure the young child that he or she will still be taken care of after a death, the friends and teachers of the school-age child may need to remind him or her of their continuing esteem and friendship. A child who is grieving the loss of a family member or friend is in a very vulnerable state and will appreciate genuine communications that recognize his or her value and importance as a person and indicate peers' intent to maintain their friendship.

Religious/Cultural Influences

In counseling a bereaved child, it is helpful to know not only what the child has been taught but also what he or she has "caught" with regard to the religious/cultural practices of his or her family. When children are confused, they combat their confusion with their own idiosyncratic logic. Thus, the child in the movie *My Girl*, whose friend died of an allergic reaction to numerous bee stings, began to feel better when she reasoned that her own mother, who had died in childbirth and who now "lived" in heaven, could take care of her recently deceased young friend.

We have learned more about the views of children following parental death from the work of Silverman and Worden (1992) and Klass, Silverman, and Nickman (1996), whose findings suggest that many bereaved children think about their deceased parent as "watching over" them from heaven. This view incorporates the concept of the parent as not only "superego" but also loving protector.

SUMMARY

The complete assessment of the bereaved child weighs the interactions between the various components of individual factors in childhood bereavement, death-related factors, and family social/religious/ cultural factors. While few therapists or counselors have *all* this information at their fingertips, they nonetheless must appreciate the power of both what they know and do not know as potentially influencing children's grief responses.

REFERENCES

American Psychiatric Association. (2000). *Diagnostic and statistical manual of mental disorders* (4th ed., text rev.). Washington, DC: Author.

Bluestone, J. (1999). School-based peer therapy to facilitate mourning in latency-age children following sudden parental death: Cases of Joan, age 10½, and Roberta age 9½, with follow-up 8 years later. In N. B. Webb (Ed.), *Play therapy with children in crisis: Individual, group, and family treatment* (2nd ed., pp. 225–251). New York: Guilford Press.

Bowen, M. (1976). Family reaction to death. In P. Guerin (Ed.), *Family therapy* (pp. 335–348). New York: Gardner Press.

Bowlby, J. (1963). Pathological mourning and childhood mourning. *Journal of the American Psychoanalytic Association, 11,* 500–541.

Bugen, L. A. (1983). Childhood bereavement: Preventability and the coping process. In J. E. Schowalter, P. R. Patterson, M. Tallmer, A. H. Kutscher, S. V. Gullo, & D. Peretz (Eds.), *The child and death* (pp. 358–365). New York: Columbia University Press.

Chess, S., & Thomas, A. (1986). *Temperament in clinical practice.* New York: Guilford Press.

Doka, K. (Ed.). (1989). *Disenfranchised grief: Recognizing hidden sorrow.* New York: Free Press.

Eth, S., & Pynoos, R. (1985). Interaction of trauma and grief in childhood.

In S. Eth & R. S. Eth (Eds.) *Post-traumatic stress disorder in children* (pp. 171–183). Washington, DC: American Psychiatric Press.

Fox, S. (1985). *Good grief: Helping groups of children when a friend dies.* Boston: New England Association for the Education of Young Children.

Goldman, L. (2001). *Breaking the silence: A guide to help children with complicated grief—suicide, homicide, AIDS, violence, and abuse* (2nd ed.). New York: Brunner-Routledge.

Gray, M. J., Prigerson, H. G., & Litz, B. T. (2004). Conceptual and definitional issues in complicated grief. In B. T. Litz (Ed.). *Early intervention and traumatic loss* (pp. 65–84). New York: Guilford Press.

Grollman, E. A. (Ed.). (1967). *Explaining death to children.* Boston: Beacon Press.

Hurley, D. J. (1991). The crisis of paternal suicide: Case of Cathy, age 4½. In N. B. Webb (Ed.), *Play therapy with children in crisis: A casebook for practitioners* (pp. 237–253). New York: Guilford Press.

Klass, D., Silverman, P. R., & Nickman, S. L. (1996). *Continuing bonds: New understandings of grief.* Washington, DC: Taylor & Francis.

Krementz, J. (1991). *How it feels when a parent dies.* New York: Knopf. (Original work published 1981)

Kübler-Ross, E. (1969). *On death and dying.* New York: Macmillan.

Lindemann, E. (1944). Symptomatology and management of acute grief. *American Journal of Psychiatry, 101,* 141–148.

Melhem, N. M., Moritz, G., Walker, M., Shear, M. K., & Brent, D. (2007). Phenomenology and correlates of complicated grief in children and adolescents. *Journal of the American Academy of Child and Adolescent Psychiatry, 46*(4), 493–499.

Mitchell, A. M., Kim, Y., Prigerson, H. G., & Martimer-Stephens, M. (2004). Complicated grief in survivors of suicide. *Crisis, 25*(1), 12–18.

Nader, K. O. (1997). Childhood traumatic loss: The interaction of trauma and grief. In C. R. Figley, B. E. Bride, & N. Mazza (Eds.), *Death and trauma: The traumatology of grieving* (pp. 17–41). Washington, DC: Taylor & Francis.

Nader, K. (2007). Assessment of the child following crisis: The challenge of differential diagnosis. In N. B. Webb (Ed.), *Play therapy with children in crisis: Individual, group, and family treatment* (3rd ed., pp. 21–44). New York: Guilford Press.

Parad, H. (Ed.). (1965). *Crisis intervention: Selected readings.* New York: Family Service Association of America.

Peck, M. L., Farberow, N. L., & Litman, R. E. (1985). *Youth suicide.* New York: Springer.

Pfeffer, C. R. (1986). *The suicidal child.* New York: Guilford Press.

Prigerson, H. G., Bierhals, A., Kasl, S., Reynolds, C., Shear, M., Day, N., et al. (1997). Traumatic grief as a disorder distinct from bereavement-related depression and anxiety: A replication study. *American Journal of Psychiatry, 154,* 616–623.

Prigerson, H. G., Frank, H., Kasl, S. V., Reynolds, C. F. III, Anderson, B., Zubenko, G. S., et al. (1995). Complicated grief and bereavement-related depression as distinct disorders: Preliminary empirical validation in elderly bereaved spouses. *American Journal of Psychiatry, 152*(1), 22–31.

Prigerson, H. G., Shear, M. K., & Jacobs, S. C. (1999). Consensus criteria for traumatic grief: A preliminary empirical test. *British Journal of Psychiatry, 174*, 67–73.

Pynoos, R. S., & Nader, K. O. (1993). Issues in the treatment of posttraumatic stress in children and adolescents. In J. P. Wilson & B. Raphael (Eds.), *International handbook of traumatic stress syndromes* (pp. 535–559). New York: Plenum Press.

Rando, T. A. (1991). *How to go on living when someone you love dies.* New York: Bantam. (Original work published 1988)

Rapoport, J. L., & Ismond, D. R. (1990). *DSM-III-R training guide for diagnosis of childhood disorders.* New York: Brunner/Mazel.

Silverman, P., & Worden, J. W. (1992). Children's reactions in the early months after the death of a parent. *American Journal of Orthopsychiatry, 62*(1), 93–104.

Walsh, F., & McGoldrick, M. (Eds.). (1991). *Living beyond loss: Death in the family.* New York: Norton.

Webb, N. B. (1991). Assessment of the child in crisis. In N. B. Webb (Ed.), *Play therapy with children in crisis: A casebook for practitioners* (pp. 3–25). New York: Guilford Press.

Webb, N. B. (1993). *Helping bereaved children. A handbook for practitioners.* New York: Guilford Press.

Webb, N. B. (Ed.). (1999). *Play therapy with children in crisis: Individual, group, and family treatment* (2nd ed.). New York: Guilford Press.

Webb, N. B. (Ed.). (2004). *Mass trauma and violence: Helping families and children cope.* New York: Guilford Press.

Webb, N. B. (Ed.). (2007). *Play therapy with children in crisis: Individual, group, and family treatment* (3rd ed.). New York: Guilford Press.

Wolfelt, A. (1983). *Helping children cope with grief.* Muncie, IN: Accelerated Development.

PART II

DEATH IN THE FAMILY

CHAPTER 3

Death of a Grandparent or a Parent

Lois Carey

This chapter focuses on the use of Sandplay in treating young children (under age 8) who have experienced the death of a grandparent or a parent. For many children, the loss of a grandparent or a pet is their first experience of death and, for some, this can be a very traumatic experience. Other children experience death through the loss of a parent. In either case, the child's age and the reactions of other family members are significant for his or her overall understanding and eventual resolution of such an event.

Children under the age of 7 or 8 have not yet developed a mature understanding of death, because they are in the preoperational stage of development, as described in the theories of Piaget (1955). This is the stage where fantasy is paramount and children view death as temporary. Because they have seen countless cartoons and videos in which the superhero returns to life after death, they have gained an unrealistic understanding of the true meaning of death. This type of fantasy can confuse a child when an actual death occurs in the family.

The death of a grandparent is often the first loss encountered by a child, so the reactions of those around him or her are paramount. Children look to their elders to understand what this loss is evoking in other family members. This leads the child either to express or repress his or her own feelings. Too many times the child's emotions are discounted when a survivor remarks, "He is too young to understand."

I recall one such incident involving a child of 4. Her mother's grandmother (her great-grandmother) and her mother's mother (the child's grandmother) had both died within 6 months of each other. This double loss had caused a severe depression that left the mother unable to attend fully to her child's needs. To complicate matters even further, within a year, the mother's only brother (the child's uncle) died at a very early age. The 5-year-old child felt completely helpless. She commented during the uncle's funeral, "I think my mother is the saddest one here." Her other grandmother, who recognized the child's unspoken grief, held her tightly to give whatever support was possible. Later that day, she and the child talked about how very sad she (the child) was.

Children who are as young as 1 year of age experience loss in ways that can undermine their coping capacities and retard their overall development. This was studied many years ago by John Bowlby (1969), who found that infants, when separated from their mothers, suffered what he identified as "anaclitic depression." Further studies led to efforts to help these children; I refer the reader to that early work for a fuller description.

Sandplay has an innate appeal to all children (Kalff, 1971; Lowenfeld, 1979; Carey, 1999), because construction of the scene can be totally nonverbal. Once the scene has been constructed, the child usually tells a story about what has been created and evoked. This verbalization allows the child to relate his or her concern through the story's use of "metaphor," the technique that allows the child to reveal feelings in a disguised form. For example, a child of 4 or 5 might say, when he or she relates a story about a bear, "The bear has gone away, but will come back later." This kind of statement is age-appropriate (for a 4-year-old), because the child is firmly convinced that the dead person will return.

The young child of today can be further confused about death when he or she sees characterized figures continuing their superhuman activities even though they are supposedly "dead." Cartoons achieve somewhat similar goals. I remember seeing movie cartoons of Daffy Duck and Tweetums when I was a young child. They were caught, thrashed, and sometimes killed, yet somehow they got the last laugh on their abusers by the end of the episode.

SANDPLAY THERAPY

Sandplay was developed in the middle of the 20th century by Dora Kalff, a Jungian psychologist. After Kalff saw a presentation about the World Technique, given by Margaret Lowenfeld (1979), a British psychiatrist, she became quite enthusiastic about this method. She discussed the possibilities she saw in this technique with Jung, who urged her to go to London to study with Dr. Lowenfeld. She did this in 1951, then returned to Switzerland to begin her practice with children. Kalff (1971/1980) added her Jungian understanding of symbols and archetypes to what she had learned, as she formulated her own theoretical base for Sandplay. Kalff had another major interest for her work: She was a believer in Zen Buddhism and added the idea of "no interpretation" when she viewed a child's Sandplay. In Zen Buddhism, when an explorer asks a question, the master turns it back to the questioner, so that he or she can then find his or her *own* answer rather than relying on someone else. She intuited, and rightly so, that if she began to interpret what she was seeing to the child, she was providing the sandplayer with the therapist's projection rather than allowing the insight to emerge from the builder. Still later, she was able to integrate the work of Erich Neumann (1973) into the overall schemas of Sandplay. She found that his theoretical stages of a child's psychological development mirrored what she was observing firsthand. The two had met and shared ideas, and had planned to do some research together; however, Neumann's death occurred before that was accomplished.

Kalff's work has spread throughout the world and is widely accepted as a major treatment of choice to help children (and adults) with their problems. The death of a parent or grandparent can often be a child's first trauma, one that lends itself to healing through the medium of sand.

SANDPLAY EQUIPMENT

The items used for this method include two sand boxes—one that contains damp sand, the other dry. A wide assortment of miniatures is also provided: humans of various ages, races and occupations; animals, wild, domestic, and prehistoric; transportation vehicles; buildings, rocks, stones, greenery, and so forth. I also have a coffin and several headstones in my collection. It is important to note that each therapist's collection is unique and reflects his or her interests and experiences. Kalff (personal communication, July 1980) always stressed that a therapist should never have any item in his or her collection to which he or she has no relation; otherwise, the item is just an item and, as such, is useless. The personal meaning of each item is where the healing potential lies.

PROCESS

When one begins individual therapy with a child, the instructions are kept simple. First, he or she is encouraged to feel the sand in both boxes to decide which one he or she wants to use. The therapist then says,

My signature below will grant permission to LOIS CAREY, LCSW, RPT-S, to use Sandplay pictures of my child or myself to illustrate any future articles or books authored by her. The child's name (or mine) is _____ and the birth date is _____.

It is my understanding that there will be no identifying features such as actual names, dates, location or photos that show the child's (or my) face.

The information will be presented in a disguised form as is generally approved in the professional literature.

PRINT NAME _____

ADDRESS _____

_____

SIGNATURE _____

DATE _____

FIGURE 3.1. Permission form for use of pictures.

"Please select as many objects as you would like and make a scene in the sand." Children younger than age 4 or 5 often take an inordinate number of figures at the first session, then become more selective after the third or fourth session. I usually tell a child that he or she will know when the scene feels complete, and that I will then take a picture of the scene. The child is next asked to tell a story about the completed scene.

One of the guidelines I discuss with the parent and the child during the intake session includes the reason for pictures (record keeping, as well as possible future use in a publication). I ask the parent to sign a permission statement that covers the possibility of future use of the pictures in an article or a book (see Figure 3.1). Confidentiality issues are also discussed at that time and the child is the one to decide if and when he or she wants the surviving parent to view the scene. A great deal more than these few remarks can provide is involved in Sandplay, so I refer the reader to several other sources (Kalff, 1971/1980; Carey, 1999; Bradway, 1981)

AGE OF THE CHILD WHEN DEATH OCCURS

Any death of a significant figure is usually traumatic for a child and, as noted earlier, is affected by the age of the child when the loss occurs. Children under the age of 8 or 9 have very limited understanding of death, and a major loss during this time period can cause a great deal of confusion for the child and his or her caretakers. Children from age 2 to age 7 do not have the reasoning power that they develop during a later developmental stage. Fantasy predominates at these early ages, and the child may believe that the person is simply away and will return. For this reason, it is helpful that the surviving relatives understand mourning stages for children of different ages so that they do not expect more than is possible for either a toddler or a teenager.

TYPICAL MOURNING BEHAVIORS OF THE YOUNG CHILD (UNDER AGE 8)

1. The child may cry sporadically and then go back to play with his or her friends.
2. There may be complaints of stomachaches or headaches with no known cause.
3. The child may regress to an earlier stage of development.
4. Quiet, well-behaved children can become aggressive and outspoken.
5. Aggressive children may begin to withdraw.
6. Children have great difficulty in telling their friends what has happened, because they fear that they will be seen as "different." Friends, also, are often at a loss as to what to say to the child, and may withdraw and no longer want to play.

Any of these behavioral changes are clues for the survivors or the child's teachers that the child might benefit from therapy.

HISTORY TAKING

When one is consulted about a child's treatment after loss, it is important to obtain a thorough history, including the period prior to the death. Nancy Boyd Webb (Chapter 2, this volume), developed the tripartite assessment of the bereaved child, which is invaluable to the practitioner in helping bereaved children. Briefly, to sum up the critical issues, one needs to explore the cause of death: whether the death was expected, sudden, accidental, a suicide, a drug overdose or a community disaster such as 9/11, a school shooting, an earthquake, a cyclone, and so forth.

Every child deserves to know the details of the death, and these must be presented according to the child's age and ability to understand. The details cannot be minimized, because the child's questions will continue until he or she can make sense of the death. The details cannot be ignored or glossed over, because, if they are, these issues will surface and may later be more difficult to resolve because of the earlier confusion. As is common to all mental health issues, early intervention is optimal.

GENOGRAMS IN THE SAND

The use of genograms in Sandplay has been adapted from McGoldrick and Gerson (1985) from a systemic family therapy (Piercy, Sprenkle, Wetchler, & Associates, 1996) model. This is a more directive approach that is well-known to family therapists and one that should be included in the repertoires of play therapists as well. This technique is successful in helping a child to visualize a traumatic event, especially the loss of a grandparent or a parent.

I have found that a very useful way to begin Sandplay with a bereaved child is to help him or her construct a genogram of the family, using animals to depict the different family members. The first step is for the therapist to draw a genogram on a large sheet of paper, then tell the child, "We are going to use some of the animals that are on the shelves and try to see which one might represent some of your relatives (i.e., mother, father, sister, brother, grandparents, aunts, uncles, and cousins). I would also like you to choose an animal for yourself."

Once the selection is made, the child is told to place each of the animals on the genogram. For example, if the child has selected a bunny for the mother, he or she places that miniature on the genogram in the appropriate spot. When the genogram is complete with the animals, the therapist then invites the child to make a scene in the sand that uses these figures, and to tell a story about what has transpired. The discussion that ensues illustrates the relationships that exist. It is also important to note whether the deceased parent or grandparent is included in the genogram and, if not, to assist the child in including him or her in some capacity.

BENEFITS OF SANDPLAY
FOR CHILDREN SUFFERING A LOSS

What are the benefits of using Sandplay with a bereaved child?

1. I believe that a child can be readily engaged with this method, which has shown positive outcomes for many children who have lost a close relative (Carey, 1990).
2. The younger the child, the more difficult it is for him or her to verbalize feelings. The feelings can be illustrated instead through

the construction of a sand picture and the storytelling about the scene that follows. This is especially true for the developmentally delayed child or a child who is on the autistic spectrum.

3. A child who has witnessed the funeral and burial has the ability to replay that painful, leave-taking event and provide some catharsis. If the child has not attended that ritual, he or she has the means at his or her disposal to make up a satisfactory answer to his or her (possible) confusion. This is where the skill of the therapist is paramount, to help the young child make sense of the insensible.

CASE VIGNETTES*

Alana S., a 6-year-old girl, was brought to therapy by her father. Her mother had died about 1 year earlier. The child had shown absolutely no reaction to this loss until shortly before her father called. She was the youngest child in the family; Alana had two teenage brothers. Alana began to experience problems at school related to her educational progress and her lack of social skills. She would suddenly burst into tears with no apparent precipitant and could not self-soothe. The history revealed that her mother had been struck by a car and was killed instantly.

Mr. S. had been quite depressed since his wife died, so part of the healing was in a family therapy format that included Mr. S. and his mother, Alana's caretaker. This set of grandparents helped out with necessary babysitting arrangements. Mr. S.'s mother prepared dinner each night for them and Alana was allowed to sleep in whichever house she chose. This pattern was continued for about the first 6 months of therapy, after which Alana slept in her own home.

The teenage brothers in this family had a different father and spent weekends and holidays with him. The father of those two boys would not give permission for therapy, so they were excluded from family sessions.

Cultural issues were important to consider with this child as well. Part of the relevant family history was that Alana's mom had been from the Caribbean, while her dad was of Norwegian descent. Her mom was in recovery from drug and alcohol abuse at the time of her death. Both of Alana's parents had severe drug histories.

This child chose to use Sandplay almost exclusively during her individual therapy hours. Her favorite animals were lions, entire families of them. She repeatedly played out the story of *The Lion King*.

---

* Cases are composites and names have been changed.

In Figure 3.2, you see the lions and other animals coming to pay their respects to the dead Father Lion buried beneath the headstone. She owned the video of this story and often watched it at home, until she felt secure enough to move on.

Family sessions that were held with Alana and her father utilized therapeutic board games. Their favorite game was Talking, Feeling and Doing, developed by Dr. Richard Gardner. I chose this intervention because I believed that both of them suffered from an undiagnosed expressive language disorder. This proved to be the case when Alana had to be tested for learning problems and required extra support in school.

One time, during a family therapy session, Alana asked her father to give mom's cross to her. It had been hanging on the wall by the parents' bed. She began to sleep with it each night thereafter, which became a part of her healing. This allowed Alana to feel close to her mom, and the cross served as a transitional object for her. Eventually, she asked that it be hung over her bed. She was able to feel her mom's presence in this way. Her grandmother was not in favor of allowing this, feeling that it was "too morbid." I supported it as a way for the child to feel some connection to her mother.

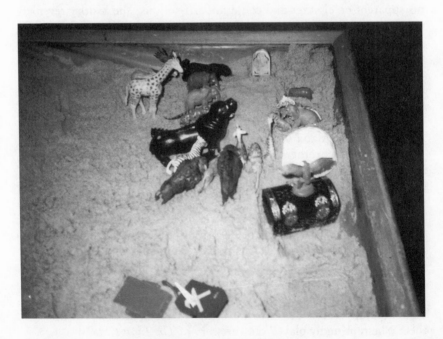

FIGURE 3.2. Alana's Sandplay picture.

The second example, a 3-year-old girl, Mary Ann Z., was the first very young child I treated with Sandplay, and her case is an example of an anticipated death. Her father had died a month or two earlier, after a lengthy battle with cancer. He had been ill for almost all of the child's life. Mrs. Z. had tried to get treatment for Mary Ann from several other therapists before she contacted me. They all told her that Mary Ann was "too young" for therapy but offered to help her instead. Mrs. Z had had her own therapy and knew instinctively that Mary Ann had her own separate problems. I explained that I had not treated such a young child, but said, "I'm game if you are." (I worked with this child for approximately 3 years after this beginning.)

This was the case of an expected death, as mentioned earlier. However, for a 3-year-old, it was much more than that. Her father's death precipitated severe reactions in this child. Mary Ann was experiencing nightmares and temper tantrums; her toilet training had regressed; and she was demanding a baby bottle several times a day and also to help her sleep. She was attending a religious nursery school that would not allow her to talk about her loss. On Parents' Night, the staff refused to post the story that she had written (dictated to her mother), because "it might upset the other children and their parents." We found another nursery school soon after that. I knew that the change would be another loss for this child, but it was nevertheless indicated, because of the long-term advantages.

Mary Ann continued to have sleep problems that were permeated with monster fears. One scene she replicated a number of times in her sessions. I made a decision to switch to a more directive approach and suggested to her that we could pretend the dinosaurs were her fearsome monsters that came to bother her at night and, if we fed them here, then that might make them content to stay on the shelves and not pursue her at home. This "clicked" with her and a ritual for her loss was developed. She and I together made "food" for the dinosaurs and fed them. They were then taken to the toy bathroom set (that had been placed in the sand), where they were toileted, bathed, and put to bed (see Figure 3.3). This ritual took place for several months.

Of particular interest was that Mary Ann always placed two other dinosaurs on top of the other sandbox. She said that one was "Daddy" and the other was "God." (She had been told that Daddy went to heaven and was now with God.) This ritual resolved most of her regressive behavior after several months. She no longer was experiencing tantrums, and she had given up the bottle and the diapers. Figure 3.4 shows another way in which Mary Ann attempted to understand death. She placed many large stones and put other stones on top of them. She placed

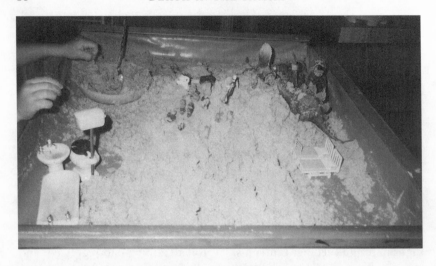

FIGURE 3.3. Mary Ann's Sandplay picture 1.

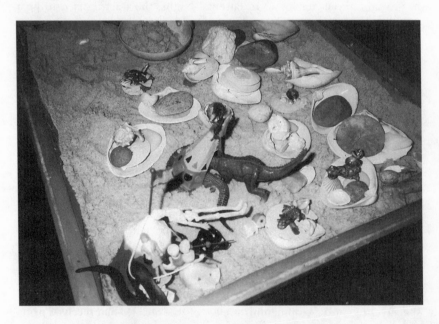

FIGURE 3.4. Mary Ann's Sandplay picture 2.

small figures between each of the stones. She said that this scene represented "All the souls in heaven." I believe that this was quite an illustration for a 3½-year-old child!

Mary Ann was a very bright, verbal child, but Sandplay allowed her
to express her fears far more effectively than any words could ever do.
Mary Ann, at 3 years of age, had no way to put these deep-seated fears
to rest, but she was able to address these issues concretely in the sand.

A few years after therapy ended, Mary Ann's mother sent me a copy
of a story Mary Ann had written for a school assignment when she was
in the fourth grade. This is taken from Carey (1999, pp. 183–184).

A Special Helper and Friend

After my dad died, I was very sorrowful. My mom took me to a special
Sand Play Therapist for kids and this helped me to learn to cope with his
death. My dad died of cancer when I was three years old. It was very sad! I
was just devastated and confused. My mom took me to a psychologist that
practices Sand Play Therapy. Her name is Lois Carey and her husband's
name is David Carey. My dad's name was David too. David Carey is a
musician. Since Lois works at home, when I went there, I sometimes got
to hear music.

Lois has a room with a sand box of wet sand and a sand box of dry
sand. When I went there, I played in the sand and made a scene with my
choice of little figures and props. She took pictures of my scene, and I told
a story about my scene that explains feelings. Sometimes I went into the
office-type room and played games, colored, or just talked and told stories.
After my dad died, I started going to Lois. I had fun with Lois and she took
my mind off my dad and convinced me that everything would be okay! She
made me feel a lot better and helped me to understand what was going on
and what had happened!

Death is very difficult for a little kid to understand. I am glad that
there are special people like Lois to help you get through it.

Another case is that of an 8-year-old boy, Jack C., with a history
of developmental delay (Carey, 1990, pp. 197–209). Jack had lost his
40-year-old father as the result of a sudden heart attack. This child
became eneuretic and encopretic after the death, and these physical
symptoms were the reason he was brought to therapy. Jack was in a
special class for developmentally delayed children and had received prior
counseling for his speech and learning problems, but the school felt
he needed more intensive treatment after this major loss. The surviving family members included his mother, who had to return to work,
and three older brothers. This was a case of an unexpected death, with
no opportunity to prepare for such a major loss. This family's religious

and cultural background was Irish Catholic. Jack's older brothers all attended a Catholic high school.

Mr. C. had died from a heart attack in the bathroom of their home. Jack, who had not yet developed a mature reasoning ability, because of his neurological impairments, now was refusing to go to the bathroom for his toileting needs. He was in the stage of preoperational functioning, as theorized by Piaget (1955).

One intervention consisted of my drawing a person that showed the digestive system. I explained to Jack some of the functions of our bodies. I showed him that food goes into the mouth, then travels through the stomach and intestines, and the waste material comes out in our bowel movements. Similarly, when we drink water or milk or soda, the fluid travels into the stomach, then is processed through the kidneys and the bladder, and expelled through the penis (on boys).

I explained to Jack that the reason his dad died in the bathroom was because when one has a heart attack, he or she feels nauseous and goes to the bathroom, thinking that he or she might throw up. However, for his dad, he had just reached the bathroom when his heart stopped working. I stressed that this was very different than needing to go to the bathroom for everyone's normal need to move his or her bowels or to urinate. This simple explanation was effective, and Jack was again able to go to the bathroom for his physical needs.

One of his sand pictures (Figure 3.5) illustrates how Jack was finally able to put his father to rest. It contains a castle with candles in the turrets, a dragon with candles in each of its two mouths, and a pyramid-shaped candle surrounded by outer-space figures. A man lay buried under the pyramid. (I moved the pyramid in order to photograph what was beneath it [see Figure 3.6].) This seemed to be a burial ritual for Jack's father, and it enabled this bereaved child to be able to put his father to rest.

Tom K., a 6-year-old boy, was brought to therapy by his clinically depressed 32-year-old mother. Her mother had just died from a sudden heart attack. The grandmother had been the sole caretaker for this boy, because his single mother was employed and they lived with her. The boy was withdrawing from all of his friends, had lost control of his bladder functioning, and had no focusing ability in school. Tom was in a frozen state, with no support from his depressed mother. There were no other close relatives; his father's whereabouts were unknown.

This case appeared to be one that required a family systems and play therapy orientation, and I presented it to the mother that way. She refused at first, saying that she didn't have time to "just play." I explained the rationale, saying that this format could help her, as well as the child,

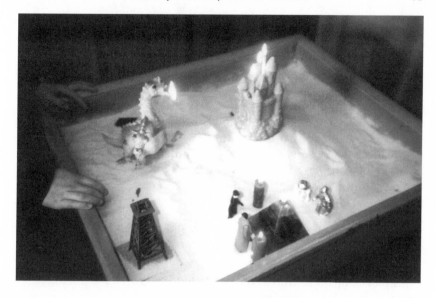

FIGURE 3.5. Jack's Sandplay picture.

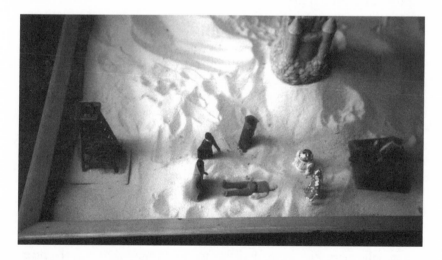

FIGURE 3.6. Jack's Sandplay picture, with the pyramid moved to reveal a buried man.

and would help in restructuring their family, now that Grandma was dead. Reluctantly, the mother agreed. In order to ensure the mother's cooperation, I suggested that they try a short-term contract of six sessions, with the option to continue should that prove necessary.

I suggested in the first session a family genogram that mother and son completed together. The mother chose a dragon for her mother, a soldier for the boy, and a kitten for herself. The boy chose a bear for Grandma, a wolf for his mother, and a lion for himself. The mother described her choice of a dragon for her mother, saying, "She was always angry and I could never find a way to please her." Her son was described as "a brave little soldier," and for herself, "the kitten was all soft and fuzzy."

The boy, in describing his choices, said, "Grandma was like a great big, lovable bear who hugged me lots." He described Mom as a snarling wolf, always angry at him and himself as the lion "like the boy in *The Lion King* story who had lost his father."

I picked up on the theme of anger from both parties and said, "You two sure have different views of Grandma! Mom, you see her as very angry, and Tom, you see her as lovable. Tell me about her as each of you saw her." In talking about Grandma, anger and tears were elicited from both mother and son, and the discussion helped each one to see Grandma in a different light. When it came to talking about themselves, Mom was able to see how deep the grieving process was for her son, and she was able to be more effective in nurturing him. I noted the absence of a figure for the father. The boy's mother said she had no idea where he might be, and that Tom had never met him. I asked each of them to pick a figure that might represent him. Mom chose a large cobra and Tom chose Superman. I made a comment about these choices: Mom sees the dad as a large poisonous snake; Tom sees him as a superhero. These choices, and the later discussion, helped them both see the father in a more realistic light. Mom's choice, the cobra, represented all that she had ever known about him. He was a one-night stand, and both were high on crack cocaine when Tom was conceived. (This fact was withheld from Tom in order to not tarnish his view of his dad. Tom was told that the father was on leave from the Army, and that he had been killed in action.) She never did see the father after that; however, it was the pregnancy that sent her to rehab. This information saddened Tom and made him wonder what his father may have been like. His fantasy life had selected Superman as a hero father, which seemed appropriate for his developmental stage. (I advised the mother to tell Tom the truth when he was older and better able to understand these facts.)

The experience with the genogram in that first session enabled us to use the information gleaned to help mother and son rebuild their lives without Grandma. Mom's depression was reduced, so that she was able to be more nurturing to Tom. Tom quickly regained control of his bladder and was again interacting positively with his peers. Grandma had left a small estate that Mom inherited and, with this added income, she was able to hire appropriate child care for Tom when she returned to work. This was a short-term contract where the set goals were achieved:

- Relieve some of Mom's depression.
- Restructure the family without Grandma.
- Allow both mother and son to mourn their loss.
- Help Tom regain control of his bodily function.
- Help Tom and his mother bond as a unit.

Another case is one that began when I received a phone call from Mrs. W., the mother of 5-year-old Gail, another example of an expected death. Mrs. W. told me that she was dying of brain cancer and asked me if I would provide therapy for her daughter. Mrs. W. was bedridden and could not come to my office for an intake, so I made a home visit to meet her and to see the child. She was indeed in the final stages of cancer. She was very frail; she had no hair, and her head was wrapped in a scarf. Our visit lasted less than half an hour because she became exhausted.

Mrs. W. was a very brave woman who had taken the time to write notes to her daughter, to be given to her at appropriate times: birthdays, graduations, sweet 16, and so forth. The notes were kept in a special place and Gail's father, Mr. W., was instructed as to when they were to be presented. This woman was setting up the process whereby the child could continue to be connected to her, even after death. The actual death occurred less than 1 week after that first meeting.

Therapy was begun with Gail shortly before Mrs. W.'s death. Family members were also included in treatment: Mr. W., the child's father, and the maternal grandparents, who were suffering from the loss of their daughter. This case is a good example of a family that had done a great deal of anticipatory mourning and had effectively planned for this young child's bereavement. Gail used sand very effectively in her individual sessions and was able to verbalize her concerns through her stories. Her stories, like those of the other children cited, were about her missing the dead parent, being angry that she no longer had a mother, and finally an eventual acceptance of the situation.

Gail's therapy might have ended within the first year except that her father remarried within 6 or 8 months of being widowed. This meant that the child needed additional treatment to accept a mother substitute so soon after her loss. She not only needed to resolve her bereavement issues, but she also had to adjust to a new family constellation. This new family also received family therapy as part of the adjustment.

This particular case therapy took place a number of years ago. Gail's grandmother has kept me apprised of her progress by sending me a new photo of the child, which she includes with a Christmas card. The most recent picture is that of a young graduate who has just completed a master's program at a prestigious university.

CONCLUSION

The challenge to help young children with the healing process after the loss of a parent or grandparent is a major one. This can be doubly challenging if the therapist had a similar loss at a similar age. One would hope that the therapist has dealt with his or her issues before treating a bereaved child; otherwise, one might be faced with difficult countertransference issues.

I have illustrated through the previous examples how these families dealt with death.

The first child, Alana S., was bicultural—Puerto Rican and Norwegian. These two cultures are widely divergent in their customs. In her mother's Latin culture, burial rites can continue for several days and the religion is Roman Catholic. Her father's family was Norwegian Protestant and much more reserved in handling of any crisis. In both of these cultures there is resistance to the whole idea of therapy: "You must be crazy if you see a therapist."

Alana was negatively impacted because of her grandmother's feelings toward Puerto Ricans. She discouraged the child from having any contact with the mother's family. This had a very undesirable side effect, because Alana knew and understood that she was bicultural, and that part of her was being rejected.

The second and fourth cases, Mary Ann Z. and Tom K., were Orthodox Jewish. There is an extended period of mourning in this community, beginning with the fact that the burial takes place within 24 hours. The family then sits *shiva* for seven days after the burial. That is the intended time for friends and family to go to the home of the deceased to express their condolences. A gift of food is offered to the family by the visitors. The final ritual occurs 1 year later, when a headstone is provided for the grave.

The third case discussed, Jack C., was of an Irish Catholic family. In this tradition, a wake takes place in the funeral home, followed by burial or cremation. A wake consists of scheduled times when the family will be present at the funeral home to greet friends and family members.

This length of time can be extremely tiring for the immediate family members, to which I can surely attest. My Protestant family has the same ritual as the Roman Catholic—1–3 days of visiting with friends and well-wishers, followed by the funeral.

The case of Tom K. illustrated a short-term contract to deal with the loss of a grandparent. This family had no active involvement with the grandmother's Catholic background, but one part of the termination session was to enroll Tom in a religious education program. His mom was able to agree, with the understanding that this could benefit him in further healing this loss.

These few examples comprise part of my professional and personal experience in providing therapy to bereaved children. The reader may have other cultural examples from his or her own practice; but regardless of the religious background of the child, it behooves all of us to pay particular attention to the cultural and religious background of each family. This is a necessity that best helps the child to incorporate the strengths found in his or her family of origin. It is doubly important that the therapist not impose his or her cultural values and/or religion into the treatment but instead be empathic and supportive to the child.

This chapter has focused on the use of Sandplay therapy for a bereaved child, primarily because that is my specialty. However, other play therapy methods can be equally effective. Techniques such as art, puppetry, and storytelling are well-utilized with a grieving child, because they do not require extensive verbalization but keep the treatment in a metaphoric milieu. This is especially true for the child under 8 years of age, who has not yet reached the age for a more intellectual understanding of death. This understanding can come later; in fact, the child may need to address various issues pertaining to the loss at different stages of life.

I believe that the most important function of therapy with a young child is to help him or her to process what has occurred at his or her level of understanding. By achieving some early resolution of the significant death, a child can then proceed with the rest of his or her developmental, educational, and social needs that certainly lie ahead, without unresolved loss issues that can be a major hindrance.

DISCUSSION QUESTIONS AND ROLE-PLAY EXERCISES

1. Describe some reactions or symptoms that might determine when a young child might benefit from bereavement counseling.
2. Who is to be the primary client—child, family, both? Why?

3. Discuss why the age of the child impacts service delivery.

4. Do you believe the loss is more significant for a child with respect to the sex of the child and the death of the same-sex parent? That is, is loss of a mother more important for a girl, and the loss of a father more important for a boy? How does one's age impact this?

5. Role play: Imagine that you are a 5-year-old boy who comes home from kindergarten and is told that his father was killed in a robbery. Pick a partner to play the part of the mother and act out two different possibilities.

REFERENCES

Bowlby, J. (1969). *Attachment and loss: Vol. 1. Attachment; Vol. 2. Loss*. London: Hogarth Press.

Bradway, K., Signell, K., Spore, G., Stewart, C., Stewart, L., & Thompson, C. (1981). *Sandplay studies: Origins, theory and practice*. San Francisco: C. G. Jung Institute.

Carey, L. (1990). Sandplay therapy with a troubled child. *The Arts in Psychotherapy, 17,* 197–209.

Carey, L. (1999). *Sandplay therapy with children and families*. Northvale, NJ: Aronson.

Gardner, R. (1973). *The Talking, Feeling, and Doing Game: A psychotherapeutic game for children*. Englewood, NJ: Creative Therapeutics.

Kalff, D. (1971/1980). *Sandplay: Mirror of a child's psyche*. San Francisco: Browser.

Lowenfeld, M. (1979). *The world technique*. London: Allen & Unwin.

McGoldrick, M., & Gerson, R. (1985). *Genograms in family assessment*. New York: Norton.

Neumann, E. (1973). *The child*. New York: Harper Colophan Books.

Piaget, J. (1955). *The child's construction of reality*. New York: Basic Books.

Piercy, F., Sprenkle, D., Wetchler, J., & Associates. (1996). *Family therapy sourcebook* (2nd ed.). New York: Guilford Press.

CHAPTER 4

The Grief of Siblings

BETTY DAVIES
RANA LIMBO

When asked what they like about their brothers or sisters, young children will often groan, "Like? I don't like anything about them!" But when questioned further, many describe positive attributes of their relationship: "He helps me with my homework" or "She talks to me about things no one else will talk about." Adolescent siblings sometimes express gratitude for the watchful eye of their older brother or sister: "He always looked out for me—made sure that I didn't get into trouble." Ambivalence often characterizes relationships between siblings. Furthermore, sibling research characterizes siblings as attachment figures, antagonists, playmates, protectors, and socializers (Davies, 1999). Through a shared history and common bonds, siblings have the potential for providing one another with intense emotional experience, support, guidance, information, and companionship. Consequently, the significance of the sibling relationship portends the profound effect that the death of one child can have upon brothers and sisters, even when the child is a baby and dies during pregnancy, at birth, or shortly after.

When a baby dies, siblings who knew about the impending birth frequently have expectations about what it will mean to be a "big sister" or "big brother." Parents, grandparents, other siblings, and even strangers help young children form images about this new baby. Technology has created the opportunity for young children to be involved early in a pregnancy. Ultrasonic images show the baby's body shape, limbs, hands and feet, and—with more sophisticated equipment—even facial features. "Knowing" an unborn or newly born sibling who dies is a significant loss for a young child as he or she tries to understand feelings of dashed expectations, sadness, and guilt—and parents who are not quite the same.

Despite the potentially traumatic effect of sibling bereavement, little attention has been directed to children's reactions to the death of a brother or sister. The earliest publication to address sibling bereavement appeared in 1943 (Rosenzweig) and discussed the relationship between sibling death and schizophrenia. This paper stood alone on the topic for two decades. Four articles appeared in the 1960s (Cain, Fast, & Erickson, 1964; Hilgard, 1969; Pollock, 1962; Rosenblatt, 1969); all focused on the effect of childhood bereavement on adults under treatment for psychiatric disorders. Authors writing on the topic in the next decade continued to be mostly psychiatrists and psychologists, who expanded beyond pathology to include the potential growth among bereaved siblings and a family perspective (Blinder, 1972; Binger, 1973; Tooley, 1973; Pollock, 1978; Nixon & Pearn, 1977; Krell & Rabkin, 1979). During the 1980s, authors represented additional health care disciplines, and a dramatic increase in the number of papers was evident. The concern shifted from consideration of sibling bereavement as a psychiatric problem to a concern for promoting children's health (Balk, 1983b; Martinson, Davies, & McClowry, 1987). As well, attention was directed toward siblings of various ages, including adolescents (Balk, 1983a, 1983b, 1996; Mufson, 1985; Hogan, 1988; Hogan & DeSantis, 1992, 1996), and toward the various factors, particularly the family, that may influence siblings' experiences (Lauer, Mulhern, Bohne, & Camitta, 1985; McCown, 1984; Davies, 1988a, 1988b). During these years, the setting shifted from psychiatry to oncology, and included the sudden death of an infant (Mandell, McAnulty, & Carlson, 1983). More recently, interest has turned to developing and testing intervention programs for bereaved siblings (Gibbons, 1992; Horsley & Patterson, 2006).

Literature specifically related to responses of siblings when a baby dies has focused more on sudden infant death syndrome than on death of the baby during pregnancy or shortly after birth (Burns, House, & Ankenbauer, 1986; Hutton & Bradley, 1994; Mandell, Dirks-Smith, & Smith, 1988; Price, 2007). According to Hughes and Riches (2003), systematic studies of siblings born prior to a stillbirth are nonexistent. Callister (2006) highlights the bereaved sibling in perinatal loss as feeling "left out" (p. 229). Pantke and Slade (2006) studied the effects on parenting from the perspective of young adults who were under 5 when a sibling died during pregnancy, at birth, or shortly thereafter. They perceived their mothers as more protective and controlling than did nonbereaved counterparts. Recent research interest focuses on children born subsequent to a perinatal death (Heller & Zeanah, 1999; O'Leary, Gaziano, & Thorwick, 2006; Pinto, Turton, Hughes, White, & Gillberg, 2006), particularly related to mother–infant attachment. Much still remains to be done to assess the complex interactions of multiple factors affecting sibling bereavement, to assess bereavement interventions for siblings and their families, and to continue the exploration of long-term effects of sibling bereavement.

SIBLING RESPONSES

Early reports in the literature provide contradictory findings with regard to children's reactions to a sibling's death. Some investigators reported disturbed reactions in the form of significant behavior problems (Cobb, 1956; Cain et al., 1964; Binger et al., 1969; Binger, 1973). In contrast, others reported no significant problems (Futterman & Hoffman, 1973; Stehbens & Lascari, 1974). A later study (Burns et al., 1986) found that length of grief response for children was similar to that of adults. The variability in findings raises questions about whether the behavior evidenced by grieving siblings represents pathology or a range of bereavement responses.

Range of Behaviors

Bereavement literature indicates that sadness, irritability, feelings of being alone, complaints of bodily discomforts, sleep disorders, and loss of appetite are common to both children and adults who are grieving. These are manifestations of normal grief, and unless they occur with severe intensity or for long periods of time, they are not necessarily indicators of maladjustment (Webb, 1993; Chapter 2, this volume). Rather than assessing children's response to a death by identifying the presence or absence of any of these behaviors, it is more important to consider the intrusiveness created by the grieving in the child's life (Webb, 1993). Moreover, the absence of typical grieving behaviors is not necessarily cause for alarm; not all children are affected in the same way or to the same degree by a sibling's death. For example, when a baby dies, each surviving sibling may have unique expectations and relationship with the anticipated baby (Limbo & Wheeler, 1986/2003). It is more likely than is the case when an older child dies that the sibling of a baby who dies in the perinatal period will be preschool age or younger. For a child who may not be able to express feelings verbally, the opportunities for play and family rituals take on added importance (Kobler, Limbo, & Kavanaugh, 2007). Parents, in fact, need to be advised that each child in the family will react differently and that some children's reactions may not become evident until later.

Absence of behavioral changes should not negate the significance of the event for siblings, since responses may be internal and not readily apparent. However, some siblings have obvious difficulty, and adults must be alert to the needs of these children. In some studies, about 25% of bereaved siblings demonstrated behavioral problems at levels comparable to those of children referred to mental health clinics; in the general population, behavior problems of only 10% of children reach this level. Unfortunately, there is no certain way to identify children whose behavior is a sign that they are in trouble, but a number of behaviors may signal which children might require further attention. Watch for children who show persistently the following signs of problematic sibling bereavement:

- Persistent sadness, unhappiness, or depression
- Persistent aggressiveness or irritability
- Loneliness and social withdrawal
- Worrying
- Persistent anxiety or nervousness
- Ongoing eating difficulties or recurrent nightmares
- Low self-esteem
- Poor school performance

It is important to remember to look for *persistent changes* in the child's behavior and for a *pattern* of problems. No single problem by itself is necessarily an indication of trouble. Though not requiring formal intervention, most bereaved siblings can benefit from opportunities to talk about their responses at the time of the death and for many years to come. If they are denied opportunities to talk about the death and their reactions, children suffer needlessly.

Duration of Bereavement

The impact of sibling bereavement lasts for a lifetime; bonds continue between siblings and even provide comfort (Packman, Horseley, Davies & Kramer, 2006). Years following the death, many bereaved siblings report that they still think about, talk to, and miss their deceased brother or sister. They often experience renewed and intense grief on occasions that would have been significant in their lives together, such as graduations, weddings, a new baby in the family, career challenges, and even retirement in their later years. It is helpful to warn parents and older siblings about the recurring grief they may experience, and to reassure them that such reactions are common and not signs of emotional disturbance.

Being a survivor from a multiple birth (e.g., a surviving twin) is a special circumstance of sibling bereavement. Survivors of a multiple birth may feel both guilty (e.g., wondering if they got all the nourishment) and special (as a twin, triplet, or higher-order multiple) (Pector & Smith-Levitin, 2002). These siblings were "wombmates," yet there may be few tangible mementoes of their relationship. Many parents choose to have photos taken of their multiples together, whether alive or dead. When one twin is stillborn, the survivor's birthday is also the deceased baby's death day. Two birthday cakes is a common way of recognizing the twin who did not survive. The juxtaposition of life and death is a lifelong awareness for the survivor. In fact, a surviving multiple sometimes feels as if part of his or her "self" is missing, or that he or she is half of something (Limbo & Wheeler, 1986/2003).

Growth Potential

A child's death may not only have potentially negative effects on surviving siblings, but psychological growth may also result. In one study, bereaved siblings scored higher than the standardized norms on a measure of self-concept (McClowry, Davies, May, Kulenkamp, & Martinson, 1987). Many siblings felt that they had matured as a result of their experience, and felt good about their ability to handle adversity. As one teenage boy commented, "I have a better outlook on life now; I mean, as a result of my sister's death, I realize how important life is." Interviews with parents also indicated that they perceive their children as more sensitive, caring individuals who have matured as a result of their experience with death. Many parents describe their children as more compassionate and aware of other people's problems. In the words of one mother about her 15-year-old daughter, "She has learned a lot from her brother's death. It hasn't been easy, but she has gained such insight about life and death. She has been exposed to things that most kids of her age are not. She had to grow up faster, and she is very sensitive and patient. She is so much more tolerant of others as well." Hogan (2008) describes the grief-to-personal-growth theory of sibling bereavement, which includes acute grief, regrieving, continuing bonds, and the impact of social support on the child's grief. The idea of the child's potential for personal growth or transformation through suffering mirrors ideas found in literature about adults (see Büchi et al., 2007; Ferrell & Coyle, 2008; Calhoun & Tedeschi, 2001).

Researchers and clinicians share the common goal of wanting to reduce as much as possible the untoward effects of sibling bereavement on children and adolescents. To this end, studies have focused on one or more influencing factors, such as age, gender, suddenness of death, self-esteem, family environment, and their effect on behavior and emotional outcomes. Though they contribute to our knowledge about sibling bereavement, such studies do not provide sufficient guidance for intervention, since a combination of factors influence how siblings respond to the death of a brother or sister.

Looking more closely at the conceptual relationships among the variables and siblings' responses provides a comprehensive description of directions to assist grieving children (Davies, 1999). The impact of a child's death on siblings results in four general responses: (1) "I hurt inside"; (2) "I do not understand"; (3) "I do not belong"; and (4) "I am not enough."

"I Hurt Inside"

This first response focuses on the emotional and psychophysiological responses normally associated with grief. These include sadness, anger, frustration, loneliness, fear, anxiety, irritability, and guilt. These responses are common to all who grieve, including children—it hurts to grieve. However, unlike adults, who more readily describe their emotions, children manifest their hurt in other ways. They may cry, withdraw, seek attention, misbehave, complain of aches and pains, pick fights easily, argue, have nightmares, fear the dark, lose their appetites, or overeat.

"I Do Not Understand"

How children begin to make sense of death depends in large part on their level of cognitive development. As children mature, they move from concrete operational ways of thinking toward more abstract or conceptual ways of thinking (see Chapter 2, this volume). For example, when a baby dies during early pregnancy (miscarriage or ectopic pregnancy), the young sibling has not had a chance to get to know the baby in any concrete way. If children are not assisted to understand and in their own way make sense of death and related events, they become very confused. Their confusion only compounds the anxiety they feel, and their anxiety in turn adds to their confusion.

"I Do Not Belong"

A death in the family disrupts the usual day-to-day activity of family life. Parents are distressed, and familiar and unfamiliar visitors invade the home. Children feel overwhelmed with the flurry of activity and the outpouring of emotions. They often feel as if they do not know what to do; they may want to help but do not know how. They may begin to feel as if they are not a part of the activity, that they do not belong. Sometimes children's unique ways of responding are not tolerated by adults. For example, a teenager who prefers to go out with friends rather than stay at home with other family members may be harshly criticized by adults who think that the family should be together during the crisis. Bereaved children frequently feel different from their peers; again, this may contribute to their feelings of not belonging.

"I Am Not Enough"

This response may result when children feel as if the child who died was a favored child. They feel that the dead child was special in some way, or in many ways, and that they themselves are not at all special. Such children may conclude that *they* should have been the one to die. No matter what they do, they are "not enough" to make their parents happy ever again. After a baby dies, a surviving sibling may have a sense of not being enough if parents' are intensely focused on getting pregnant again.

Sibling Responses in Context

Siblings' reactions to the death of a brother or sister do not occur in isolation. Characteristics of the children themselves, the circumstances surrounding the death, and environmental factors play a role. These various factors, characterized as individual, situational, and environmental characteristics, interact with one another to impact siblings' responses to the death of a brother or sister (E. Davies, 1983; B. Davies, 1995, 1999; Hunter & Smith, 2008; see Figure 4.1).

Paying attention to individual characteristics is basic to perceiving each child as being his or her own person. It requires knowing what makes each sibling unique and the factors that influence the child's vulnerabilities to loss. Individual characteristics include physical aspects (e.g., gender and age, dependence, and health status), coping style, socioemotional aspects (e.g., as temperament and self-concept), and experience with death and loss.

The circumstances surrounding the death also contribute to how siblings respond. These variables include the cause of death, the duration of illness preceding the death, the place of death, the time elapsed since the death, and the extent of involvement in the death and death-related events.

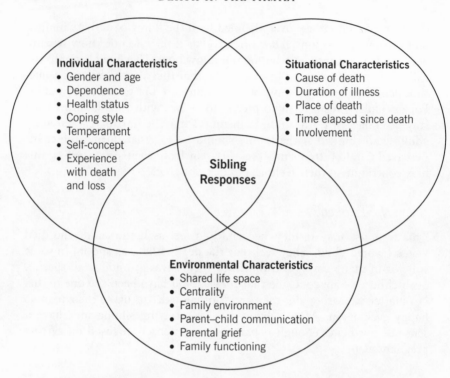

FIGURE 4.1. Mediating variables impacting upon sibling bereavement. From Davies (1999). Copyright 1999 by Taylor and Francis, Inc. Reprinted by permission of Taylor and Francis, Inc., *www.routledge-ny.com.*

Environmental variables constitute the third category; these are factors that contribute to the socioemotional atmosphere of the child's context. The nature of the predeath relationship between siblings is of significance. The closer the relationship between two siblings, the more difficulty the surviving child will have after the other's death. Closeness may override age and gender differences. Family environment, particularly family social climate, level of functioning within the family, and parental grief responses, also are instrumental in sibling bereavement response. Children react strongly to these factors, since they are dependent on their families for the information and support they receive. Families characterized by open communication about the death and about feelings tend to provide environments that are supportive of grieving children. Children learn from their parents and from other adults about death and grief, and how to deal with them. If children see their parents openly sharing their own sorrow, if they hear conversations in which their parents talk about their sadness and confusion and how to deal with these reactions, then children are more likely to learn effective ways of expressing and managing their own sadness.

The cause of death (whether the death is sudden and unexpected or follows a downhill illness trajectory) is one situational factor commonly viewed as significant to bereavement outcome. Literature on adult bereavement widely documents that sudden death results in more intense grief of longer duration (Ball, 1976–1977; Carey, 1977; Fulton & Fulton, 1971; Parkes, 1975; Vachon, 1976); this applies to sibling bereavement as well. Regardless of the cause of death, all siblings require a clear understanding of what happened. In cases of accidental or violent death, however, issues of fault or preventability come into play, often resulting in family members', including siblings, feelings of responsibility (Kaplan & Joslin, 1993). In addition, elements of trauma and violence raise children's anxiety levels, since they may fear a similar fate. When the death is a result of suicide, surviving children are at risk for disturbed grief reactions (Stephenson, 1986; Brent et al., 1993), since they must cope with their grief, possible feelings of rejection by the deceased child, and the negative and social stigma that accompanies suicide (Doka, 1989).

The death of a child from a long-term illness implies that the surviving children have had the opportunity to learn about the disease and to prepare for the ill child's eventual death. The assumed benefit of anticipatory grief making grief easier for these families is not the case. All parents hope that their child will be the miracle child who recovers at the last moment. They struggle to put aside their fears of death. Siblings also tend to appraise the situation in positive ways (Brett & Davies, 1988). As a result, there is always an element of the unexpected in a child's death. Moreover, the stress of a long-term illness on families is profound. As a result, siblings may experience the death with a "backlog" of unmet needs and feelings of resentment, because their parents have had little time to spend with them. Each family's situation and the experience of each surviving sibling must be assessed individually.

Perinatal loss (miscarriage, ectopic pregnancy, stillbirth, or the death of a newborn) is more common than most people realize. There are over 1 million miscarriages, approximately 43,000 ectopic pregnancies, 26,000 stillbirths, and 18,000 newborn deaths (death in the first month of life) each year in the United States. In almost all instances, the event is sudden and unexpected. Exceptions include infants in a neonatal intensive care unit (NICU), whose death is expected (e.g., a baby born at the margin of viability), or a baby diagnosed during pregnancy with a life-limiting condition (e.g., trisomy 18 or hypoplastic heart).

Sibling responses occur within a larger familial and social context as well. Cultural and community values and priorities also contribute to the experiences of bereaved siblings. Within their immediate family, or within their extended families and communities, the interactions siblings have with the significant adults in their lives are integral to how they manage and adapt to the death of a brother or sister.

A STILLBIRTH TOUCHES A YOUNG SIBLING

Carrie listened to the 40-year-old woman tell her story. This was a panel discussion of adults, reflecting back on their childhood experience of having a sibling die during the mother's pregnancy or shortly after birth. As a bereavement coordinator and bereaved parent herself, Carrie found that panel discussions were always interesting, usually engaging her both personally and professionally. The woman on the panel described herself as being 8 years old when her brother died right after birth from severe congenital anomalies. Then the panel member said something that caught Carrie's attention: The last time she had seen her mother happy was before her brother was born. Carrie recalls being "dumbfounded" by that observation. And where her thoughts went next would be life changing: "I wondered how my own children had perceived me after the loss of my babies." Here is the rest of Carrie's story.

> "After the panel, I called my son Colin in New York, where he was attending college, to tell him what the woman said. I asked him about his recollections and feelings surrounding the deaths of his brother Adam in 1997 and sister Meg in 1998, both of whom were born too prematurely to survive. I wondered if he remembered and if he still felt the impact. His answers brought tears to me:
>
> " 'Oh, my gosh, Mom. Yeah, it was terrible. After Adam, everything was different. You were never happy, you stopped being a room mother or participating with any of our sports teams. You cried all the time. We didn't go to St. Thomas [the family's church] anymore.'
>
> "We changed churches a few months after we lost Adam because we didn't feel our priest supported or responded to our grief. Not going to St. Thomas meant giving up the camp Colin had attended every summer for 7 years. He also recalled that we didn't 'hang out' with some of the families we had always spent time with, and I can say we had many relationships that changed if people couldn't deal with our grief, or we couldn't deal with their responses. He also remembered me being 'obsessed' with having a baby, and that I couldn't go back to work because I was so 'upset.' That led to expensive fertility treatments instead of expensive private sporting

leagues. We eventually adopted our daughter Caroline—but I had to work full time to help recover from all of the spending, so again, I missed school and athletic events. Looking back, I know that none of us would change the way things went, as Caroline is truly the perfect fit for our family, and both of her brothers are crazy about her. But the magnitude of impact that perinatal loss has on *all* members of a family can shape the future for those it touches, often in ways that we won't know until the 'touched' grow up."

Comments

What lessons can we learn from Carrie's story? Children generally move on faster than do adults in their grief work. With perinatal loss, a young child may have patted his or her mommy's tummy, talked to the baby, and shared in the family's anticipation of the birth. The expectation of being a "big brother" or "big sister" is a powerful imagining for a young child. Yet young children are also "in the moment" creatures. Their day-to-day life of play, sleep, socialization, and eating remains important after the baby's death, sometimes, as in Carrie and her husband Rex's case, more important than parents are able to realize at the time. This illustrates how bereaved children carry the loss with them, with the need to reprocess the loss as they grow, develop, and mature. It also illustrates that the perception and experiences of the child can be dramatically different from those of the parent and need to be drawn out.

ADULT INTERACTIONS WITH BEREAVED SIBLINGS

The four major sibling responses listed earlier can serve as a guide to adults who are striving to help grieving children (Davies, 1999). For children who are "hurting inside," the goal for parents and other adults is to comfort and console. Adults must accept the child's feelings and behaviors as normal manifestations of grief. They must be patient in allowing children to express their own thoughts and feelings in their own time, and in their own ways. Adults who endeavor to share their own thoughts and feelings with children instill a sense of being with them and offer hope for feeling better in the future. On the other hand, when adults limit expression of feelings, children may conclude that there is something wrong with their feelings. In such situations, children frequently learn to stifle their feelings.

Parents and other adults play a major role in helping children who "don't understand." Adults must explain and interpret all that is happening. Adults need to remember that confusion and ignorance contribute to additional hurt. Therefore, adults must provide honest information in ways that children can understand. They must provide explanations and offer information ahead of time, so that children know what to expect. Children learn that it is OK to ask questions, if they have adults in their lives who offer explanations of feelings and not just events, and who help them to interpret their own feelings and reactions. They also learn that not all questions have answers; in the company of understanding parents, they learn to accept the uncertainties of life.

Adults can do much to prevent bereaved siblings from feeling as though they "don't belong," if they include and validate the children. When children are included in what is happening, when they have an active role to play in plans and activities, when they are prepared in advance for what is happening, children can manage very well. They feel as if they are part of the family, as if they have valuable contributions to make. On the other hand, when children are excluded from the plans and activities, when they are not given a choice about the nature of their involvement, or when they are not adequately prepared for what to expect, they feel as if they do not belong; their presence and contributions are invalidated. Such children often seek attention through acting out, risk taking, avoiding home, or withdrawing into themselves or their schoolwork.

When children hurt inside, feel as if they are stupid because they do not or cannot understand what has happened, or perceive that they do not belong, their feelings of "I am not enough" are enhanced. This response can be lessened by adults who reassure and confirm through both word and deed that the children are indeed special. Through both verbal and nonverbal messages from adults, children must be made to feel that they are loved, appreciated, and valued. Children who feel that they are not enough may deal with their feelings of inadequacy and inferiority by overachieving, taking on the identity or characteristics of their deceased sibling, excelling at meeting the needs of others, or becoming unrealistically good.

A child's death has lifelong implications for that child's brothers and sisters. However, siblings who are comforted, taught, included, and validated feel that they learn from their experience. They feel that they have become better people, are better able to help others who are grieving, and are better prepared to handle death in the future. Siblings who are belittled, disregarded, left out, or shamed live with feelings of regret and remorse, and feel that nothing good came of their experience. Of course, the experience of any sibling is not entirely one way or the other, but the goal of helping bereaved siblings is to help them to integrate their losses in ways that are regenerative rather than degenerative in the continual unfolding of their lives.

IMPACT OF A SIBLING DEATH IN EARLY CHILDHOOD

When Jan Thomas, age 18, was interviewed for one of my (B. D.) research projects about sibling bereavement, she had just completed her first year of study at the local university, majoring in philosophy. She lived at home with her parents. Jan was the youngest of three siblings. Her older sister, Julia, age 23, attended college in another state. When Jan was 5 years old, her brother Mark died at age 11, one year after being diagnosed with a brain tumor. The interview was tape-recorded and transcribed; excerpts appear below.* Jan described her initial response to her brother's death:

> "I guess my first childhood memory, the first thing I can remember, as far back as I go without people actually telling me what happened, is the viewing of the body at my brother's funeral. It's probably one of the worst memories I have, too, because I can remember standing there and looking at my brother and I can remember feeling no remorse, nothing. I think it's because I was so young, I didn't even know what was going on. . . . "

Jan began to think about her earlier experience in seventh grade, when she was asked to present the annual award that had been established in her brother's name:

> "Yeah, that's what got me started thinking about it. We never talked about it as a family, so I went on just trying to, trying to figure out what it all meant. . . . I wanted to know what it was and why my brother died. . . . "

Jan struggled alone with her grief; her thoughts and feelings in response to her brother's illness and death were not addressed by the significant adults in her life:

> "Growing up, right through junior high and high school, I would never bring it up to my parents. [My dad] had a lot of deaths in his family that affected him, and he doesn't let his emotions out. And we never talked about it. I can never remember talking about it as a family. They told me that we never did even when I was little. Occasionally you might talk about something he did, but you never

---

* Names and identifying information have been altered to protect the anonymity of Jan and her family.

talked, you never mentioned that he died. . . . I was just scared to talk to them about it."

In recent conversations with her mother (e.g., *"Mom said that she would have liked for me to talk to her about it earlier on, but I was just a little kid when it happened so I couldn't really be the one to set the stage"*), Jan could remember some of the times that might have been opportunities for discussion: *"Like when something Mark made had broken and Mom would break down,"* but Jan's mother did not talk about her own grief or talk to Jan about what she may have been feeling.

Jan perceived that other people did not seem to understand her need to learn more, and she *"didn't feel right"* talking to anyone other than her parents, because *"I was also brought up in a family where problems within the family stay in the family, and that's how things are dealt with."* In high school, Jan attended classes at her church and found *"a lot of inner connections between death and religion."*

> "I think that's an effect my brother's death had on me. . . . Anytime I look at a religion, I base my thoughts on my brother's death to see if that religion can justify it. I stopped being active in the Christian religion, I stopped believing in a Christian God, because I felt that it couldn't justify my brother's death. And I held that against Christianity, and I still do. So his death has led me to the way I live now."

Jan's desire "to find out why my brother had to die, especially at such a young age" resulted in her spending time reading all she could about death. She realized she was different from her schoolmates:

> "I never felt ashamed to go into class, having a book on death and reading it before class. In junior high especially is the time where kids see you're reading a book on death, and they have their preconceived ideas about how weird that is. So, I never had close people through school. I played basketball in school and I had friends there, but there was never anybody that I felt I could call up on the weekend and say 'Why don't we all go to the movie' or 'Why don't we do something.' I just felt different than the other kids somehow, and I think it was because I was always thinking about Mark. Later on, I felt more comfortable with people I didn't go to school with. I got a job at 16, and I used to love to go to work because nobody knew who I was. They didn't know about Mark and about what I was interested in. That's where I met my friend. She was starting to work there, too, and she was the first person

that I felt I could open to and talk to. She was the first person I talked to about Mark."

Jan found that a death and dying class she took her freshman year in college served as a catalyst for doing things she had wanted to do for a long time, such as visiting the cemetery:

"That's something [going to the cemetery] that I had wanted to do. It was 6 years [since seventh grade] that I was thinking about my brother's death and thinking of all these questions that I could never find an answer for. . . . I couldn't go to the cemetery because I didn't have my driver's license. I knew the cemetery, but I didn't know where in the cemetery [Mark was buried] because I had never been there. I got my license and felt I could go out and do something on my own. That was two summers ago. That's when I went and saw the grave, so it was something that I had wanted to do but I never felt I could until then."

The course also facilitated Jan's talking with her parents:

"My mom knew I was taking the class. . . . I was reluctant to let her read my papers, but then I decided to let her read the first group of papers and then I got to talking with my mom about it . . . [and] started to get some answers."

Jan used the class also to develop a strategy for connecting with her father. In her final paper, she wrote about wanting to talk with her dad: "I took it home and I left it somewhere, and he found it and read it." Ultimately, he wrote back to her, telling of his own grief when his mother died while he was fighting in the Vietnam War.

"He didn't really know her before he went off to war, and then she died before he had a chance to get to know her. He explained to me how all of these things affected him and that's why he is the way he is now. So I was finally able to talk to my dad—it was the first time that I ever saw him be emotional."

Jan's older sister Julia had a different experience.

"Julia is a lot like my father. They both have the problem where they can't be open about this. . . . I've talked to my sister only a few times. . . . She sees how Mark was. Mark was a perfect child, and Julia thought she was always judged against Mark. Mark was always a straight A student, and he was sociable. He was real popular with everybody, and everybody liked him. Julia always felt that my parents judged her against that. Then I came along, and I was good in school, too. Julia felt like she was stuck in the middle. She feels that she can't be good enough, that she can't match up to Mark. She can only remember me and Mark being together all the time and being the best of friends and she was left out. She has a resentment to Mark."

Jan concluded her interview with advice for others:

"The most important thing is to talk to kids, tell them what's happening—at the time and later, too, all the time. Don't try to hide them from death and from all the emotions. Because if you keep things in the closet when kids are little, you just have to clean it out later, and by then there's an awful lot of junk stored in that closet."

Comments

Jan's story highlights the experience of many bereaved siblings. At the time of Mark's death and afterward, there was little discussion in the Thomas family about what had happened. In families, when a child's death is not discussed openly, the surviving children are often left with unanswered questions about what happened, and oftentimes about their role in and responsibility for what happened. Jan did not seem to feel responsible in any way for her brother's death, but she did not have a clear understanding of the illness that caused his death. Because Mark's name was seldom mentioned, Jan was left with the impression that she "should" not talk about him. Moreover, Jan felt that to raise the subject carried the potential of upsetting her mother or making her father angry. In such families, children tend to keep their thoughts and feelings to themselves, and are thereby deprived of the information and comfort that parents might be able to offer. But the parents, too, are distressed, and often, out of their perceived need to protect their surviving children from additional distress, they try to hide their own sadness—as Mr. and Mrs. Thomas did when they took turns going upstairs to cry away from the children. When families can openly talk about what happened and about their reactions to events, children learn that sadness is a normal and natural response, and that there is comfort in sharing the sadness.

Jan's story, and that of her sister Julia, exemplify how the quality of the relationship between siblings affects the bereavement experience of the surviving child. Jan had a close relationship with Mark. Even though Jan and Mark were neither close in age nor the same gender, they shared a special bond. She found comfort in learning more about Mark's death. Julia, on the other hand, had felt "left out" of the special relationship Mark and Jan had shared; Julia resented her two siblings. Moreover, Mark was a good student, an accomplished athlete, and popular, and Julia felt inadequate by comparison. Her sense of inadequacy persisted after his death to the point of her stating that she wished *she* had been the one to die. Her father was very dismayed over this comment, but the lack of open communication and reassurance to Julia that she was special in her parents' eyes more than likely contributed to her feelings of "I am not enough."

In my interviews with other siblings who have experienced the death of a brother or sister in their childhood, I learned that some of them continued to have their questions unanswered throughout many years of their lives. Then, by attending a lecture or presentation on sibling bereavement, or reflecting on their inner lives with a counselor for some seemingly unrelated reason, they realize the impact of their sibling's death. Jan showed remarkable persistence and determination, knowing at some level that finding out the answers to her questions was important for her. She experienced greater peace of mind, as many bereaved siblings do when they have the opportunity to examine their earlier experiences.

CONCLUDING COMMENTS

My interview with Jan was for research purposes. However, as a clinician who has worked with and talked to many bereaved siblings, I have learned that such interviews also serve therapeutic purposes. At the conclusion of each research interview, after the tape has been turned off, I ask about the experience of participating in the study. Frequently, people indicate that this is the first time they have ever told their story; such was the case with Jan, though she had written about various aspects of her experience in the class on death and dying. More often than not, individuals say that they enjoyed the opportunity just to "tell their story" and to have someone be "interested in what I have to say." Through telling their story, they often gain new insights and perspectives. Jan felt that the interview had been another step in "cleaning out the closet." And, as is the motivation for many siblings who participate in a research project of this type, Jan hoped that sharing her experience would somehow benefit other children, so they would have "less junk stored in the closet."

DISCUSSION QUESTIONS

Carrie's Story

1. Colin had just entered his teen years when Adam died. What people, events, and concerns tend to be important to a child at that age?

2. Related to question 1, what points in Colin's story illustrate the multiple losses he experienced as a bereaved sibling?

3. What impact might the death of two siblings so close together have on a family's life?

Jan's Story

1. Discuss some of the typical reactions of a 5-year-old to death. How do Jan's memories of her brother's death resemble or differ from these?

2. Since different family members often have very different responses and feelings about the death of a child or sibling, what type of counseling is appropriate? Discuss the pros and cons of family–individual and group counseling with regard to Jan's family.

3. How would you assess Jan's capacity for dealing with future losses? Do you consider her to be "at risk," and why or why not?

4. How could Jan's experience be used to provide guidance to parents about how to support their well children when another child is seriously ill? About how to support their bereaved children following the ill child's death?

5. What approach might be appropriate in helping Julia, Jan's older sister, in dealing with her experience of sibling bereavement?

REFERENCES

Balk, D. (1983a). Effects of sibling death on teenagers. *Journal of School Health, 53*(1), 14–18.

Balk, D. (1983b). Adolescents' grief reactions and self-concept perceptions following sibling death: A study of 33 teenagers. *Journal of Youth and Adolescence 12*, 137–161.

Balk, D. (1996). Attachment and the nations of bereaved college students: A longitudinal study. In D. Klass & P. Silverman (Eds.), *Continuing bonds: New understandings of grief* (pp. 311–328). Washington, DC: Taylor & Francis.

Ball, J. (1976–1977). Widow's grief: The impact of age and mode of death. *Omega: Journal of Death and Dying, 7*, 307–333.

Binger, C. M. (1973). Childhood leukemia: Emotional impact on siblings. In J. E. Anthony & C. Koupernick (Eds.), *The child and his family: The impact of disease and death* (pp. 195–209). New York: Wiley.

Binger, C. M., Ablin, A., Feuerstein, R., Kushner, J., Zoger, S., & Mikkelsen, C. (1969). Childhood leukemia: Emotional impact on patient and family. *New England Journal of Medicine, 2804,* 414–418.

Blinder, B. J. (1972). Sibling death in childhood. *Child Psychiatry and Human Development, 2,* 1969–1975.

Brent, D. A., Perper, J. A., Moritz, G., Liotos, L., Schweers, J., Roth, C., et al. (1993). Psychiatric impact of the loss of an adolescent sibling to suicide. *Journal of Affective Disorders, 28,* 249–256.

Brett, K., & Davies, B. (1988). What does it mean?: Sibling and parental appraisals of childhood leukemia. *Cancer Nursing, 11*(6), 329–338.

Büchi, S., Mörgeli, H., Schnyder, U., Jenewein, J., Hepp, R., Jina, E., et al. (2007). Grief and post-traumatic growth in parents 2–6 years after the death of their extremely premature baby. *Psychotherapy and Psychosomatics, 76,* 106–114.

Burns, E. A., House, J. D., & Ankenbauer, M. R. (1986). Sibling grief in reaction to sudden infant death syndrome. *Pediatrics, 78*(3), 485–487.

Cain, A., Fast, I., & Erickson, M. (1964). Children's disturbed reactions to the death of a sibling. *American Journal of Orthopsychiatry, 34,* 741–745.

Calhoun, L. G., & Tedeschi, R. G. (2001). Postraumatic growth: The positive lessons of loss. In R. A. Neimeyer (Ed.), *Meaning reconstruction and the experience of loss* (pp. 157–172). Washington, DC: American Psychological Association.

Callister, L. C. (2006). Perinatal loss: A family perspective. *Journal of Perinatal and Neonatal Nursing, 20*(3), 227–234.

Carey, R. G. (1977). The widowed: A year later. *Journal of Counseling Psychology, 24,* 125–131.

Cobb, B. (1956). Psychological impact of long-term illness and death of a child in the family circle. *Journal of Pediatrics, 49,* 746–751.

Davies, B. (1988a). Shared life space and sibling bereavement responses. *Cancer Nursing, 11,* 339–347.

Davies, B. (1988b). The family environment in bereaved families and its relationship to surviving sibling behavior. *Children's Health Care, 17,* 22–31.

Davies, B. (1995). Sibling bereavement research: State of the art. In I. Corless, B. Germino, & M. Pittman (Eds.), *A challenge for living: Death, dying and bereavement* (Vol. 2, pp. 173–202). Boston: Jones & Bartlett.

Davies, B. (1999). *Shadows in the sun: The experiences of sibling bereavement in childhood.* Philadelphia: Brunner/Mazel.

Davies, E. (1983). *Behavioral response of children to the death of a sibling.* Unpublished doctoral dissertation, University of Washington, Seattle.

Doka, K. (Ed.). (1989). *Disenfranchised grief: Recognizing hidden sorrow.* New York: Free Press.

Ferrell, B. R., & Coyle, N. (2008). *The nature of suffering and the goals of nursing.* Oxford, UK: Oxford University Press.

Fulton, R., & Fulton, J. (1971). A psychosocial aspect of terminal care: Anticipatory grief. *Omega: Journal of Death and Dying, 2,* 91–100.

Futterman, F. H., & Hoffman, I. (1973). Crisis and adaptation in the families of fatally ill children. In E. F. Anthony & C. Koupernick (Eds.), *The child and his family: The impact of disease and death* (Vol. 2, pp. 121–138). New York: Wiley.

Gibbons, M. B. (1992). A child dies, a child survives: The impact of sibling loss. *Journal of Pediatric Health Care, 6,* 65–72.

Heller, S. S., & Zeanah, C. H. (1999). Attachment disturbances in infants orn subsequent to perinatal loss: A pilot study. *Infant Mental Health Journal, 20*(2), 188–199.

Hilgard, J. R. (1969). Depressive and psychotic states as anniversaries to sibling death in childhood. *International Psychiatry Clinics, 6,* 197–207.

Hogan, N. S. (1988). Understanding sibling bereavement. *The Forum, 12,* 4–5.

Hogan, N. S. (2008). Sibling loss: Issues for children and adolescents. In K. J. Doka & A. S. Tucci (Eds.), *Living with grief: Children and adolescents* (pp. 159–174). Washington, DC: Hospice Foundation of America.

Hogan, N. S., & DeSantis, L. (1992). Things that help and hinder adolescent sibling bereavement, *Western Journal of Nursing Research, 16,* 132–153.

Hogan, N. S., & DeSantis, L. (1996). Adolescent sibling bereavement: Toward a new theory. In C. Corr (Ed.), *Handbook of adolescent death and bereavement* (pp. 173–195). New York: Springer.

Horsley, H., & Patterson, T. (2006). The effects of a parent guidance intervention on communication among adolescents who have experienced the sudden death of a sibling. *American Journal of Family Therapy, 34*(2), 119–137.

Hughes, P., & Riches, S. (2003). Psychological aspects of perinatal loss. *Current Opinion in Obstetrics and Gynecology, 15*(2), 107–111.

Hunter, S. B., & Smith, D. E. (2008). Predictors of children's understandings of death: Age, cognitive ability, death experience and maternal communicative competence. *Omega: Journal of Death and Dying, 57*(2), 143–162.

Hutton, C. J., & Bradley, B. S. (1994). Effects of sudden infant death on bereaved siblings: A comparative study. *Journal of Child Psychology and Psychiatry, 35*(4), 723–732.

Kaplan, C. P., & Joslin, H. (1993). Accidental sibling death: Case of Peter, age 6. In N. B. Webb (Ed.), *Helping bereaved children: A handbook for practitioners* (pp. 118–136). New York: Guilford Press.

Kobler, K., Limbo, R., & Kavanaugh, K. (2007). Meaningful moments: The use of ritual in perinatal and pediatric death. *MCN: The American Journal of Maternal Child Nursing, 32*(5), 288–295.

Krell, R., & Rabkin, L. (1979). The effects of sibling death on the surviving child: A family perspective. *Family Process, 18,* 471–477.

Lauer, M. E., Mulhem, R. K., Bohne, J. B., & Camitta, B. M. (1985). Children's perceptions of their sibling's death at home or in hospital: The precursors of differential adjustment. *Cancer Nursing, 8,* 21–27.

Limbo, R. K., & Wheeler, S. R. (2003). *When a baby dies: A handbook for healing and helping.* La Crosse, WI: Gundersen Lutheran Medical Foundation. (Original work published 1986)

Mandell, F., Dirks-Smith, T., & Smith, M. F. (1988). The surviving child in the SIDS family. *Pediatrician, 15*(4), 217–221.

Mandell, F., McAnulty, E. H., & Carlson, A. (1983). Unexpected death of an infant sibling. *Pediatrics, 72*(5), 652–657.

Martinson, I., Davies, B., & McClowry, S. (1987). The long-term effects of sibling death on self-concept. *Journal of Pediatric Nursing, 2*, 227–235.

McClowry, S., Davies, B., May, K., Kulenkamp, E., & Martinson, I. (1987). The empty space phenomenon: The process of grief in the bereaved family. *Death Studies, 11*, 361–374.

McCown, D. (1984). Funeral attendance, cremation and young siblings. *Death Education, 8*, 349–363.

Mufson, T. (1985). Issues surrounding sibling death during adolescence. *Child and Adolescent Social Work Journal, 2*, 204–218.

Nixon, J., & Pearn, J. (1977). Emotional sequelae of parents and siblings following the drowning or near-drowning of a child. *Australian and New Zealand Journal of Psychiatry, 11*, 265–268.

O'Leary, J. M., Gaziano, C., & Thorwick, C. (2006). Born after loss: The invisible child in adulthood. *Journal of Prenatal and Perinatal Psychology and Health, 21*(1), 3–23.

Packman, W., Horsley, H., Davies, B., & Kramer, R. (2006). Sibling bereavement and continuing bonds. *Death Studies, 30*(9), 817–841.

Pantke, R., & Slade, P. (2006). Remembered parenting style and psychological well-being in young adults whose parents had experienced early child loss. *Psychology and Psychotherapy, 79*(1), 69–81.

Parkes, C. M. (1975). Determinants of outcome following bereavement. *Omega: Journal of Death and Dying, 6*, 303–323.

Pector, E. A., & Smith-Levitin, M. (2002). Mourning and psychological issues in multiple birth loss. *Seminars in Neonatology, 7*(3), 247–256.

Pinto, C., Turton, P., Hughes, P., White, S., & Gillberg, C. (2006). ADHD and infant disorganized attachment: A prospective study of children next-born after stillbirth. *Journal of Attention Disorders, 10*(1), 83–91.

Pollock, G. (1962). Childhood parent and sibling loss in adult patients. *Archives of General Psychiatry, 7*, 295–305.

Pollock, G. (1978). On siblings, childhood sibling loss and creativity. *Annual of Psychoanalysis, 6*, 443–481.

Price, S. K. (2007). Social work, siblings, and SIDS: Conceptual and case-based guidance for family system intervention. *Journal of Social Work in End-of-Life and Palliative Care, 3*(3), 81–101.

Rosenblatt, B. (1969). A young boy's reaction to the death of his sister. *Journal of the American Academy of Child Psychiatry, 8*, 321–335.

Rosenzweig, S. (1943). Sibling death as a psychological experience with reference to schizophrenia. *Psychoanalytic Review, 30*, 177–186.

Stehbens, J. A., & Lascari, A. D. (1974). Psychological follow-up of families with childhood leukemia. *Journal of Clinical Psychology, 30*, 394–397.

Stephenson, J. (1986). Grief of siblings. In T. A. Rando (Ed.), *Parental loss of a child* (pp. 321–338). Champaign, IL: Research Press.

Tooley, K. (1973). The choice of a surviving sibling as "scapegoat" in some cases of maternal bereavement: A case report. *Journal of Child Psychology and Psychiatry, 16,* 331–339.

Vachon, M. (1976). Stress reactions to bereavement. *Essence, 1,* 23.

Webb, N. B. (1993). Assessment of the bereaved child. In N. B. Webb (Ed.), *Helping bereaved children: A handbook for practitioners* (pp. 19–42). New York: Guilford Press.

CHAPTER 5

The Disenfranchised Grief of Children

DAVID A. CRENSHAW
JENNIFER LEE

"Disenfranchised grief" is a term introduced by Kenneth Doka (1989, 2002) to describe grief that is not acknowledged by society and not viewed as legitimate. The concept of disenfranchised grief has also been applied to children (Crenshaw, 2002). Examples of disenfranchised grief for children are the loss of a pet or even a fictional character, or a cherished object like an old, worn out blanket that young children carry with them as a transitional object. These losses, while significant to the child, may be viewed as inconsequential by adults. The grief of young children in general may be disenfranchised because adults are reluctant to believe that young children can comprehend death. It reaches the absurd extreme at times when preschool children receive more preparation, explanation, and emotional support in preparing for a shot at the pediatrician's office than they do when their mother or father dies. Parents will say, "Oh, she is only 4, she doesn't understand." Any 4-year-old will notice right away that her mother is gone and everyone else in the family is distressed, but sadly, in these cases, no one is talking to the child. This is an unintended example of disenfranchised grief in children.

The reason that parents sometimes do not talk to young children about a death in the family goes beyond their beliefs that such a young child cannot possibly understand such matters. It causes unbearable pain in adult family members at a time when they are already grief stricken to see the pain of a young child when told of the death of a family member. They therefore avoid it and rationalize that the child is too young to understand anyway. While this is understandable in human terms, it is misguided, because the child suffers without adult guidance, comfort, and support.

Many examples of disenfranchised grief arise in clinical practice. When separation and divorce occurs, the loss the child feels for the absent parent may be devalued by the parent who is present at the time. It is quite common when divorced parents start dating that the children become attached to one or more of the dating partners. If the relationship dissolves, the grief of the child may be unrecognized, or even forbidden, if the parent is angry with the former lover. Often the grief that children experience on the death of a pet is not respected or honored by adults who may be insensitive to the magnitude of the loss for the child. The adults might comment, "Oh, it was just a 'critter.' No need to be upset." Missed in such comments is that for the child not only was it not just a "critter," but the death of a pet is often the child's first encounter with death, and it can hit with great emotional impact.

The devastation that children feel when a good friend moves away is often underestimated by adults. Children may be particularly bereft if they feel they have lost their best friend. Children in out-of-home placement often are moved from home to home in the foster care system, sometimes on short notice, with little time to say adequate good-byes. These children leave behind a trail of broken relationships and a huge reservoir of disenfranchised grief. Adolescents form intense but often brief romantic relationships and when they break up, one or both partners may experience acute grief. Adults tend to minimize the grief, because they consider it just "puppy love." The loneliness, pain, and grief of children who habitually are socially rejected are often not recognized. Yet the suffering of these youngsters is intense. Although we can cite many more examples, the types of disenfranchised grief experienced by children can be grouped into disenfranchised grief within the family, disenfranchised grief within the community, disenfranchised grief within the culture, and disenfranchised grief within the self.

DISENFRANCHISED GRIEF WITHIN THE FAMILY

As mentioned previously, the grief of young children often is ignored because of the misguided belief that the child is simply too young to understand. In that case, the child may have no one to ask questions about the loved one or, in extreme cases, the name of the deceased family member may not even be mentioned in the presence of the child.

In the case of the death of a divorced parent, the other parent may be unable to support or sanction the grief of the children because he or she cannot tolerate such expressions of grief related to the ex-spouse. In less extreme cases, the death of the ex-spouse may cause the other parent to minimize the grief of the children or try to move them past it before they are ready to do so.

In some families the significance of the loss for a child may be minimized if the child had a conflictual relationship with the now deceased family member. In fact, in such a case, the child may suffer more, not less. Not only is the child faced with enormous loss, but also guilt that cannot easily be resolved, a rupture in a relationship that he or she has no opportunity to repair, and longing for the kind of relationship with the deceased that now can never happen.

Pauline Boss (2006) discussed the concept of "ambiguous loss," which she defined as a loss that remains unclear. The uncertainty or a lack of information about the whereabouts or status of a loved one as absent or present, as dead or alive, can be traumatizing for families. Ambiguous loss may be experienced in families due to military casualties, natural disasters, or terrorist events in which the body of the deceased is never located or recovered. But within the family there may also be significant differences in the tolerance for ambiguity; thus, some children may not feel sanctioned in their grief, because the adults in the family may still not recognize or accept the death of the loved one.

The very manner in which children react to the death of a family member may contribute to the disenfranchisement of their grief. In a study of the reactions of children to the death of a sibling, the Child Behavior Checklist (CBCL) revealed behavior problems in 50% of the total sample of 42 boys and 48 girls, ages 4–16 years, whose siblings had died 2–24 months earlier (McCown & Davies, 1995). The predominant behavior problems fell into the Aggression subscale of the CBCL. When children are acting out aggressively it may be difficult for parents to be attuned to the underlying pain of their grief, particularly when the parents are grieving the death of a child.

Another common reaction of children and adolescents to death is avoidance (Swihart, Silliman, & McNeil, 1992). When children are deeply affected by the death of a family member but their way of coping is avoidance of any remembrance, discussion, or commemoration of the deceased, they may mislead the rest of the family. The family may feel they are not hurting, or even worse, that they do not care. The latter perception may lead to angry accusations, such as "How could you be so cold and unfeeling?" Usually children avoid their grief in desperation. They fear being overwhelmed and engulfed, like being swept up in a tidal wave, if they focus on their grief. These children may not be internally strong enough to withstand the taxing emotional demands of overt grief. Of course, we know that children in general tend to approach their grief in measured steps, because they simply do not have the psychological resources to immerse themselves in grief as do adults in the mourning process. Understanding this difference in the way children grieve compared to adults may help parents to be more supportive and empathetic with the plight of their grieving child or teen.

Still another source of disenfranchised grief in the family is the failure to understand the importance of the child's continuing bond and attachment to a deceased sibling or parent. It is not surprising that families may be unaware of the child's need for a continuing attachment to a deceased loved one, since only in the last two decades in the bereavement field have professionals fully appreciated the importance of this bond (Hogan & DeSantis, 1992; Rubin, 1999). Although Nagera (1981) discussed the need for continuing bonds with the deceased parent in psychoanalytic writing much earlier, it seems to have had little impact on the field.

Nagera (1981) especially emphasized that children need this continuing relationship with their deceased parent to complete the unfinished tasks of development. Until the last two decades, however, the bereavement field largely adopted the prevalent view of bereavement in medical science that grief is time bound, and healthy recovery depends on severance of emotional bonds with the deceased (Hogan & DeSantis, 1992). It is small wonder given the debate and confusion in the field that well-meaning parents sometimes give the stern message to their bereaved children—"Enough already! It is time to get over it and let your mother go." When children are told to sever the emotional bonds with their deceased parent that are vital for the successful completion of development, their grief is not honored, not understood, and both their grief and developmental needs are disenfranchised.

DISENFRANCHISED GRIEF IN THE COMMUNITY

When a family member dies, the grief of a child may not be recognized or adequately supported within the community. This is particularly true if the family member's death was stigmatized in some way, such as death by suicide or AIDS. Also, in the case of traumatic death, the horror of the manner of death may serve to frighten or inhibit surrounding community members from offering the usual measure of support and concern, partly because friends and neighbors may not know what to say or how to respond in such traumatic circumstances. The tendency is to avoid or distance themselves from such painful tragedies, and even if the family is adequately supported in the immediate aftermath, family members may quickly find themselves isolated and cut off from the community as friends and neighbors distance themselves from the overwhelming grief and pain of the family. While the distancing is understandable, it comes at the worst possible time for the grieving family members, at the very time when they most need the support and caring of the surrounding community.

The emotional support of peers is critical when an adolescent experiences death in the family, but teens do not always know how to act in such circumstances. Due to their own lack of comfort and preparation in death-related matters, peers may not know how to respond to a bereaved adolescent in a supportive or consoling way. Gordon (1986) reported that one high school boy's friends were afraid to tell jokes in his presence or invite him to parties after his father died. Fortunately, this is not always the case, but the lack of such support can increase the sense of isolation and marginalization of a grieving teen.

It is common for teens to grieve with their peers rather than with their families. Adolescents do this because turning to their family at a time of significant emotional devastation would threaten their fragile sense of emerging autonomy. Typically teens cluster and huddle together after a tragic or major loss, sometimes moving from family to family like nomadic tribes so as to not become too dependent on any one family. The failure of the community, the schools, or the parents to understand this as a developmentally appropriate form of coping can lead to misunderstandings or harsh criticisms at a time when teens need all the support they can accept in a face-saving way. Thus, the school community and the community at large can be helped to understand that adolescent bereavement has to be viewed in the context of the importance of peer relationships during this developmental stage. Regardless of how supportive the peer group is, teens still need the sensitive understanding and support of the school community, their teachers and coaches, as well as their parents, because the journey through grief, especially in the case of a parent or sibling, is a long road.

The deaths of youngsters and family members in the inner-city war zones, where exposure to violence can be a daily part of the lives of many children and families, are not accorded the same respect and honor they receive in more affluent and privileged communities. A school shooting in a suburban community is sure to command headlines, while a shooting in an inner-city school is often treated with a shrug and an attitude of "What do you expect?" These deaths and devastating losses are devalued and trivialized by the larger community and society as a whole, but the devastation to poor families is no less than that in affluent families. People who are marginalized in life are equally devalued in death. But the life of an impoverished family member is of no less value, importance, or meaning than the life of a person in an upper-class family. In previous writing, Crenshaw (2008a) told the story of his great-grandparents providing a home to an African American woman who was a former slave. When she died in the early 1900s, members of the church that the family attended would not allow them to bury her in the church cemetery. The family could not get an undertaker to transport the body, so they placed the body on the back of a horse-drawn wagon and traveled to a neighboring town, where there was a cemetery just for "blacks."

Communities in America that reflect the prevailing cultural attitudes surely have come a long way over the past century, but issues of race and class still serve to marginalize children and families not only in life but also in death.

DISENFRANCHISED GRIEF WITHIN THE CULTURE

Ethnic/minority children, adolescents, and their families may experience disenfranchised grief when their cultural practices are not recognized or respected by the majority culture. As stated earlier, one source of disenfranchised grief in the family can be promulgated by developmental assumptions that a child is too young to understand the meaning of death, and the failure to recognize the child's need for continuing bonds with the deceased. Yet even when a child's grief is supported and validated within the family, the dominant majority culture can be a source of disenfranchised grief when the expressions of grief in a minority culture are ignored and invalidated.

Reactions and responses to death are shaped by our cultural context. Mainstream American culture tends to focus on the individual rather than the collective, to deny the importance of continuing bonds, and to identify atypical grief reactions as pathological (Shapiro, 1996). Individuals who have suffered the loss of a loved one are expected to display certain levels of emotional expression, usually in the form of sadness and depression, over a typical length of time in order to grieve "properly." These norms constitute "valid" responses to death, and reactions that deviate from the norm are considered excessive, pathological, or inappropriate. However, ethnic/minority families may subscribe to vastly different norms. Culture-bound reactions to death are then challenged when a minority culture is enfolded within a majority culture, and normal expressions of grief are limited when they are not sanctioned by the society at large.

Cultures vary in their definitions for "acceptable" expressions of grief. For some cultures, subdued emotional expressivity or stoicism is appropriate, while for others, overt, intense emotional displays are expected. African Americans tend to be more expressive than European Americans at funerals and to grieve more openly for the departed (Rosenblatt & Wallace, 2005). In other cultures, like the Irish, humor takes center stage in rituals around death and dying. Irish funerals may sometimes resemble a celebration, where attendants tell stories and jokes about the deceased over drinks, displaying little or no overt expressions of grief (McGoldrick et al., 1991).

Cultures also differ in their perspectives of life after death and the need for continuing bonds with the deceased. The cultivation of strong bonds with the departed signifies the endurance of the community beyond the material world. In some Mexican American communities, individuals may celebrate the Day of the Dead (*el Día de los Muertos*), visiting cemeteries to communicate with the souls of those who died, and erecting private altars containing favorite foods, flowers, and personal memorabilia (Moore, 1980). These offerings encourage spirits to visit and hear the prayers of the living. Some Asian cultures also emphasize the importance of carrying out rituals to revere ancestors. In Japanese culture, cabinets called *butsudans,* holding incense burners, candles, and photographs, are displayed in the home as an act of veneration for ancestral spirits (Klass, 2001). Similarly, in Korea, *chae-sa* is a ceremonial rite in which families welcome in the spirits of deceased relatives and share prepared food offerings (Grayson, 1989). Although the ceremony is performed every year, the most elaborate rites are the three annual rites following the person's death. After the execution of the third rite, the spirit is then presumed to go permanently to the next world, and the formal period of mourning is concluded. In such instances, when the need to forge continuing bonds is a culturally sanctioned act of grieving within the family, yet disregarded by the majority culture, the child and the family are left to grieve in silence.

Culture not only defines expressions of grief, it also influences patterns of attachment and kinship. Yet societal expectations draw limits on appropriate responses to loss, not only in terms of emotional expressivity and length of mourning but also by way of the child's relationship to the deceased. The death of a mother or father is expected to be more devastating to a child than the death of an unrelated friend of the family. When a child creates strong attachments with adult figures, but those relationships are not regarded with the same respect and validation as relationships within one's family, the child's sense of loss may be minimized and belittled. Some may assume, "She was only a friend of the family. It's not like she lost her own mother."

In some cultures, the bonds of *fictive kinship* are critical in the raising of children. In Hispanic families, a child may develop mutual attachments with his or her *compadre* and *comadre,* godparents who play significant roles in the child's upbringing (Doka & Martin, 2002; Doka & Tucci, 2008). In contrast, the role of a godparent in other societies may be minimal and only significant at the time of the child's baptism. In the African American community, families are also defined by an "extended kinship system," which consists of adult role models, including deacons, ministers, and friends of the family granted honorary titles, such as "aunt" and "uncle," all of whom play an important part in the life of a child (Doka & Tucci, 2008; Hines & Boyd-Franklin, 1996). African American families can be further described as three-generational systems that comprise a grandmother, a mother, and her child (Nichols, 2008). Under certain circumstances, the grandmother may take on a parental role, and act as the primary caregiver. In such cultures, where extended kin are central to the life of the child, the death of a godparent, a family friend, or a grandparent can be equally as intense and devastating as the death of a parent. Through the loss of a parental figure, who may or may not be related to the family, a child becomes disenfranchised when that loss is not given the same respect and honor as that of an immediate family member.

Ethnic/minority children and adolescents may also be faced with the added tension of growing up in a traditional family that maintains strong cultural ties to its country of origin, while navigating the process of acculturation into mainstream society. In essence, these youth often have to negotiate between two vastly different worlds—the world of their parents and that of their peers. In adopting Western values, ethnic/minority adolescents may seek comfort and identify with their peer groups at school, yet family ties and cultural expectations may exert an equally strong influence. Children or adolescents who experience a loss may find themselves caught in a conflict, straddling differing generational, cultural, and societal expectations related to the loss.

Perhaps one of the most poignant examples of disenfranchised grief within the culture is illustrated by the tragic story of Lia Lee in Anne Fadiman's book *The Spirit Catches You and You Fall Down* (1997), which describes Hmong immigrants in the United States and their catastrophic collision as a minority family with the expectations of Western medicine in the treatment of their young daughter. When Lia was brought into the hospital after a seizure, her doctors diagnosed her with a severe case of epilepsy. However, her parents believed that her problem was *qaug dab peg,* the Hmong name for "the spirit catches you and you fall down," caused by the flight of Lia's soul from her body. In this moving narrative, Fadiman describes the tragic consequences that befall families when indigenous healing practices come into direct conflict with the prevailing norms of Western society. She also points to the assumptions of Western societies regarding the seemingly incomprehensible rituals of foreign cultures around death and dying. The Hmong have important shamanistic rituals that may involve days of drumming, chanting, and animal sacrifices, in the midst of large clan gatherings. These rituals hold tremendous significance in the spiritual lives of traditional Hmong people. For some cultures, like the Hmong, the inability to carry out such rituals and mourn in accordance with their cultural norms may induce anxiety and fear, and may even be considered dangerous to oneself, the family, or the spirit of the deceased. Rosenblatt (2007) stated, "Despite the demands of a surrounding culture, people in a minority culture need to grieve . . . their way. Anything less than that disenfranchises them ethically, violates their human rights, and may have dire consequences for the course of their grieving and their spiritual well-being" (p. 118).

DISENFRANCHISEMENT OF GRIEF WITHIN THE SELF

The grief when a family member dies may be so overwhelming to children that they must deny or fail to acknowledge their grief to prevent psychological collapse (Crenshaw, 2002; Kauffman, 1989). It is not unusual even in adults that grief is so intense that they fear "losing their minds." Grief, when it is most acute and intense, can be a frightening experience; this is especially true of children whose coping resources are still in the process of development.

In the case of the death of multiple family members caused by acts of war, terrorist attacks, or natural disasters, children may not feel that they have the "luxury to grieve" (Crenshaw & Hill, 2008). Partly this may be due to the overwhelming nature of the losses and accompanying grief that may also threaten their "survival orientation" (Hardy & Laszloffy, 2005). The urgent tasks of survival at such a time may consume psychological resources to the point that grieving becomes a luxury that the child simply cannot afford.

The more vulnerable and fragile the child is prior to the loss, as indicated by psychiatric disorders, prior losses or exposure to trauma, and factors related to social toxicity (e.g., poverty, academic failures, or learning disorders), the more at risk the child will be to disenfranchisement of grief within the self. It is critical in school-based and community outreach programs to identify children with these risk factors, so that additional supports can be offered to them and to surviving family members. If the death was either traumatic or associated with stigma, shame, or secrecy, the child may be especially prone to self-disenfranchisement of grief.

A child who is unable to face grief for fear of being overwhelmed may suffer additional stress within the family, because family members may not understand the true nature of the problem, may blame the child for being cold and indifferent, and may hurl accusations, such as "Don't you even care that your brother died?" A crucial intervention, then, is to educate the family about individual differences and some of the developmental factors that impede the child from grieving overtly as some of the siblings may be able to do.

CASE EXAMPLE

Child's name: Rodney
Age: 7 years old
Family: Mother (Roxanne, age 37)
             Father (deceased)
             Sister (Becky, age 9)
             Brother (Ricky, age 4)

Rodney's father was killed in an attempted robbery when he was accosted in a parking lot after working late in a major city. The shock of the father's death jolted not only the family but also the small community, where the father was employed as a security officer at a hotel. The family was active in church and school-related activities, and received a huge outpouring of support and concern at the time of the father's death.

Rodney was referred for therapy when 2 months into his second-grade year, 5 months after his father's sudden death, he began to act out aggressively toward other children. He would push them out of line in the hallway and knock them down on the playground, without apparent provocation. His mother Roxanne, faced with extremely difficult financial concerns and raising three young children on her own, was anxious and overwhelmed. She was concerned about all of her children but particularly about Rodney. Becky, the oldest child, on the surface appeared to be doing well, but both her mother and therapist wondered if she was "overreaching"—trying hard to be grown-up and to help her mother but in the process denying the true measure of her grief. The youngest child, Ricky, most of the time appeared to be oblivious to what was going on, but this impression was contradicted by occasional questions to his mom, such as "When is Daddy coming home?" or "Can we go visit Daddy in heaven?" These questions broke Roxanne's heart and served as a startling reminder that even preschool children struggle with understanding the mysteries of death. The implication is that parents need assistance from therapists in the form of coaching on how to talk with young children about death in the family (Crenshaw, 2006). In a family session, *The Bramley Stories* (Crenshaw, 2006) were read by the mother and the therapist one episode at a time to allow the children to ask questions and absorb the emotional impact of the information. These stories about a rabbit whose father dies suddenly were written for preschool children and their parents to create dialogue about these sensitive and emotional issues, so that young children are not left to grapple alone with the mysteries of death. All three children were mesmerized by the stories and asked questions about Bramley and his Uncle Benny, who tried to help Bramley cope with his grief. The mother expressed relief after the family sessions that the stories enabled even her youngest son Ricky to participate in the discussion and ask questions.

The mother was most concerned about Rodney, because he and his father had an extremely conflictual relationship. Roxanne described Rodney as a child with a difficult temperament pattern from the day he was born. Unlike her other two children, she had observed Rodney to be irritable, quick to anger, and impulsive, with both feeding and sleeping difficulties during infancy. He was hard to console and to soothe. He did not like to be cuddled or held. Roxanne reported that, based on discussions with the father's mother, the father had had a similar temperament pattern as a little boy. In fact, the mother often wondered whether the basic problem in the relationship between Rodney and his father was that Rodney reminded the father of himself in early life. She shared with the therapist that her husband was determined "to straighten that boy [Rodney] out." But Rodney was willful and would respond to his father's increasingly sharp criticism by acting out in more extreme ways, such as punching his little brother or breaking things belonging to his brother or sister. It became a vicious, self-sustaining cycle.

In the first therapy session with Rodney and his mother present in the room, Rodney was immediately drawn to the alligator puppet and began attacking the other puppets and the therapist with such force and intensity that the therapist had to set limits, because he inflicted pain on the therapist. The therapist said, "It is OK for the alligator to be mad but I won't let him hurt me. Here, perhaps he can express his anger at the dinosaur." It was only occasionally necessary after that moment to remind Rodney of the limits, and he accepted the redirection without breaking the momentum of the play. During subsequent sessions that usually, but not always, included his mother, the therapist noted a pattern of decreasing rage. In addition to the alligator puppet, Rodney used the soldiers, tanks, and artillery to enact battle scenes to express his fury symbolically. But as the therapy progressed, he was less and less interested in the battle per se, and became more involved with the creative aspects of staging the battles. This developmental progression in the containment of aggression has been observed repeatedly in our clinical experience and attests to the healing power of therapeutic play.

Rodney had good reasons to be enraged. As a 7-year-old boy he had lost a lot: He no longer had a father; he had lost any chance of resolving the conflict with his father, he had lost the hope of ever having the relationship he longed for with his father; and he had lost a sense of virtue, something every child needs (Kagan, 1998). Rodney blamed himself for his father's criticalness. He experienced a sense of shame and "badness," because he felt he could never live up to what his dad expected of him. The therapist addressed the issue of devastating loss in therapy by frequent reflections, such as "It is hard enough to lose your dad at any age, but when you are only 7, that really hurts" and "It can also make a young boy very angry, because it seems so unfair that other kids have their dads but you don't."

Rodney was the kind of child often seen in the therapist's office. He was practically nonverbal when it came to feelings but very expressive in action. While his sister Becky was articulate in expressing her feelings, the best that could be hoped for was that Rodney would be able to express his emotions through the symbolic action of his play, and that the therapist, through reflections, could validate the feelings Rodney could never verbalize directly.

It was also important in the therapy to address the issue of shame and "badness" in relation to the father's death. Not until the 12th session was Rodney able to acknowledge that when his father stayed late at work, he thought it was because his dad did not want to come home, because of so much yelling due to Rodney's behavior. Rodney had decided that if he had not caused so much trouble at home, his father would not have stayed so late the night he was killed; therefore, he (Rodney) was to blame for his father's death. What a terrible burden for a 7-year-old child secretly to carry! The therapist preferred to have the mother present in the sessions for multiple reasons. One was to highlight for the child the availability and presence of his surviving parent. But another important reason related to Rodney's revelation that he felt responsible for his dad's death. The therapist could certainly challenge and dispute this faulty notion. But more importantly, Rodney needed to know that he was not responsible for his father's death in the eyes of his mother, the most essential remaining person in his life. The presence of his mother at the precise moment that Rodney revealed this burdensome secret and her strong, genuine rebuttal was more healing than anything the therapist could have said. It should be noted that parents are not always included in the play sessions, and there may be some cases in which their presence would be contraindicated, but in our clinical experience, their participation typically facilitates the therapy process.

Rodney suffered disenfranchised grief because the trying behavior that intensified after his father's sudden, traumatic death diverted both him and others from the true source of the pain that drove his intense acting-out behavior. Even his supportive and sympathetic teachers were extremely frustrated and worn down by his aggressive and what appeared to be mean-spirited behaviors. At home, he never seemed to tire of aggravating his mom and siblings in endless ways. It is hard to keep in mind the inner pain of a child who is constantly provoking even his or her most faithful and loving supporters.

Rodney enacted precisely the painful pattern of his interpersonal life in a family play therapy session in which he refused to participate. He was sitting off to the side of his mother, who was encouraging him to join in as his brother and sister played out a scene with the puppets. The therapist combined strength with the mother and cajoled Rodney into engaging in the family puppet drama, in which he played a leading role and in fact took on the role of healer in the form of a doctor attempting to take care of an eagle with a broken wing. The "broken wing" was a rich metaphor for this family's struggle to get airborne after a devastating crash. Rodney enacted the role that caused him such great pain, "the child who did not fit in." He did not fit in the family because he was the object of his father's sharp criticism, even though his father meant well. He was the one who did not fit in because of his difficult temperament pattern. He made sure he did not fit in at school either by provoking and doing mean-spirited things to other kids that were sure to result in rejection from his peers and criticism from his teachers. He was the one who "did not fit" at first in the family session, by refusing to join in with the others, by sitting off in the corner, and by mumbling angry comments. When the mother and therapist together were able to persuade Rodney to participate, they essentially conveyed to him that they did not buy into the notion that "he did not fit." His siblings welcomed him when he joined in the play and were quite willing to let him take a leading, constructive, healing role.

Eventually, the idea that he was "the child who did not fit" no longer had a defining role in Rodney's life either at home or at school. He enjoyed greater acceptance among his peers and was more integrated into his family. Another important task in the therapy was to help Rodney appreciate that even though his dad was misguided in the way he went about it, he had been very concerned about Rodney and wanted him to have an easier time in life than had his father. Although his dad was quite hard on Rodney, he felt he could spare Rodney later pain by trying to "shape him up," much as is done with strict discipline in the military. Rodney's intense interest in the military made this notion meaningful to him, and he began to think of his dad as trying to help him be a "good soldier" to prepare him for the battles he would face in his life. Even though Rodney would have appreciated a dad who could more easily express warmth, approval, and affection, at least he could draw on the comfort that his dad really cared about him and was doing what he thought Rodney needed. This step was critical in enabling Rodney gradually to relinquish not only his shame and sense of "badness" but also his anger and rage toward his father.

As a final task to facilitate family healing, the children worked together on a memory album honoring their father. They included photos, stories, drawings, and collages that captured some of the happier times they spent together as a family. Rodney participated readily in this family project. His grief was no longer hidden, no longer disenfranchised.

CONCLUDING COMMENTS

When children and adolescents are faced with the death of a family member, recognition of their intrapsychic dynamics and developmental issues augments our understanding of their individual expressions of grief. We also acknowledge the impact of the external environments that children must navigate, whether at home with their families, at school with their peers, or in their neighborhood or communities. Furthermore, one of the greatest challenges we face as practitioners is striving to understand the grief expressions and rituals of another culture, when our tendency is to hold fast to familiar, biased, and conventional worldviews. The subtle nuances, the changes due to acculturation, and the individual differences within cultures add to the complexity of understanding how children and families within a culture deal with loss. In the multicultural fabric of our society, we are called upon to challenge and expand our majority worldviews of "normality" and honor the traditional practices of ethnic/ minority children and their families.

We mainly have discussed the different ways in which a child's grief may be disenfranchised outside of the therapy room. It is important to note, however, the possibility of ignoring or minimizing the child's grief reaction within a therapeutic context. As therapists, we are not infallible when we inadvertently contribute to the further disenfranchisement of grief. We note the potential hazards involved in grief and trauma work—through vicarious traumatization or the immunity we develop to defend against threats to our own psyches—and the importance of self-awareness of our limits (Crenshaw, 2008b). It is the delicate balance we strive to master by being engaged, empathetic, and compassionate as we enter the subjective world of our clients, while also maintaining enough therapeutic distance to be objective. We dive in with our clients, while holding onto a lifesaver floating at the surface of the ocean. At times, we lose our grip on the lifesaver in our desire to be fully present and connected with our clients; at other times, we cling on too strongly when we are overwhelmed by the prospect of losing perspective. We may vacillate between these opposing forces, yet we know in the end that the balancing act is difficult to achieve on our own. Just as we help our clients draw upon available resources within their families, schools, and neighborhoods, we help ourselves by making connections within our professional communities, with the support of our colleagues and other mental health professionals.

In this chapter, we have highlighted the different situations in which a child may experience disenfranchised grief within the self, the family, the community, and the culture. Armed with the awareness of the various contexts and expressions of grief, we may feel overwhelmed by the myriad pathways that lead to disenfranchised grief. Yet we are wise to recognize also the resilience of the human spirit and the potential for children's natural healing capacities. From the child who needs to work through grief in an active way to the child who needs a few words of support, we are called upon to listen. By listening to the stories that children and their families tell us, we work to understand their experiences, as told through the various perspectives of the self, the family, the community, and the culture. As therapists, it is the nature of our intention and our genuine desire to understand and help our clients that often sets up the necessary conditions for the healing process to unfold.

DISCUSSION QUESTIONS AND ROLE-PLAY EXERCISES

1. Why is it important to acknowledge variations and individual differences within the self? Discuss this issue from a developmental perspective and how young children may differ from older children in their expressions of grief.

2. Facilitate a discussion about other examples of disenfranchised grief, as experienced within the self, the family, the community, or the culture. Ask students to draw upon their personal experiences or clinical case examples.

3. In the case of Rodney, the therapist facilitated healing by having family members create a memory album in honor of their deceased father. What are some other therapeutic techniques or family projects that could be utilized in a case like this?

4. Facilitate a discussion about the cross-cultural differences in grief reactions. Describe typical or "normal" reactions to death, as expected in American culture. How do these cultural norms around death and dying differ from those in other cultures? Ask students to think about examples from their personal experiences and their clinical work.

5. Facilitate a discussion about the rewards and challenges therapists may face in their work with children who suffer from disenfranchised grief.

6. Role play: Ask four students to volunteer in a role-playing exercise in which two students play the parents, one student plays a 10-year-old boy, and another plays the therapist. The 10-year-old boy has become increasingly angry since the death of his dog Rusty, who was killed by a car. The child accidentally left the backyard gate open, allowing Rusty to roam the streets, and now feels responsible for the death. Even though the parents acknowledge Rusty's death and repeatedly tell their son that it was not his fault, they do not understand why he is having such a difficult time dealing with the loss. Every time they hint at their plans to get a new dog, the 10-year-old boy gets upset, tells his parents that no one understands, and then retreats to his room. In this role play, have the therapist facilitate a family session to address the disenfranchised grief experienced by the young boy. At the end of the role play, elicit reactions from each of the family members, and discuss specific therapeutic interventions made by the therapist.

REFERENCES

Boss, P. (2006). *Loss, trauma, and resilience: Therapeutic work with ambiguous loss.* New York: Norton.

Crenshaw, D. A. (2002). Disenfranchised grief of children. In K. J. Doka (Ed.), *Disenfranchised grief: New directions, challenges, and strategies for practice* (pp. 293–306). Champaign, IL: Research Press.

Crenshaw, D. A. (2006). *Evocative strategies in child and adolescent psychotherapy.* Lanham, MD: Aronson/Rowman & Littlefield.

Crenshaw, D. A. (2008a). *Therapeutic engagement of children and adolescents: Play, symbol, drawing, and storytelling strategies.* Lanham, MD: Aronson/Rowman & Littlefield.

Crenshaw, D. A. (2008b). Therapist healing and use of self. In D. A. Crenshaw (Ed.), *Child and adolescent psychotherapy: Wounded spirits and healing paths* (pp. 123–140). Lanham, MD: Lexington/Rowman & Littlefield.

Crenshaw, D. A., & Hill, L. (2008). When grief is a luxury, children can't afford. In D. A. Crenshaw (Ed.), *Child and adolescent psychotherapy: Wounded spirits and healing paths.* Lanham, MD: Lexington/Rowman & Littlefield.

Doka, K. J. (Ed.). (1989). *Disenfranchised grief: Recognizing hidden sorrow.* Lexington, MA: Lexington.

Doka, K. J. (Ed.). (2002). *Disenfranchised grief: New directions, challenges, and strategies for practice.* Champaign, IL: Research Press.

Doka, K. J., & Martin, T. L. (2002). How we grieve: Culture, class, and gender. In K. J. Doka (Ed.) *Disenfranchised grief: New directions, challenges, and strategies for practice* (pp. 337–347). Champaign, IL: Research Press.

Doka, K. J., & Tucci, A. S. (Eds.). (2008). *Living with grief: Children and adolescents.* Washington, DC: Hospice Foundation of America.

Fadiman, A. (1997). *The spirit catches you and you fall down.* Stanford, CA: Stanford University Press.

Gordon, A. K. (1986). The tattered cloak of immortality. In C. A. Corr & J. N. McNeil (Eds.), *Adolescence and death* (pp. 16–21). New York: Springer.

Grayson, J. H. (1989). *Korea: A religious history.* New York: Oxford University Press.

Hardy, K. V., & Laszloffy, T. (2005). *Teens who hurt: Clinical interventions to break the cycle of adolescent violence.* New York: Guilford Press.

Hines, P. M., & Boyd-Franklin, N. (1996). African American families. In M. McGoldrick, J. K. Pierce, & J. Giordano (Eds.), *Ethnicity and family therapy* (2nd ed., pp. 66–84). New York: Guilford Press.

Hogan, N., & DeSantis, L. (1992). Adolescent sibling bereavement: An ongoing attachment. *Qualitative Health Research, 2,* 159–177.

Kagan, J. (1998). *Three seductive ideas.* Cambridge, MA: Harvard University Press.

Kauffman, J. (1989). Intrapsychic dimensions of disenfranchised grief. In K. J. Doka (Ed.), *Disenfranchised grief: Recognizing hidden sorrow* (pp. 25–29). Lexington, MA: Lexington.

Klass, D. (2001). Continuing bonds in the resolution of grief in Japan and North America. *American Behavioral Scientist, 44,* 742–763.

McCown, D. E., & Davies, B. (1995). Patterns of grief in young children following the death of a sibling. *Death Studies, 19,* 41–53.

McGoldrick, M., Almeida, R., Hines, P. M., Rosen, E., Garcia-Preto, N., & Lee, E. (1991). Mourning in different cultures. In F. Walsh & M. McGoldrick (Eds.), *Living beyond loss: Death in the family* (pp. 176–206). New York: Norton.

Moore, J. (1980). The death culture of Mexico and Mexican Americans. In R. Kalish (Ed.), *Death and dying: Views from many cultures* (pp. 56–61). New York: Baywood.

Nagera, H. (1981). *The developmental approach to childhood psychopathology.* New York: Aronson.

Nichols, M. P. (2008). *Family therapy: Concepts and methods* (8th ed.). Boston: Allyn & Bacon.

Rosenblatt, P. C. (2007). Culture, socialization, and loss, grief, and mourning. In D. Balk, C. Wogrin, G. Thornton, & D. Meagher (Eds.), *Handbook of thanatology* (pp. 115–119). Northbrook, IL: Association for Death Education and Counseling, Thanatology Association.

Rosenblatt, P. C., & Wallace, B. R. (2005). *African American grief.* New York: Routledge.

Rubin, S. S. (1999). The two-track model of bereavement: Overview, retrospect, and prospect. *Death Studies, 23,* 681–714.

Shapiro, E. R. (1996). Family bereavement and cultural diversity: A social developmental perspective. *Family Process, 35,* 313–332.

Swihart, J., Stillman, B., & McNeil, J. (1992). Death of a student: Implications for secondary school counselors. *School Counselor, 40,* 55–60.

CHAPTER 6

Suicide in the Family

Helping Child and Adolescent Survivors

CYNTHIA McCORMACK
NANCY BOYD WEBB

Survivors of suicide are not alone. It is estimated every suicide leaves behind at least six survivors, creating approximately 200,000 new survivors in the United States every year. In 2005, one in every 65 Americans was a suicide survivor (Kung, Hoyert, Xu, & Murphy, 2008). Unfortunately there are no data available on the specific number of children and adolescent survivors, although we know there are many. Research on children and suicide has focused primarily on prevention of the suicide act; however, recently, more attention has been directed toward survivors and how to help those left behind. Since 2000, an increasing number of worldwide studies has been completed on children and adolescents bereaved by suicide, yet researchers agree that more studies are needed (Cain, 2002; Dyregrov & Dyregrov, 2005; Jordan & McMenamy, 2004; Parrish & Tunkle, 2003; Ratnarajah & Schofield, 2007; Sethi & Bhargava, 2003).

This chapter reviews the impact of a suicidal death in the family on child and adolescent survivors, and discusses the special challenges, including complicated and disenfranchised grief associated with suicidal deaths. Case vignettes of children and adolescents at different developmental stages illustrate typical responses and treatment approaches.

OVERVIEW OF THE TOPIC

Of the thousands bereaved by suicide, it has been found that bereaved children and adolescents are at increased risk for developing psychiatric disorders, such as major depressive disorder, posttraumatic stress disorder (PTSD), and panic and conduct disorders (Melhem, Moritz, Walker, Shear, & Brent, 2007; Ratnarajah & Schofield, 2007; Pfeffer et al., 1997; Sethi & Bhargava, 2003; Mitchell, Kim, Prigerson, & Mortimer-Stephens, 2004; Mitchell et al., 2006). Children bereaved by suicide may have greater difficulty dealing with peers at school and in other social settings (Sethi & Bhargava, 2003). Additionally, bereaved children and adolescents have been found to be at greater risk for complicated grief (CG; Mitchell et al., 2004) and for committing suicide themselves (Sethi & Bhargava, 2003; Jordan, 2001).

Complicated Grief

Originally studied in adults, CG has emerged as a syndrome in both children and adolescents. Found to be separate and distinct from major depression, anxiety, and PTSD (Melhem et al., 2007), CG has been identified as a group of depression and grief-related symptoms that interfere with an individual's ability to return to his or her life after a period of "normal" grieving (Mitchell et al., 2004; Prigerson et al., 1995). For example, if after approximately 14 months, a grieving individual has difficulty accepting the death; isolates him- or herself; is preoccupied with thoughts of the deceased; feels stunned, numb, angry or bitter; and experiences disproportionate longing and yearning for the loved one, he or she may fit the CG criteria (Horowitz et al., 1997). Goldman (2001) describes children with CG as caught in "frozen blocks of time," unable to move through the grief process because of overwhelming feelings. Children, Goldman says, can become "imprisoned in these feelings if they are not given the freedom to work through their grief" (p. 10). She further states that to help children grieve, mental health professionals, caretakers, and parents need to facilitate a "meltdown process" for the bereaved child. The meltdown involves creating a safe holding environment in which the child can reexperience the loss of the loved one and all the accompanying feelings associated with it, without shame or fear of judgment.

Researchers have recently developed a promising assessment tool to identify CG in children and adolescents, the Inventory of Complicated Grief—Revised (ICG-R; Melhem et al., 2007). Since CG has been strongly correlated with increased risk for suicide in adolescents bereaved by the loss of a peer, early identification of CG is crucial (Melhem, Day, Shear, & Day, 2004). Pfeffer et al. (1997) found that additional factors, such as poor parental psychosocial functioning and pre- and postsuicide family stressors, increase difficulties for children following a death from suicide. Therefore, after a death from suicide, it is important to assess the needs of parents and caretakers ultimately to aid the recovery of the children.

The Nature of Suicide Bereavement

Researchers have long debated whether suicide bereavement is different from other types of grief, such as bereavement from illness or accident (Cerel, Fristad, Weller, & Weller, 1999; Jordan, 2001; Ratnarajah & Schofield, 2007). Studies to date have yielded conflicting opinions. Melhem et al. (2007) concluded that CG scores of children bereaved by suicide were no different than CG scores of children bereaved by accidental or sudden natural deaths. It is possible, however, that the unexpected nature of suicidal, accidental, and sudden natural deaths may have accounted for the similarity in CG scores.

Most of the recent literature in fact does suggest that suicide bereavement differs in many ways from other types of grief in terms of not only suicide survivors' increased risk for psychopathology or poor social functioning but also the potential stigma, shame, and isolation associated with suicide bereavement (Cerel et al., 1999; Jordan, 2001; Mitchell et al., 2006; Sethi & Bhargava, 2003). Additionally, finding meaning from a suicidal death is more challenging than finding meaning following deaths from other causes. Jordan (2001) points out that some common survivor questions, such as "Why did they do it?", "Why didn't I prevent it?", and "How could they do this to me?", set suicide bereavement apart and "may distinguish it from other losses, regardless of the measured intensity of the grief or psychiatric symptoms" (p. 92). Last, suicide bereavement is a form of "disenfranchised grief," a term created by Kenneth Doka (1989) to refer to a type of grief that people experience when a death cannot be "openly acknowledged, publicly mourned, or socially supported" (1989, p. 4). Substantial evidence indicates that mourners bereaved by suicide feel stigmatized and may be looked upon more negatively by their peers and social group (Jordan, 2001). Survivors bereaved by suicide may be perceived as being more emotionally dysfunctional, more ashamed, more depressed, more often blamed, and more in need of psychological counseling than other mourners (Jordan, 2001). When a death, such as a completed suicide, is not publicly acknowledged or socially accepted, the survivors suffer great isolation and a lack of community support. Despite the similarities in all grief experiences, these unique circumstances set suicide bereavement apart from other types of grieving.

CHILDREN'S BEREAVEMENT AFTER SUICIDE

The topic of child and adolescent survivors of suicide deserves special attention, because children grieve differently from adults and uniquely within their age group, depending on their level of cognitive development and ability to verbalize. These developmental differences were reviewed in Chapter 1, this volume, and will not be repeated here.

We know that children as young as 6 years understand what it means to "kill oneself," even if they do not understand the word "suicide." By third grade, children are capable of fully comprehending a death from suicide. Children ages 6–12 reported that they learned about suicide from peers, through the media (e.g., TV depictions), and by overhearing adult conversations (Mishara, 1999). Although many adults believe that children do not understand what suicide is, clearly this is not true. It is important, therefore, to speak openly and directly about suicide, so that children are able to grieve fully this type of loss. Denying or withholding the truth about a death from suicide may interfere with a child's grief process and make it more difficult or impossible to process his or her feelings about the death (Goldman, 2001)

As discussed in Chapter 1, this volume, most children do not fully understand the meaning and implications of death until approximately ages 7–12 years. Many parents and caregivers feel confused about how to address suicide with their preschoolers, because children at this age do not understand the finality of death. However, the children are aware that something important has happened, and they may ask questions related to the absence of the dead person. It is important to address children's questions in simple, straightforward ways that give honest answers yet do not overburden them with information they cannot yet comprehend (Requarth, 2006). As children mature, they will need additional information about the suicide, so that they can work through their feelings at each new stage of emotional, physical, and cognitive development.

Adolescents bereaved by suicide may experience many conflicting emotions. They may cry a lot or not at all; they may try to act more mature than their years or regress to younger behavior; they may withdraw and isolate or want to be with their peers. Teens, having full knowledge of suicide, struggle to find meaning in the death. Because adolescents are often in conflict with their parents, siblings, and friends, it is not uncommon for a teen to feel excessive guilt after a death from suicide, especially if he or she had a recent argument with the person who died. Teens need lots of support and reassurance while grieving a loss from suicide (Doka, 2000; Requarth, 2006; American Academy of Pediatrics, 2000; Rando, 1991).

Most research on children and adolescents bereaved by suicide focuses on the loss of a parent; however, it is evident from the research that bereavement from the suicide of a sibling or peer can also be quite devastating for young people. Because youth bereaved by a sibling or peer suicide may not be acknowledged and noticed in the same way as those bereaved by a parent's suicide, grieving may be more difficult. For example, in a 2005 study of siblings after suicide, Dyregrov and Dyregrov found that because parents were so distraught themselves following their child's suicide, siblings were left alone and felt isolated. In fact, "parents confirmed that the bereaved siblings were "forgotten" in the hours and days following the suicide" (p. 719). Months passed before siblings felt they could rely on their parents for support. Parents were found to experience intensified fears that something might happen to the surviving children and became over protective. Siblings expressed difficulty with talking to their parents about their feelings for fear of stirring up parental grief. Research has confirmed that siblings who live at home experience greater difficulties than older siblings living out of the house or even the parents themselves (Dyregrov & Dyregrov, 2005). Therefore, support from others in the community, such as friends, relatives, teachers and counselors, is critical for children and adolescents bereaved by a sibling's suicide (Dyregrov & Dyregrov, 2005; Parrish & Tunkle, 2003).

How to Talk about a Suicide in the Family

Telling a child or teen that his or her parent, sibling, or friend has committed suicide is a formidable task. It is important that caregivers communicate about suicide in an age-appropriate, clear manner, using language the child can understand (Mitchell et al., 2006). If parents or caretakers use an inaccurate expression, such as (the person) "passed into eternity" instead of "died from suicide," then it may have later repercussions as the child struggles to comprehend what actually happened. The word "suicide" should be used in an age-appropriate way, with proper explanations that provide the information children need for grieving at their particular stage of development. It has been suggested that a parent may explain to the child that the dead person was feeling very sad and did not know how to stop the sad feelings, so he or she (shot and killed him- or herself; took a lot of medicine, etc.) to stop the pain. An older child might benefit from further explanations such as the fact that the person was very depressed and did not know about special medications that might have helped him or her feel better (The Dougy Center, 2001).

For some families, avoiding the truth may seem preferable to telling, because of the stigma associated with a death from suicide. For others, the very concept of suicide may challenge the family's religious or cultural belief system, making suicide difficult to acknowledge. Researchers agree, however, that hiding the truth and creating a family secret is harmful to children and adolescents (Cain, 2002; Mitchell et al., 2006; Webb, 1993). Children who are uncertain of the facts surrounding a death from suicide may fabricate their own story. "Such self-explanations can create even more confusion, fear, and isolation" (Requarth, 2006, p. 16). Therefore, age-appropriate information given by a loving parent or family member or friend in a safe environment is best (Requarth, 2006). Experts agree that children's questions should be answered at the age- and developmentally appropriate level for the child, with no more detailed information than is necessary. Sometimes, in talking to very young children, information related to their basic needs, such as the need to know they are safe, that they will be taken care of, and assurance they are loved, may take precedence over knowing details about the death. Early childhood basic needs include the need to know who will help them get dressed in the morning, walk them to school, make them dinner, help them if they are sick, and put them to bed. These needs may be initially more important to a very young child than the need to know specifics about the death (Cain, 2002). As previously mentioned, the age and developmental stage of the child are critical factors in determining how much a child should be told about a suicidal death, but they are not the only factors to consider. The individual child's maturity, ability to cope with emotions, and even the child's interest or disinterest in knowing about the death, are additional factors to consider before talking with a child about suicide (Cain, 2002).

Parents should try to take some time to sort out what they want to say before initiating a discussion with children or adolescents about a suicidal death (Requarth, 2006). In fact, it has been reported that some parents do not tell their children right away because of needed time to cope with their own emotions, to accept the fact of their situation, and to regain some confidence in their ability to parent (Cain, 2002). For support, some parents may want to have a family member, close adult friend, or grief counselor with them when they talk to the children. Additionally, Requarth explains the value in using language the child will understand, which includes defining terms when necessary. For example, if a child does not understand the word "died," then the parent needs to educate him or her about death, using simple language and examples from the child's life experience, such as the death of a grandparent or pet. Parents with young children should be prepared to repeat explanations and information over and over, as repetition is the normal way children begin to understand concepts such as "dead." See Requarth (2006, pp. 18–19) for a case example of a parent talking to her 5- and 12-year-old children after their father had completed suicide.

Parents who have difficulty speaking honestly and directly with their children or teenagers may benefit from individual counseling. Therapists trained in bereavement counseling may use techniques such as role playing or letter writing to help a parent begin the process of facing fears about telling the child. In Goldman's (2001) book *Breaking the Silence,* she demonstrates the use of both these techniques in the case of Steve, whose wife died by suicide, and his son Justin, age 9, who had not been told how his mother died. Goldman's example stresses the importance of getting help from professional counselors when a parent simply cannot face telling his or her children. Furthermore, some parents try to tell their children of a death by suicide only to be rebuffed by a child who prefers to remain in a state of denial (Cain, 2002). This type of challenge may best be handled with the help of a mental health professional. In addition, it is important to obtain immediate crisis intervention if a child has witnessed the death by suicide, since there is greater risk for the child to develop posttraumatic stress syndrome or complicated grieving after such a disturbing experience (Requarth, 2006).

TREATMENT CONSIDERATIONS AND OPTIONS

The goal of treatment for children and adolescents bereaved by suicide is to facilitate the mourning process and to foster resilience. Not all grieving children need professional support (Webb, 1993); however, children bereaved by *suicide* should receive professional attention, since they are at greater risk for developing PTSD, complicated grief, anxiety, and major depression (Melhem et al., 2007; Mitchell et al., 2004, 2006; Pfeffer et al., 1997; Ratnarajah & Schofield, 2007; Requarth, 2006; Sethi & Bhargava, 2003). Therefore, they should be given a thorough assessment to determine whether individual counseling, family therapy, or group intervention is advisable. When planning a particular treatment method for a child or adolescent, the child's age and stage of development should be considered, together with the nature of the suicide and the child's overall reaction to the death. Especially important is the degree to which the child (and family) regard the death as shameful (or sinful). Obviously, in circumstances in which the family and child feel shamed, it is very difficult for them to talk about the nature of the death with other people, and this may argue for either individual or family treatment rather than group approaches, especially soon after the death.

Following a suicide in the family, every family member needs support and care, perhaps most especially the children and adolescents, who may sometimes go unnoticed in the crisis. We mentioned previously that parents may overlook their children's response to a suicidal loss because of their own pain and compromised psychological state (Dyregrov & Dyregrov, 2005). Therefore, it is important that others, such as relatives, teachers, religious leaders, or friends surrounding the bereaved family, pay attention to any difficulties children or teens may be experiencing. Parrish and Tunkle (2003) recommend that interventions with those bereaved by suicide begin as soon as possible. Kaslow and Aronson (2004) recommend that therapists working with families bereaved by suicide assess *all* family members for their own unique needs as a guide to choosing the proper intervention for each. Treatment options include individual therapy, family therapy, and group counseling. These are discussed below, with case examples illustrating various interventions.

Family Therapy

Some practitioners consider that family therapy alone or in conjunction with other types of therapy, such as individual or group therapy, may be the best choice of treatment for suicide survivors (Kaslow & Aronson, 2004). "The goal in bringing the family together after a death is to facilitate the grieving process through active reminiscing about both positive and negative characteristics of the deceased" (Webb, 1993, p. 144). Later, the family therapy technique of creating a shared suicide story exemplifies a way to reach this goal. However, suicide can cast an entire family system into turmoil, and different members respond differently, so the therapist needs to assess and monitor individual needs, together with the responses of the family as a group. Researchers have recommended an integrative family therapy approach, "devoted to altering and improving the destabilized system" (Kaslow & Aronson, 2004, p. 240). The suggested integrative approach is based on systems theory, attachment theory, and narrative intervention, and includes a psychoeducational component (Kaslow & Aronson, 2004).

When working with a family bereaved by suicide, Kaslow and Aronson (2004) assert that therapists must take time to create a safe holding environment in which family members can express their feelings. "Children should be encouraged to talk about the deceased; be involved in rituals related to the deceased; and be supported in resuming normal peer, school, and extracurricular activities" (p. 242). Concurrently, therapists need to normalize the grief process, to emphasize that grief will resolve in time, and to teach family members how to cope with their complex emotions and thoughts. "Members need to be encouraged to improve their awareness, insight, understanding, and acceptance of the emotional fluctuations they are likely to experience in their recovery" (p. 242).

Helping family members to talk about their loved one who completed suicide is important in the therapeutic process (Webb, 1993). Communication between and among family members bereaved by suicide may be encouraged by creating a suicide narrative or story, with the help of a family therapist. "This technique helps families find an understanding that preserves each person's self-esteem, satisfies their search for meaning, and creates a contextual framework for the suicide within the family" (Kaslow & Aronson, 2004, p. 244). Creating a narrative of this type involves a family discussion of the events leading up to the suicide. While creating the shared version of the experience, the therapist must also allow for each family member to "develop his or her unique interpretation of the consequences of the act" (p. 244). This way, members can hold on to their autonomy while participating in the creation of the family's shared story. Kaslow and Aronson point out that therapists using this technique must be aware of the cultural influences and religious values of the family. Some believe suicide is unacceptable, a sin, in which case this type of treatment may not be appropriate. The therapist might attempt to help such a family by explaining how depression can interfere with an individual's judgment thereby reframing the "sinful" behavior as a "mental illness." Often it is helpful for family members to find a way to forgive the person who committed suicide; understanding the possible role of depression in precipitating the death may encourage feelings of forgiveness.

Parrish and Tunkle (2003) also suggest that therapists be prepared to address the vast array of feelings family members may have toward the deceased, such as anger, ambivalence, and relief. They further state that communication between family members may be problematic because of feelings of guilt, shame, and blame. Therapists should pay close attention to the family dynamics, reminding members that grieving need not be overpowering or be kept secret (Parrish & Tunkle, 2003). Therapists must also acknowledge the different ways family members grieve a loss and help them to accept each other's unique grief process (Kaslow & Aronson, 2004; Parrish & Tunkle, 2003). Very small children may cry more than usual and need reassurance that they will continue to be cared for after the death. Elementary school-age children may want to draw pictures, read books, or create a memorial for the person who died. Teenagers may withdraw, go out more with friends, feel numb and embarrassed, or distract themselves with activities. These examples of different grieving styles at different stages of development demonstrate the vast range of responses to a death from suicide that may be expressed in family therapy sessions.

There are some circumstances when family therapy may be contra-indicated or should be delayed until after parents gain support through individual therapy. For example in her 2001 book, *A Special Scar: The Experiences of People Bereaved by Suicide*, Allison Wertheimer writes:

> Non-communication between family members is not uncommon; after both of Marjorie's sisters had committed suicide, she became increasingly upset when her mother, Eileen, refused to talk to her about the twins and their deaths. After another member of the family had pointed this out to her, Eileen decided to seek help from a counselor. This not only helped her to deal with her guilt, but enabled her to start talking with her surviving daughter about the twins' deaths. Counseling can help to re-open channels of communication which may have become blocked or distorted. (p. 143)

Another example when family therapy may be contraindicated is when a spouse is very angry because his or her partner completed suicide. The bereavement counselor must evaluate the extent to which it might be harmful for the children to witness their surviving parent expressing rage directed toward the deceased family member. Although feelings of anger are normal and need to be expressed, intense anger might be more effectively addressed in individual therapy rather than in family sessions that include children. In circumstances like this, family sessions might be better planned to occur *after* an interval of time, following a period of individual counseling for the parent.

Group Treatment

Support groups for bereavement can offer a variety of benefits to children and adolescents (as well as to the adults in the family). A support group can offer children and adolescents bereaved by suicide respite from isolation, a shared experience, a safe place to express thoughts and feelings, support from others like themselves and a normalizing experience and role models for survival (Werthheimer, 2001). Although there is a lack of research on support group interventions for children and adolescents bereaved by suicide (Mitchell et al., 2007; Pfeffer, Jiang, Kakuma, Hwang, & Metsch, 2002) a study by Pfeffer et al. found that group treatment reduced anxiety and symptoms of depression in children ages 6–15 bereaved by suicide of a parent or sibling.

Experts disagree on whether suicide survivors should be integrated into groups for those bereaved by other types of deaths. Some believe that benefits can be attained from involvement in a general bereavement support group (Requarth, 2006), while others feel that the better choice is a suicide-specific group (Webb, 1993, 2005, 2007). Webb (2007) pointed out the potential dangers of placing a child in a bereavement group for those bereaved by other types of deaths, because of the nature of suicide and the potential for stigmatization and shame associated with it. Webb pointed out that the benefits of group participation for children can be undone by the potential difficulties. In addition, other children in the group might become frightened hearing about the details of a suicidal death. Requarth (2006) counters that although children may be asked awkward questions regarding the death of their parent who completed suicide, integrating a child into a general bereavement group, with proper preparation, could offer a child the opportunity to become more comfortable with peer social interactions around the death from suicide. Assessing a child's readiness for a support group intervention of any type is important and should be done on a case-by-case basis to be sure this type of treatment is appropriate for the child. Webb suggests that in situations with insufficient numbers of similar-age children bereaved by suicide, an effort should be made to pair up at least *two* suicide bereaved children in a bereavement group.

Teens may or may not respond well to the idea of a support group for those bereaved by suicide. Adolescents can be inquisitive or shy, and each may need to find what works best for him or her. Teens may be more amenable to joining a group after first meeting with the group facilitator and being informed about the confidentiality of a support group (Requarth, 2006). "Teens are curious about their peers. They may consent to attending a group if they have information about how the group works and have the option to stop if they are not benefiting" (p. 145).

Case Example: A Teen's Response to the Suicidal Death of a Parent*

PRESENTING PROBLEM

Michael, age 17, lived with his mother following his parents' divorce 5 years earlier. He saw his father every other weekend; his father had remarried and lived in a neighboring town. Michael's mother, a nurse, worked full time in the local hospital. Michael had a part-time job after school and was looking forward to going away to college the coming fall. Michael's relationship with his mother was not close; he did not know

---

* This is a fictional case, based on a composite of several cases; it is also discussed in Webb (2010).

that she had recently been diagnosed with inoperable cancer. One day when he returned home from his afterschool job, his father was there and told him that his mother had taken an overdose of medication, then had sat in her car with the motor running in the garage until she died.

Michael was distraught and blamed himself for not realizing that his mother was depressed. His father, a physician, made arrangements for Michael to move in with him and to attend a bereavement group at the local hospice.

ISSUES IN THERAPY

In the group, Michael keep repeating how he could not believe that his mother was dead and that she had actually killed herself. He also kept wondering why she had not told him about her diagnosis. He kept asking why he had not noticed that she was worried or depressed. Because both of his parents were in the medical field, he had grown up with the idea that illnesses were curable. He could not understand how this had happened to his mother without any warning.

The group members were sympathetic to Michael's questions. One member commented that even though Michael was almost 18, his mother still considered him her child and probably did not want to cause him worry. Michael's mother had left a note addressed to him. She said that when she found out her condition was not treatable, she had begun to make plans to die. She had arranged for Michael to inherit her pension so that he would have money for his school books and other needs. In her note she expressed her love for Michael and her wish to spare him the grief of watching her die gradually. She said that she had seen many patients waste away, and that she did not want to inflict that on herself or on Michael.

When Michael read the note, he felt weak and looked for some alcohol to give him strength. He told the group that he thought he needed the alcohol to keep him strong. A group member whose parents were alcoholics mentioned that alcohol can be a trap, and once a person starts drinking it, he or she cannot stop. This kid Danny warned and even begged Michael not to fall into the trap.

SUMMARY OF THERAPEUTIC THEMES

Membership in the bereavement group soon after his mother's death proved to be extremely supportive for Michael. Although he had not been particularly close to his mother, he knew he could count on her if he needed anything, and now he felt alone. The group members spoke about their relationships with other family members, and Michael realized that he wanted to get to know his father better. Because of the bitterness of the divorce, Michael had not wanted to take sides, and he tried to distance himself from both parents. Now he realized that he could share some activities and develop a relationship with his father. Additionally, he gradually made friends with some of the group members who understood the pain of his loss and wanted to support him. He began to spend time with Danny, whose father had died from the consequences of alcoholism. After the group concluded when the school year ended, Michael remained in contact with Danny and with several other members who had become his friends.

COMMENTS

It is clear how beneficial the group therapy experience was for this very lonely young man. It not only offered him the chance for friendship but it also provided support and guidance. Because adolescents are very peer-oriented, a group is often the treatment of choice, even when the youth bereaved by suicide is the only group member with this particular life experience.

Individual Therapy

As previously indicated, each family member should be assessed individually following the suicidal death of another family member. The assessment evaluates the person's own strengths and vulnerabilities, in addition to his or her views about why the loved one made the decision to end his or her life. The assessment helps to determine the appropriate type of treatment. In Michael's case, it is doubtful that he would have felt the same degree of support had his school counselor recommended a family approach, and although Michael did have individual issues related to his mother's decision, it is not clear that he would received the same feeling of shared support with an individual therapist. Michael was able to share his concerns with his peers in the group, thereby receiving group support from the various members. Had Michael appeared to be depressed, or if he had seemed to question his future plans, then a referral for individual therapy would have been appropriate.

This chapter focuses on children and adolescents. Their ability to understand and make sense of the suicide depends on developmental factors, family factors, and the particulars of the suicide itself (the tripartite assessment; see Webb, Chapter 2, this volume). For example, the response to a deliberate overdose of medication resulting in the death of a mother with terminal cancer (as in Michael's case) would probably be experienced very differently by family members than would a similar death following news of a job loss. Some situations lend themselves to greater sympathy on the part of family survivors of suicide. We must acknowledge that suicide does not occur in a vacuum, and often it is the "last straw" in a series of disturbing and escalating events. All family members seek to understand "why" the person chose to die, but the ages of children and adolescents may affect their abilities to comprehend the various contributing factors. Often children are not privy to family secrets (e.g., that Daddy has had many affairs or that Mommy and Daddy do not love one another anymore). Children, of course, pick up tensions in the family, but they may not understand the source of tensions that might lead to a suicide. Furthermore, young children do not have words to express their confused feelings, and this is why play therapy is a useful method to help them sort out and clarify their feelings (Webb, 2007). It is most helpful to work with young children on an individual basis, as we demonstrate in the following case examples.†

A Preschooler Tries to Understand
Her Father's Suicidal Death: Case of Cathy, age 4½‡

PRESENTING PROBLEM

Cathy, a 4½-year-old girl, was referred for therapy 1 month after her father's suicide (by gunshot) related to a psychotic depressive episode. Cathy's behavior regressed following her father's death and included frequent crying and clinging, sulking, and insisting on sleeping with her mother.

ISSUES IN PLAY THERAPY WITH CATHY

The play materials most frequently chosen by this child were dolls and plasticine (Play-Doh). She washed the dolls carefully and arranged them lovingly in their beds. This type of age-appropriate play seemed to give her a sense of comfort, control, and safety in the knowledge that she could take care of the dolls in a competent manner. The play therapist commented to Cathy that she seemed to like to have the dolls safe in their beds.

In contrast, Cathy's play with the Play-Doh revealed some spontaneous trauma reenactment. She created five "cookie faces," with the last one having only one eye and no mouth. Ideally the therapist might make some reference to the cookie that was disfigured, by saying something to

---

†Two of the cases were previously published in books edited by Webb. They are summarized here with permission of the original authors/child therapists. The examples have also been included in Webb (2010).

‡Adapted from Hurley (1991).

Cathy, such as "That poor cookie, what happened to his face?" By keeping the dialogue in the realm of fantasy, the child could explain her view of what happened to her father (i.e. "The cookie got hurt; a gun shot his eye" or some such explanation). This then would allow the therapist to express empathy ("Oh, that's too bad !") and to refer to the other cookies' grief ("They must be very sad about this").

The important point about play therapy is that it allows young children to express fears–anxieties–beliefs in a *displaced and disguised* manner, so that confusion and emotion can be expressed through the play object, using children's imagination and ability to project. In contrast, had the therapist made the direct connection to Cathy's own personal experience, she probably would have become quite anxious and reluctant to continue the play.

A different play episode occurred when Cathy found a toy male figure in the sandbox. This stimulated her to talk about people ("like my dad") who are buried. Since the child herself made the connection to her father's death, this time the therapist engaged Cathy in a discussion about her father's body in the ground, and her wish to be able to see her father again. She wondered whether her father could come back or not, and how he died. Cathy knew her father had shot himself, but she was not clear about the permanence of death. The therapist clarified to the child, "When a person is dead, they cannot come back, even if they want to."

This description presents a brief snapshot about how play therapy can assist a young suicide survivor in dealing with some of her worries and grief about her father's suicidal death. The play therapy continued for several months and 1 year later, the therapist reported that Cathy was more independent of her mother, crying less, and preparing to enter kindergarten.

The next case example reworks similar bereavement themes with older school-age children.

A Fourth-Grader Tries to Understand Her Mother's Suicidal Death: Case of Rosa, Age 9½§

PRESENTING PROBLEM

Rosa's mother, who had been previously psychiatrically hospitalized and expressed suicidal thoughts daily, shot herself at the beginning of the school year. After about a month of weekly individual therapy with the

---

§ Adapted from Bluestone (1991, 1999).

school social worker, Rosa expressed interest in talking to other children who had had a parent die, and the social worker decided to offer peer therapy to Rosa and to Cindy, whose father had died suddenly of a heart attack. Rosa and Cindy were seen together, because both had similar fears about the death and about the possible disappearance of their single surviving parent, and both also were having difficulties with peer relationships and with their schoolwork.

ISSUES IN THERAPY

As weekly sessions progressed, the girls spoke openly about missing their deceased parents, and about how these feelings intensified when they were in bed and often caused them to cry themselves to sleep. The girls both spoke longingly of the dead parent but resisted the therapist's attempt to have them elaborate further on their feelings. Instead, they spontaneously decided to put on a puppet show, because "we don't want to *talk* anymore"!

The theme of the puppet show involved puppet characters who sold drugs that eventually killed all the various puppet characters. The show thereby symbolically continued to deal with the topic of death in the girls' chosen play scenario.

The next week, the play therapist suggested that some of the characters who died in the previous show could come back to life. The girls immediately verbalized their wish that they could see their dead parents again and acted out a scene in which (in the role of puppets) they went to heaven and visited their dead parents. This was a very emotional and meaningful enactment of the children's natural wishes to be reunited with their parents, *even for one day* (as the script specified). They continued the same play the following week, in which there was more expression of open grief and the desire to remain in heaven to stay with their dead parents. In this scene, the therapist took the role of Rosa's mother and expressed not only her ongoing love but also her wish to have her daughter return to her "home on earth and be happy with her friends." After a very powerful farewell scene, the puppets sang a goodbye song and hugged each other.

SUMMARY OF PLAY THERAPY THEMES

Although these girls were fourth graders, it was too difficult for them to speak at length about their feelings of longing for their deceased parents. However, they needed to work on these feelings and used play effectively to help them deal with their emotional issues. After they had developed a degree of comfort with the therapist and with each other, the girls spontaneously created a puppet play that expressed the themes of death and an imagined visit to heaven, so they could have contact with their parents who died. They were able to convey their questions and their wishes more effectively through the play enactment than either girl could have done by verbal means alone. It also seems evident that each girl benefited from the support of the other, and that their shared experience of suffering the loss of a parent through death gave them a meaningful bonding relationship that they could not have had in one-to-one, individual counseling. Thus, this case (together with the others in this chapter) demonstrates the value of matching the type of intervention with the specific needs of each bereaved child.

SUMMARY

Children bereaved by suicide are at greater risk for developing psychological disorders, such as anxiety, depression, and PTSD. Although not a universally accepted disorder, CG has been found to be a separate and distinct syndrome for which children bereaved by suicide are at risk. Although all types of bereavement share some commonalities, recent literature describes bereavement from suicide as different from other grief. In addition to the stigma, shame, and blame associated with suicide, survivors often have difficulty finding meaning in the death. These factors separate suicide mourning from other types of bereavement. Additionally, bereavement in children and adolescents differs at varying ages and stages of development. These are also important factors to consider when counseling children and adolescents mourning a loss from suicide.

When the loss is a sibling, grieving may be complicated if the parents are grief stricken and unable to attend to the surviving child's needs. Attention should be paid to surviving siblings by other family members, close friends, and counselors to be sure they are not slipping under the radar. Siblings and peers are also at risk for CG reactions. Children and adolescents bereaved by suicide often need the support and care of a mental health professional in the form of individual counseling, family therapy, or supportive group treatment. Finding the best intervention for a child depends on many factors, including the child's age, maturity, psychological status prior to the death, family support, and so forth. All members of a family bereaved by suicide may need help to understand and accept such a difficult death.

When possible, a loving adult should talk with children and adolescents about death from suicide in a direct, open, and honest way in a safe environment. Information should be given using language appropriate for each age group. Last, in view of the fact that keeping secrets has been proven to be detrimental to the grief process, when parents or other adults are unable to talk with children and adolescents about suicide, they should seek help from a mental health professional.

Suicide presents great challenges for those who knew and loved the deceased, and they must find a way to navigate their mourning process with the added burden of thinking that this act might somehow have been prevented. Acceptance of the reality of what happened must be coupled with forgiveness and compassion for the victim and all the survivors.

DISCUSSION QUESTIONS AND ROLE-PLAY EXERCISES

1. In the case of Cathy, this preschooler knows that her father shot himself, but she did not know the word "suicide." Do you think that it is important for the therapist to advise the mother to use the word "suicide"? At what age? Why?, Why not?

2. What factors would you consider in determining whether to recommend family, individual, or group therapy for a preschool child? For an elementary-school-age child or an adolescent? How would you explain to a family member the value of such treatment and what they might say to the child/adolescent about the referral.

3. Discuss how you might explain to a 9-year-old boy that his father committed suicide. How would you help the boy explain his father's death to his friends?

4. Role play: Role play a disagreement in an adolescent bereavement group over the issue of how obligated a teen son should be to check up on his mother's health and mental state, when the two of them are living together following the parents' divorce.

REFERENCES

American Academy of Pediatrics: Committee on Psychosocial Aspects of Child and Family Health. (2000). The pediatrician and childhood bereavement. *Pediatrics, 105*(2).

Bluestone, J. (1991). School-based peer therapy to facilitate mourning in latency-age children following sudden parental death: The cases of Cindy age 10½, and Rosa T., age 9½. In N. B. Webb (Ed.), *Play therapy with children in crisis: Individual, group, and family treatment* (pp. 258–275). New York: Guilford Press.

Bluestone, J. (1999). School-based peer therapy to facilitate mourning in latency-age children following sudden parental death: Cases of Joan, age 10½, and

Roberta, age 9½, with follow-up 8 years later. In N. B. Webb (Ed.), *Play therapy with children in crisis* (2nd ed., pp. 225–251). New York: Guilford Press.

Cain, A. C. (2002). Children of suicide: The telling and the knowing. *Psychiatry: Interpersonal and Biological Processes, 65*(2), 124–136.

Cerel, J., Fristad, M. A., Weller, E. B., & Weller, R. A. (1999). Suicide-bereaved children and adolescents: A controlled longitudinal examination. *Journal of the American Academy of Child and Adolescent Psychiatry, 38*(6), 672–679.

Doka, K. J. (Ed.). (1989). *Disenfranchised grief: Recognizing hidden sorrow.* New York: Free Press.

Doka, K. J. (Ed.). (2000). *Living with grief: Children, adolescents, and loss.* Washington, DC: Hospice Foundation of America.

Dougy Center, The. (2001). *After a suicide. An activity book for grieving kids.* Portland, OR: Author.

Dyregrov, K., & Dyregrov, A. (2005). Siblings after suicide—"the forgotten bereaved." *Suicide and Life-Threatening Behavior, 35*(6), 714–724.

Goldman, L. (2001). *Breaking the silence: A guide to help children with complicated grief—suicide, homicide, AIDS, violence, and abuse* (2nd ed.). New York: Brunner/Routledge.

Horowitz, M. J., Siegel, B., Holen, A., Bonanno, G. A., Milbrath, C., & Stinson, C. H. (1997). Diagnostic criteria for complicated grief disorder. *American Journal of Psychiatry, 154,* 904–910.

Hurley, D. J. (1991). The crisis of paternal suicide: Case of Cathy, age 4½. In N. B. Webb (Ed.), *Play therapy with children in crisis: Individual, group, and family treatment* (pp. 237–253). New York: Guilford Press.

Jordan, J. R. (2001). Is suicide bereavement different?: A reassessment of the literature. *Suicide and Life-Threatening Behavior, 31*(1), 91–103.

Jordan, J. R., & McMenamy, J. (2004). Interventions for suicide survivors: A review of the literature. *Suicide and Life-Threatening Behavior, 34*(4), 337–350.

Kaslow, N. J., & Aronson, S. (2004). Recommendations for family interventions following a suicide. *Professional Psychology: Research and Practice, 35*(3), 240–247.

Kung, H.-S., Hoyert, D. L., Xu, J., & Murphy, S. L. (2008, January). Deaths: Final draft for 2005. *National Vital Statistics Reports, 56*(10). Retrieved January 16, 2008, from *www.cdc.gov/nchs/data/nvsr56_10.pdf.*

Melhem, N. M., Day, N., Shear, M. K., & Day, R. (2004). Traumatic grief among adolescents exposed to a peer's suicide. *American Journal of Psychiatry, 161*(8), 1411–1417.

Melhem, N. M., Moritz, G., Walker, M., Shear, M. K., & Brent, D. (2007). Phenomenology and correlates of complicated grief in children and adolescents. *Journal of the American Academy of Child and Adolescent Psychiatry, 46*(4), 493–499.

Mishara, B. L. (1999). Conceptions of death and suicide in children ages 6–12 and their implications for suicide prevention. *Suicide and Life-Threatening Behavior, 29*(2), 105–118.

Mitchell, A. M., Kim, Y., Prigerson, H. G., & Martimer-Stephens, M. (2004). Complicated grief in survivors of suicide. *Crisis, 25*(1), 12–18.

Mitchell, A. M., Wesner, S., Brownson, L., Gale, D., Garand, L., & Havill, A. (2006). Effective communication with bereaved child survivors of suicide. *Journal of Child and Adolescent Psychiatric Nursing, 19*(3), 130–136.

Mitchell, A. M., Wesner, S., Garand, L., Gale, D., Havill, A., & Brownson, L. (2007). A support group intervention for children bereaved by parental suicide. *Journal of Child and Adolescent Psychiatric Nursing, 20*(1), 3–13.

Parrish, M., & Tunkle, J. (2003). Working with families following their child's suicide. *Family Therapy, 30*(2), 63–76.

Pfeffer, C. R., Jiang, H., Kakuma, T., Hwang, J., & Metsch, M. (2002). Group intervention for children bereaved by the suicide of a relative. *Journal of the American Academy of Child and Adolescent Psychiatry, 41*(5), 505–513.

Pfeffer, C. R., Martins, P., Mann, J., Sunkenberg, M., Ice, A., Damore, J. P., et al. (1997). Child survivors of suicide: Psychosocial characteristics. *Journal of the American Academy of Child and Adolescent Psychiatry, 36*(1), 65–74.

Prigerson, H. G., Frank, H., Kasl, S. V., Reynolds, C. F., et al. (1995). Complicated grief and bereavement-related depression as distinct disorder: Preliminary empirical validation in elderly bereaved spouses, *American Journal of Psychiatry, 152*(1), 22–31.

Rando, T. A. (1991). *How to go on living when someone you love dies.* New York: Bantam Books.

Ratnarajah, D., & Schofield, M. J. (2007). Parental suicide and its aftermath: A review. *Journal of Family Studies, 13*(1), 78–93.

Requarth, M. (2006). *After a parent's suicide: Helping children heal.* Sebastopol, CA: Healing Hearts Press.

Sethi, S., & Bhargava, S. C. (2003). Child and adolescent survivors of suicide. *Journal of Crisis Intervention and Suicide Prevention, 24*(1), 4–6.

Webb, N. B. (Ed.). (1993). *Helping bereaved children: A handbook for practitioners.* New York: Guilford Press.

Webb, N. B. (Ed.). (2005). *Helping bereaved children: A handbook for practitioners* (2nd ed.). New York: Guilford Press.

Webb, N. B. (Ed.). (2007). *Play therapy with children in crisis: Individual, group, and family treatment* (3rd ed.). New York: Guilford Press.

Webb, N. B. (2010). Grief counseling with child and adolescent survivors of parental suicide. In J. R. Jordan & J. L. McIntosh (Eds.), *Grief after suicide: Understanding the consequences and caring for the survivors.* New York: Routledge.

Wertheimer, A. (2001). *A special scar: The experience of people bereaved by suicide* (2nd ed.). East Sussex, UK: Brunner/Routledge.

CHAPTER 7

The Loss and Death of a Pet

SHARON M. MCMAHON

Our modern lives are complex and many life events come and go, and little do we realize the impact of the stress and emotional toll that these experiences have upon our lives (Lee & Lee, 1992). Such is the situation in which a child finds that a much loved animal companion (pet, animal friend, confidant, or assistant–service helpmate) reaches a natural end of life and dies of old age or becomes critically ill, or has been injured beyond survival, stolen, or the victim of an environmental trauma or disaster, or somehow becomes lost or separated from the child forever. The euthanasia of a beloved pet is one aspect of the human–companion animal relationship that can be particularly complicated for adults, as well as for children (Kay et al., 1988). We can only imagine the degree of emotional anguish that such events have for children of all ages (Quackenbush & Graveline, 1985). In the past, adults devalued grief and mourning for pets; pet bereavement used to be considered a form of disenfranchised grief (Doka, 1989; Lee & Lee, 1992; Quackenbush & Graveline, 1985).Today, we realize that children's grief for their pets is legitimate, painful, intense, and real (Fitzgerald, 1994, p. 140). Children express their grief differently then do adults, and with growing complexity across the ages and stages of development (Quackenbush & Graveline, 1985; Wolfelt, 1991; Lee & Lee, 1992; Webb, 1993, 2002). It is our ability to empathize that urges us to reach out to youngsters to help them cope at such sad and tragic times. Many may want to help, but not everyone knows how ((Grollman, 1976). I hope the guidelines in this chapter can be of help. Further scientific inquiry into the growing field of scholarly research in juvenile grief, bereavement, and mourning is left to other scholars, such as those contributing to this book.

It is without debate that the death of a beloved pet creates grief and great sadness. My goal in this chapter is to help practitioners help youth to understand, cope, and heal in a healthy manner. I begin with the recognition that children have a cultural identity and place within families, among friends, and in the greater community, in which concepts of who they are become shaped by the attitudes, values, beliefs, behaviors, roles, and relationships embedded into their daily lives (McNamara, 2000). Children are exposed to daily hassles, tensions, fears, worries, stress, and challenges counterbalanced by: sustainable and unconditional love; healthful and benevolent resources and messages; uplifting and resilience-building activities; inspirational and compassionate mentors; and positive role examples, behaviors, attitudes, lessons and problem-solving strategies demonstrated and shared by others who care about their well-being ((Goldstein & Brooks, 2005). As I explore strategies and give suggestions designed to help youth cope with the death of a pet, keep in mind the continuous influence of culture, through the healthful traditions, rituals, meanings, and ceremonies, as both the foundation and the fabric of protective factors for resilience that may counteract trauma and ameliorate devastating emotions and experiences (Goldstein & Brooks, 2005, p. 30). Modern grief therapies are built around the scientific evidence and understanding of the waves of change and processes that foster healthy adaptation and resilience of the child within the context of society, as well as the practice of informed therapeutic interventions designed to (1) prevent fear and traumatic outcomes; (2) reduce risk-taking behaviors, delinquency, and destructive behaviors; (3) promote and integrate natural developmental stages and activities, skills, and knowledge levels; (4) avoid adversity, mental health concerns, issues, and interpersonal problems, and pathological grief; (5) foster coping strategies that are compatible with the ongoing lived experiences of children and youth; and (6) empower the family and care providers to foster a loving milieu in which the child may safely, honestly, and confidently experience compassion, understanding, and acceptance, learn positive coping strategies and memorialize in meaningful ways the death of a pet (Bertman, 1999; Fiorini & Mullen, 2006; Goldstein & Brooks, 2005; Hughes, 1995; Monbourquette, 1994; Munroe & Kraus, 2005; Seibert, Drolet, & Fetro, 2003; Turner, 2005; Wass & Corr, 1982).

Helping children and adolescents through their journey of grief requires that adults be attuned to preverbal, nonverbal, and symbolic communication (Di Ciacco, 2008). At the core of any attempt to soothe and comfort the griever, no matter the age, is the realization that words alone cannot heal the pains or speed the process and steps of mourning. It takes an interpersonal harmony of feelings, emotions, needs, questions, sounds, stories, play, action–reaction cycles, tears, fears, pictures, dreams, and the ongoing attentiveness of significant caretakers over time. The uniqueness of childhood bereavement and mourning reflects a lack of language to voice feelings, worries, loss and separation, aloneness, and vulnerability. Young children lack experience with emotional regulation strategies, and they are unfamiliar with aloneness and separation. They can neither anticipate danger nor understand the distinction between sleep and death. They also have no appreciation of the concepts of universality versus self-centeredness. Development of the child physically, emotionally, psychologically, cognitively, spiritually, morally, and socially occurs gradually since the young child lacks logic and mature cognition. Chapters 1 and 2 in this volume discuss this more fully.

Children may get stuck in their grief due to a lack of appropriate orientation processes and skills to resolve their loss and engage in restoration (Di Ciacco, 2008). It is important for any care provider to explore the developmental stage of the child who is grieving or experiencing a loss or permanent separation so as to understand the impact of age-appropriate growth and development on tasks, competencies, skills, cognitive capabilities, thoughts, behaviors, problem-solving approaches, likely strengths, and coping strategies in creating a useful helping strategy (Pearson, 2004). The ongoing interpersonal support and assistance of adults helps children clearly and accurately identify their feelings and learn healthy ways to express these feelings. This constitutes the socioemotional learning (SEL) that is vital to the ongoing understanding and mastery of the rainbow of feelings associated with loss. Often, adults' lack of patience and devalued respect for or acknowledgment of the depth and strength of the emotion attached to pet loss, hinders their ability to support the development of a child's emotional understanding and personal resolution of mourning, grief, and bereavement.

STEPS IN HELPING THE CHILD GRIEVE A LOSS

The first step to helping any child is to create a safe and genuine environment in which the young person may express feelings; create and use art, and fine and gross motor activity; listen to and tell stories; play; make and listen to music; reflect on and share pictures; employ tradition and ritual; and engage in meaningful ways to create memories (Sorensen, 2008). Each child is unique, and his or her experience with the death and loss of a pet is also unique. Keeping this in mind, all adults should attempt to provide patient and gentle contact, active listening, unhurried time line, and easy support. Adults should be open to opportunities to teach expressions, variations, and meanings of intense, strong, weak, subtle, and unclear emotions, as well as facial and body language, responses, and sensations associated with the loss of a pet (Sorensen, 2008).

CASE EXAMPLE

Jeffrey, a bright, energetic, and healthy infant, was adored and protected by Farlie, the golden retriever, from the moment of his arrival into the family. Farlie had been the four-footed, sole "surrogate child" of Patty and Josh for 8 years. Their newborn son Jeffrey had now come to share life with Patty and Josh—and, of course, Farlie (see Figure 7.1).

When Jeffrey was 11 months old, Farlie was hit by a car and died. Jeffrey did not witness this, but all of a sudden, he sensed that his mother was rushed, tense, and would not sit and play with him anymore, and she did not want to breast-feed him like before. Jeffrey missed the warm unhurried rocking, the assistance to get up that Farlie provided, the clean licking of his fingers, and the sharp bark when Patty or Josh wanted to run or speed up with the stroller. Life was not the same. Jeffrey started to cry in the middle of the night, was not getting enough to eat, and wondered why Farlie was not coming to nap- or bedtime. No one told him

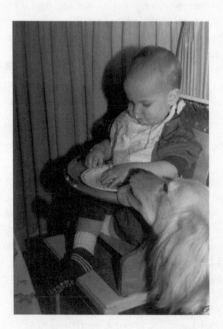

FIGURE 7.1. Farlie and Jeffrey.

anything. The doggie toys disappeared; the old soft blanket from the couch was put away, and no one wanted to go for walks anymore. Something was wrong, but Jeffrey could not understand what his parents were saying. Their faces looked mean and stern, like when he did something naughty. What could he have done to make them so angry? What could a baby do to let them know he was upset too, besides clinging to Mommy and Daddy, crying and kicking, refusing to eat, or stiffening when he got his face and hands washed with a cold towel?

Jeffrey began to get colds and was not gaining weight. He stopped talking and began to cry at the least frustration. Patty started to yell and always wanted to sleep, and Josh went to the garage and fixed things. The house was quiet, and no one called for Farlie anymore; no barks echoed into the laundry room or playroom. Soon Patty and Jeffrey were away from home more often, separated from each other for a long time each day as Patty had to return to work. Jeffrey did not seem to adjust to this separation, especially without Farlie. He cried and looked for Mama, Dada, and Doggy from the moment they dropped him off with the babysitter. This went on all winter.

In the spring, Patty and Josh decided that they would like to add other members to the family—canine companions. This time, two English setters that needed a home were selected from the animal rescue shelter. Jeffrey was very attracted to them both right away. From the start, these dogs returned the attachment. Jeffrey felt more settled, happier, started to regain weight, had fewer colds, slept better, started talking, cried less, and responded to the gentler and calmer body language and facial expressions of his parents. They began smiling again and getting out for exercise, and they took the dogs for a walk with them as well. In spite of dramatic differences in his behaviors and health, no one ever recognized that Jeffrey had been grieving for Farlie.

When Jeffrey was 9 yeas old, Max, one of their doggy duo, died. Things were different then, too, but Jeffrey understood sadness this time. It was expected that Jeffrey knew that life and death were part of the cycle of life, consisting of seasons, old age, death, and loss. Winnie remained the lone pet for this family. Winnie died 3 years later when Jeffrey was 12 years old. At this age, he understood that all living things die, including himself and his parents, when it was their time. Jeffrey demonstrated understanding of the elements of universality. He looked back in his baby book and album to his photos with Farlie, Max, and Winnie, stating that he remembered them and would always love them, even though he could neither show nor tell anyone how much Farlie had meant to him at the time.

From his various experiences, Jeffrey was able to help his friends learn about ways to show grief and feelings of loneliness, separation, and loss through the memory tree at school during the week dedicated to empathy-building activities to show kindness for animals (Figure 7.2). Some friends suggested that they would like to learn about funerals; others thought prayers, as well as rituals, were important and wanted to plan and prepare for a role-playing drama of a play funeral with their stuffed animals to symbolize their loved pets (see Figure 7.3). These activities fostered role playing and allowed the children to control and prepare for a future eventuality. Others wanted to bring in pennies for cat food and dog biscuits to support a charitable cause, such as the pets of homeless persons, in memory of some deceased pet, or one that was indeed still very much a part of the child's life (in gratitude for its non-judgmental friendship). Still others painted and created clay models and made picture frames from yarn and sticks to adorn photos of their beloved animal friends, alive and dead, to give as testimonials to special people who would appreciate the love behind the creativity. The teacher invited the class to create poems or letters that could be sent to beloved pets and family members in heaven, by attaching them to lighter-than-air balloons (see Figure 7.4). These were released on the field trip to the zoo, shortly after the first rainbow was reported in the weather news in class.

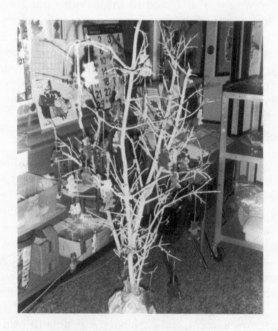

FIGURE 7.2. The memory tree.

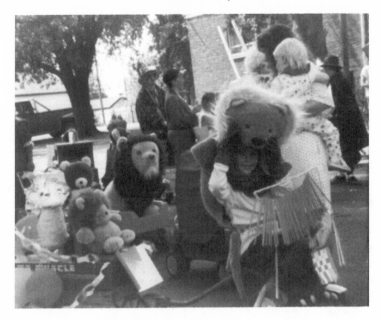

FIGURE 7.3. Role playing a funeral.

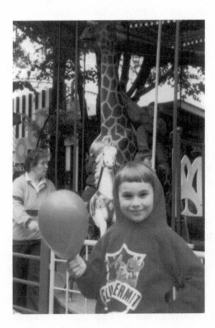

FIGURE 7.4. Balloon messages to the heavens.

All these were ways to help Jeffrey and his friends transform pet death and loss into meaningful, age-appropriate experiences and provided them with meaningful and respectful transitions from life to death that included life lessons in resilience and positive coping. The grief of these children was accepted as real, and their feelings were respected. Their curiosity about death and dying was not disenfranchised. Together they explored the changes between being alive and dead, the natural way that bodies return to the earth, and they listened to many philosophies and cultural beliefs about what happens in a spiritual sense after the physical body dies. Time with social workers, grief counselors, and aftercare workers was provided to help the class learn about and understand the feelings, beliefs, and behaviors associated with the process of grieving. The adults in Jeffrey's life supported each child by fostering personal meanings from deaths that each child had experienced. Through the collective activities of friends and classmates, each child felt that he or she could speak out, sharing thoughts, fears, rituals, and ideas, as well as asking questions, creating memories and traditions, and rehearsing roles that all would need in the future as the cycles of life and death move around each and every child.

In this case example, Patty and Josh would have been more helpful to Jeffrey if they had appreciated that their grief was shared by their son, even though he was too young to express verbally his anxiety, separation, and attachment confusion, loss, and fear of abandonment. The lack of language was a developmental barrier that prevented Jeffrey from expressing his feelings. Even though he could detect parental anxiety and tension, he was unable to comprehend his feelings due to his lack of world experiences and understanding of the complexities of time, relationships, and daily schedules. Patty and Josh made the mistake that many do, namely, to think that their infant would not understand or realize that there was something different, wrong, unsettled, and unfamiliar. Patty and Josh needed help with their own grief, and they should have been encouraged to explain and reinforce how they *all* missed Farlie, and to label clearly their feelings, expressions, and moods. As a child becomes more verbal, parents may ask how he or she is feeling and spend unrushed time listening to his or her stories, and provide craft and drawing materials for self-expression plus storytelling. These are healthy ways to encourage young children to transform their sad feelings and grief, and to mourn the loss, separation, and death of a beloved pet.

Adults can help throughout childhood. Consideration of the child's developmental stage and age, capabilities, and resources helps adults to mentor and guide children though their grief and mourning. The following list of helping methods can be integrated into a comforting and compassionate plan of communication with children and adolescents as they seek to understand, and find meaning, in the death, loss, or separation from a beloved pet. These suggestions demonstrate that there are many appropriate ways for adults to help children mourn the death of a pet.

1. Maintain the child's usual routine and pattern of eating, sleeping, play, school, and activities.

2. Provide soothing activities—relaxation, meditation, special foods, rocking, and contact time.

3. Expect temporary regression or a desire for simpler, more familiar situations, and maintain safety.

4. Promote activities to foster successful, safe, and restorative self-care behaviors.

5. Prevent unnecessary separations from important care providers and family.

6. Be calm and avoid reminders of the traumatic situation (e.g., on TV, in video games, or DVD's), especially if the child witnessed the traumatic death.

7. Provide creative crafts and drawing, sculpting, woodworking, and other materials, and give children sufficient unrushed time and a quiet and safe place to create meaningful symbolic expressions of feelings, rituals, and memories. Drawing and art by children can have great representational, symbolic, and communicative qualities even prior to language proficiency (Milbrath & Trautner, 2008, pp. 28–30, 43–49). It is useful to help young children express unknown feelings and experiences. One does not care about the perfection of the drawing, for it is in the action of creating images that healing is found.

8. Offer play materials, figures, and toys, and allow for children's undisturbed imaginative play alone or with others, but remain close by in case there are questions or fears that arise. Children should lead the way. There is no prescribed way to safely play, except in a manner that results in no harm to others and no destruction of common play materials.

9. Clearly set limits on hurtful and scary play, and on harmful risk-taking behavior, such as choking games or other attempts to experience what it is like to be dead or united with the deceased.

10. Help children learn to express emotions (e.g., happiness, anger, fear, frustration, and sadness).

11. Teach children to solve problems logically; remove threats and fears, and relieve, eliminate, or prevent worry.

12. When children are older and words become tools for expression, listen patiently to the retelling of stories from the past related to the beloved pet, including the death, loss, or separation tales.

13. Be prepared for short, intense bursts of questions about dead

things, what makes something dead, and what it is like to be dead, and clarify the difference between the finality of death and sleep or coma.

14. Give children honest answers and practical observations that differentiate between being alive and dead—breath, heartbeat, eating, sleeping, making sounds, moving, elimination, reproduction, and bodily warmth.

15. Use the Internet and other computer social contacts with care and supervision, and explore the feelings and experiences of others through secure, approved, and quality chat lines, such as the Canadian Association for Child and Play Therapy (*www.cacpt.com*), *www.allaboutpets.org.uk*, *www.dmoz.org/kids_and_teens*, *pbssmail@bluecross.org.uk*, *www.sharegrief.com/resources*, or Kids Health (*www.kidshealth.org*), griefblog.com, *www.compendium.com*, the Child Bereavement Network (CBN; e-mail: *cbn@ncb.org.uk*), the Child Bereavement Trust (CBT; *www.childbereavement.org.uk*), or the Association for Pet Loss and Bereavement (*www.aplb.org*). Other resources are pet loss and bereavement counselors, such as "Angie Rupra" (*angie.rupra@petvethospitals.ca*; personal communication, April 24, 2009) and international pet loss bereavement support accessed through the Calgary Humane Society Pet Bereavement Group (*www.surpriseyourpetlinks.com/results.html?query=calgary%20humane%20society%20pet%20bereavement%20group*).

16. Seek assistance from a local librarian and/or consult the Appendix of this book for other resources about grief, mourning, and pet death, separation, and loss. The use of bibliotherapy can be an excellent, focused, bonding activity between an adult and a grieving child or adolescent. It is appropriate for all ages, since books are selected with respect to language and cognitive level, and with typical interests and questions in mind (Fiorini & Mullen, 2006; Jones, 2001; Leaman, 1995; Markell & Markell, 2008; Seibert et al., 2003; Sorensen, 2008).

17. Other suggestions to assist with transitions to healing pet-associated grief include creating a memory box in either a wooden, plastic, or cardboard shoebox format, into which the child can place a collection of special items from the deceased or create a montage of memorabilia, such as photos, cards, notes, toys, and keepsake talismans (e.g., locks of hair).

18. Sending goodbye letters to the beloved, burying or burning notes of goodbye and special messages, or sending notes aloft can help people feel their messages are reaching beyond the limits of *terra firma*. A class or family or individual may wish to create and forward notes of thankfulness for care and attention to care providers such as veterinarians, veterinary technicians, office staff, and even animal care students through posters or letters to a veterinary college or office, indicating

support, understanding and gratitude for their special skills, especially in situations of euthanasia.

19. Wash an old blanket or bedding box and donate it to a local humane shelter or animal protection society for another animal needing love and warmth.

20. Plant a tree, flowers, bulbs, or seeds locally in honor of the beloved pet.

21. Create a CD/DVD of images and recordings of family and friends telling stories about the beloved pet.

22. Create a Memory Tree from a pruned limb painted a favorite color. Then invite others to write about the beloved pet and make an ornament that can be hung on the tree and be displayed.

23. Compile scrapbooks of thoughts and memories, with input from all sources, cards, Internet connections, pictures, collages, tags, or other memorabilia assembled in a storable format to be shared in the future or downloaded as PDF images into a DVD.

24. Apply the principles of aromatherapy to foster relaxation by sprinkling lavender fragrance onto a piece of fabric, or as a lotion for skin massage. Other botanicals provide therapeutic support for life processes, spirit, mood, and emotional healing. Care, guidance, and the advice of experts are essential for safe, alternative stress-reducing botanical products, oils, and essences in helping bereaved children (Turner, 2005).

25. Dance, rhythmics, and music blend activity with expression. Children love activity, from the use of large exercise/yoga balls to those that are palm size to squeeze as a stress reducer. The giant-size balls can be used as drums and to dance around, and lifted in dance and free expression. Other sources of musical sound, rhythm, percussion, and singing can be healthful and expressive in releasing inner emotions and applying the benefits of movement in an energizing and safe manner.

26. Many cultures have oral histories and alternative forms of storytelling, such as the use of puppets and inanimate objects (e.g., stones, water, or animals) to convey emotions and social/life lessons. Imaginary integration of other voices can help children tell their stories of grief in a transitional, third-party voice, not necessarily their own. This distance allows the transfer of a lesson or meaningful message to others without personal attribution that might be pain-filled and arouse anxiety. It is the human-to-human connection that is vital. Media, keyboards, and screens may provide periods of distraction, but they do not promote the exchange, sharing, or humanization of emotional pain that is so often associated with loss, grief, and mourning.

27. Create a game or a puzzle from a copy of a favorite photo of the beloved; this can help with the concept of creating memories from bits

and pieces and help the child see how to put pieces together in an orderly fashion that results in an image of the loved one.

28. Older adolescents need to be able to express the importance of the pet bond and relationship to their peers. One creative method is to share cell phone pictures of the beloved pet with others who also loved the pet. Music composed of ring tones can also be meaningful. A digital photo key chain is another way to keep memories and cherished moments literally in one's hand.

29. Submitting a photo obituary to a local newspaper for publication or posting a notice on a bereavement-focused website serves as a public declaration of the special relationship and a way to express the very special bond with the pet.

30. Building a cohort of supportive and empathetic friends does much to heal the additional emptiness, loneliness, and separation that may arise from the death of a beloved pet. The computer may help teens connect through social networks via safe and supportive chat rooms, with links to professionals who may provide suggestions and reflections when invited, or when they notice that the topics and moods are becoming dark and depressive, dangerous and unhealthy.

31. Some teens may wish to get a tattoo of the pet's name or some other symbolic image. Those who have made this choice suggest that a temporary tattoo may serve the purpose of grieving, without the permanence of a lifetime commitment.

32. When the pet dies after the young adult moves away from home, he or she should still be included in the information, plans, and final decision making regarding euthanasia, services, handling of the body, and ways of memorializing (e.g., a candlelight ceremony), and have a say in distribution of objects associated with the pet. Often licenses and tags are seen as cherished jewelry and reminders of the unconditional love given by the animal companion across the childhood years. Parents must be respectful and supportive of their child's emotional needs across the miles, and keep the doors of the family home and lines of communication open (Munroe & Kraus, 2005; Di Ciacco, 2008).

33. Special mail or parcels that connect the student or young working adult with his or her childhood home and pet can be bittersweet, and not always helpful or positive. Sometimes thoughts about moving away from the pet can arouse guilt. Counseling may be needed to help refocus and create healthy closure (Brown, 2005; Di Ciacco, 2008; Fiorini & Mullen, 2006; Sorensen, 2008; Association for Pet Loss and Bereavement, 2008; Travis, 2008; Joshua, 2007).

34. Mature ways of dealing with the intense emotions of grief for a pet or a human loss include journal keeping, letter writing, poetry composition, and composing a song or creating a drama.

35. Be alert for signs of depressive or dark thoughts and seek psychological and medical help, if necessary.

36. Encourage exercise and group activities that promote endorphin release in the brain that promotes feelings of accomplishment and enjoyment, happiness, and stress relief.

37. Fostering meditation and relaxation skills, perhaps martial arts and yoga as forms of mind–body connection and anger management, can help children to heal, while promoting brain growth, insight into healthy therapeutic relationships, self-esteem, and diversion, which can foster multiple strategies for grief work (Munroe & Kraus, 2005).

38. Support or therapy groups may help individuals, as well as groups of children, who share the experience and challenge of the death of a beloved pet. Mental health facilities, funeral homes, and aftercare professionals may sponsor day camps or weekly social get-togethers and specialized play groups to provide fellowship, group support, and the power of friendship as healing energies for grief (Wolfelt, 1992; Travis, 2008).

39. Integrate faith and cultural practices into traditions that facilitate the healthy resolution of grief over a pet (Joshua, 2007; Shaw, 2006).

40. Keep alert to new and innovative programs and services designed to facilitate grief in children and adolescents associated with pet death, loss, or separation (Brown, 2005).

CONCLUDING COMMENTS

These suggestions are far too numerous for the therapist, counselor, or parent to use with any one child. The variety of suggestions here permit the reader to choose responses and activities that fit the particular bereaved child mourning the loss of a pet. When a particular approach seems to be ineffective, then another approach may be chosen.

In summary, children, like adults, need to be respected and supported in their grief whenever it presents itself. The emotions associated with a pet's death may reappear from time to time as the growing child attempts to reexamine his or her understanding of old experiences through newfound reasoning skills, language, knowledge, and observations. Children must find their way through the darkness of sorrow and endings. Classical books and research articles, as well as person-to-person storytelling and the Internet, provide suggestions, guidelines, and supportive ideas for resolving grief. The Internet can assist with understanding and be a source of ongoing support, so that children do not feel they are alone or rushed, or disenfranchised in their grief. Helping children and youth in their grief work after the death of a family pet requires sensitivity, respect, and personal validation of the child. Take time to listen and follow the pace of the child, regardless of age. Mental health is promoted through kindness and universal, inclusionary, and positive social support for the transitions associated with pet death and childhood grief. Sensitive adults are essential to help bring adjustment, wellness, and normalization to this process. Healthy grieving is work that no one can or should undertake alone.

DISCUSSION QUESTIONS AND ROLE-PLAY EXERCISES

In the following section, I present several scenarios that are common to childhood pet bereavement experiences. Each has several questions to help readers reflect and discuss positive and healthful adaptive responses to the situations described. There may be a number of ways of responding, and dialogue with others may help to expand the repertoire of support strategies and skills that might be of benefit to children of any age and their significant care providers. The vignettes may be used for both role playing and discussion.

Scenario 1: Riva and Goldie

Riva, 4 years old, comes down for breakfast and finds Goldie on the kitchen floor, dry and stiff, and not moving. Goldie has never been out of the aquarium before, except when her dad helps to clean the tank. Riva gently picks Goldie up and places her in the tank. Dad comes into the kitchen. Goldie is floating on top of the water.

> What should Dad do next?
> How would you help Riva understand what has happened to Goldie?
> How can the family dispose of Goldie's body in a respectful manner?
> What role can Riva take in helping with the final handling Goldie's remains?
> If you were a teacher's aide in Riva's preschool class, what would you say to Riva when you learn that her goldfish has died?

Scenario 2: José and Chico

José is 7 years old. He has just moved with his parents and two older siblings. They had to leave his beloved pet guinea pig Chico back home with a stranger, who bought Chico during their "selling up" sale. The family speaks Spanish fluently but only a little English. José has started in grade 1, but he seems sad, refuses to come and play at recess, has nothing to eat for snack or lunchtime, and does not want to join in the circle time for show and tell. He rocks and keeps whispering, "Chico, Chico." Describe what José might be thinking and feeling.

What signs of grieving does José show us?
If you were the teacher, what would you do?
How can José's parents and family help him?
When would you suggest working with an interpreter, and how?

Role Playing: D'wan and the Storm

D'wan was 14 when the brutal storm ravaged his beachside community. There was extensive property damage all over the area. D'wan's family had the roof of their home blown off, while waves and water demolished their front yard, washing out the electricity poles and ending the power. There was no safe drinking water because of all the flooded land and broken water mains. The family was ordered to be evacuated as soon as the rescue personnel could come by boat. The family of five persons was forced either to leave their pets or release them, because not all pets could come with them. After much discussion, they released the singing finches. Spike, the green iguana, was set free in the back garden near the bamboo bushes. Beau, the dog, and Felix, the cat, were crated up and placed in a separate rescue boat, apart from D'wan and the rest of the family. D'wan insisted on bringing his backpack. Inside was a secret traveler—Rosey, "the big hairy spider." D'wan never let that pack out of his hands. At the relocation and refuge center, D'wan began to ask about Beau and Felix, looking for them all over the site. They were not there. D'wan began to run around, looking and calling for them. He tried to return home, but the police brought him back to the center. D'wan could not sleep that night and began to use other people's Internet connections to follow up on suggestions from the aid workers. After 3 days of frantic searching, disheartened family members walked to the shelter over 10 miles away. They found their beloved pets, and the family gave praise and thanks. D'wan was relieved but angry that no one had followed up, as promised. The pets were reunited with their family members, and Rosey made her appearance.

You may take the roles of the family members, the rescue personnel, and D'wan to act out the scenarios and create healthful responses to the questions posed for reflection.

What effect did this storm have on D'wan and his family regarding losses, separation, death, and emotional stress?
What losses, separations, and anticipated deaths did they experience? Would you anticipate that others might have had similar experiences? Is this important to expect? Why or why not?
Discuss how families need to prepare for disaster care of pets and prevent unnecessary separation, abandonment, death, and loss.
What plans can be developed by communities to reduce the trauma of people–pet separation and animal abandonment and/or death?
Which of D'wan's skills and characteristics helped him cope with this trauma?

How can you help teens with grief associated with pet death, disappear-ance, and separation?

Role Playing: Charity and MzT

Charity and Jo are 18 and 19 years old. Charity has just become emanci-pated from her family. She and Jo are going on the road to sing with their band. Charity's parents are not very happy with this new relationship and the open-ended plans. Charity had planned to go to college in the fall. All that has been put aside. Charity is upset because she must leave MzT, because Jo is allergic to cats, and they cannot include this long-lived childhood pet in the bus accommodations. Charity's parents reluctantly agree to look after MzT, secretly hoping that MzT will be a bridge that encourages Charity to call and to see or talk to the cat whenever she can. After 3 weeks, Charity finally calls from several hundred miles away, only to learn that MzT died 48 hours before she called. Charity hangs up the pay phone, speechless and in tears.

Role-play the principal characters in this story, dramatizing the emo-tional tensions and conflicts that Charity is trying to manage in her life, including the final end of MzT, the 17-year-old kitty companion.

As Charity's parents, what would you do now?
Would you have told Charity about MzT right away when she called for the first time?
How would you have handled the situation?
How do you think Charity is feeling? What might she be thinking?
How would you help her during her grieving?
What words and actions would be supportive in this situation?

ACKNOWLEDGMENT

Dedicated to the memory of Dr. W. G. A. Brack, D. V. M., "the James Herriott of Essex County, Ontario, Canada," who died in the summer of 2009 after a long battle with cancer: inspiration, dedication, and compassion are his legacy.

REFERENCES

Association for Pet Loss and Bereavement. (2008). *Children and pet loss.* Retrieved August 2, 2008, from *www.aplb.org/services/shildren.html*.
Bertman, S. L. (Ed.). (1999). *Grief and the healing arts.* New York: Baywood.
Brown, R. J. (2005). *How to ROAR: Recovering from the grief of pet loss.* Ath-ens, GA: Spring Water. Retrieved August 7, 2008, from *momslifeline.com/ petloss/index.php?id=A5&gclid=cpiM6uuitpqcfqayqaodtd5h*.
Di Ciacco, J. A. (2008). *The colors of grief: Understanding a child's journey through loss from birth to adulthood.* London: Jessica Kingsley.

Doka, E. (Ed.). (1989). *Disenfranchised grief: Recognizing hidden sorrow.* Lexington, MA: Heath.

Fiorini, J. J., & Mullen, J. A. (2006). *Counselling children and adolescents through grief and loss.* Champaign, IL: Research Press.

Fitzgerald, H. (1994).*The mourning handbook: A fireside book.* New York: Simon & Schuster.

Goldstein, S., & Brooks, R. B. (Eds.). (2005). *Handbook of resilience in children.* New York: Springer Science + Business Media.

Grollman, E. (1976). *Talking about death: A dialogue between parent and child.* Boston: Beacon Press.

Hughes, M. (1995). *Bereavement and support: Healing in a group environment.* Washington DC: Taylor & Francis.

Jones, E. H. (2001). *Bibliotherapy for bereaved children: Healing reading.* London: Jessica Kingsley.

Joshua, S. R. (2007). *Children and pet loss: How to help your child and teen cope with the loss of the family's pet.* Retrieved August 2, 2008, from *www.shirijoshua.com.*

Kay, W. J., Cohen, S. P., Fudin, C. E., Kutscher, A. H., Neiburg, H. A., Grey, R. E., et al. (Eds.). (1988). *Euthanasia of the companion animal.* Philadelphia: Charles Press.

Leaman, O. (1995). *Death and loss: Compassionate approaches in the classroom.* London: Cassell/Wellington House.

Lee, L., & Lee, M. (1992). *Absent friend: Coping with the loss of a treasured pet.* Bucks, UK: Henston.

Markell, K. A., & Markell, M. A. (2008). *The children who lived.* New York: Routledge/Taylor & Francis.

McNamara, S. (2000). *Stress in young people: What's new and what can we do?* London: Continuum.

Milbrath, C., & Trautner, H. M. (Eds.). (2008). *Children's understanding and production of pictures, drawings and art.* Cambridge, MA: Hogrefe & Huber.

Monbourquette, J. (1994). *Growing through loss: A handbook of grief support groups.* Toronto: Novalis.

Munroe, B., & Kraus, F. (Eds.). (2005). *Brief interventions with bereaved children.* Oxford, UK: Oxford University Press.

Pearson, M. (2004). *Emotional healing and self-esteem: Inner-life skills of relaxation, visualization and meditation for children and adolescents.* London: Jessica Kingsley.

Quackenbush, J., & Graveline, D. (1985). *When your pet dies: How to cope with your feelings.* New York: Simon & Schuster.

Seibert, D., Drolet, J. C., & Fetro, J. V. (2003). *Helping children live with death and loss.* Carbondale and Edwardsville: Southern Illinois University Press.

Shaw, M. (2006). *Interfaith memorial service suggestions for a young child's pet.* Association of Pet Loss and Bereavement. Retrieved August 7, 2008, from *www.interfaithofficiants.com/companionanimalpages/companion-animalclergysamp.*

Sorensen, J. (2008). *Overcoming loss: Activities and stories to help transform children's grief and loss*. London: Jessica Kingsley.

Travis, H. (2008). *Coming to terms with grief—2007, information topic sheet #1: Child Bereavement Charity*. Retrieved August 7, 2008, from *www. childbereavement.org.uk*.

Turner, M. (2005). *Someone very important has just died: Immediate help for people caring for children of all ages at the time of a close bereavement*. London: Jessica Kingsley.

Wass, H. & Corr, C. A. (1982). *Helping children cope with death: Guidelines and resources*. Washington, DC: Hemisphere.

Webb, N. B. (Ed.). (1993). *Helping bereaved children: A handbook for practitioners*. New York: Guilford Press.

Webb, N. B. (Ed.). (2002). *Helping bereaved children: A handbook for practitioners* (2nd ed.). New York: Guilford Press.

Wolfelt, A. (1991). *A child's view of grief*. Fort Collins, OH: Center of Loss and Life Transition.

Wolfelt, A. D. (1992). *Helping children cope with grief*. Batesville Management Service, available through the Morris Sutton Funeral Home and Chapel, Windsor, Ontario, Canada.

CHAPTER 8

War-Related Deaths in the Family

DIANE L. SCOTT

Images of a military sedan pulling up in the driveway, a child peeking out from behind the curtains in a window of the house, two military service members emerging from the sedan wearing their dress uniforms, and the ringing of the doorbell are scenes that remind many American citizens of wars past. In the days since September 11, 2001, families who have a service member serving in the Global War on Terrorism era live in hope that the reality of those images will not manifest itself in their neighborhood. The war efforts and other peacekeeping missions have reached beyond the insulated environments of military installations to almost every community in the United States with the widespread use of Reserve and National Guard units. The increased tempo of deployments means that both military and civilian families are being impacted by the war, and many of them in the most extreme way, with the death of a family member in the military. Although social workers and mental health practitioners are unable to undo or change the facts surrounding the service member's death, it is possible to intervene to help children grieve and adjust to the loss of a loved one.

Current war activities are one cause of deaths, but military life has always had risk of death or injury from training accidents in preparation for war, personal factors, and weapons and artillery (Daley, 1999). Children in military families have a heightened sense of awareness of war-related issues and risk factors their active duty parent routinely face (Cozza & Lieberman, 2007; Gorman & Fitzgerald, 2007). Children in active duty military families or families with a Reserve or National Guard member live in environments that may include a parent who is physically absent but psychologically present because of deployment-related life cycles (Gorman & Fitzgerald, 2007). Despite children's knowledge of the risk factors, there is a scarcity of data regarding the impact of war-related death on children in military families (Cozza, Chun, & Polo, 2005; Cozza & Lieberman, 2007) or children in families with a parent in the Reserves or National Guard.

Several models depict the deployment cycle that encompasses the lives of military families (see Figure 8.1). Expanded from an earlier three-stage cycle of deployment that included predeployment, deployment, and postdeployment (Logan, 1987, as cited in Stafford & Grady, 2003), the five-stage (Deployment Health and Family Readiness Library, 2006) and seven-stage (Pincus, House, Christenson, & Adler, n.d.) models reflect longer deployments and successive deployments that include relatively short turnaround time at home before redeployment. Children with deployed family members react to the family stressors and parental emotional responses in ways that are consistent with their ages and developmental levels. It is helpful to remember that despite the additional stressors, most military families cope well during deployments and many emerge stronger and develop new skills (Cozza & Lieberman, 2007).

The behavioral and emotional issues in the five- and seven-stage models are similar and provide a useful framework to help families understand and manage the dynamics around deployment. The five-stage model includes predeployment, deployment, sustainment, redeployment, and postdeployment (Pincus et al., n.d.). The seven-stage model includes anticipation of departure, detachment and withdrawal, emotional disorganization, recovery and stabilization, anticipation of return, return adjustment and renegotiation, and reintegration and stabilization (Deployment Health and Readiness Library, 2006). The models and their tasks are reflected in Figure 8.1 and reinforce how family members and children face the separations with a clearly anticipated return of the service member.

During deployments, children behave and respond to the changes and loss in the family in ways that correspond with their developmental age, and they adapt to the stress based upon their resilience and coping skills (Murray, 2002; Pincus et al., n.d.; Rice & Groves, 2005). Pincus et al. (n.d.) advise that infants under 1 year of age need continual care and nurturing to thrive, but toddlers, preschoolers, and older children take some of their cues from their caregivers and remaining parent. Adhering to family routines as much as possible provides stability and reassurance to children (Murray, 2002). Regression from age-appropriate

Three-stage model	Five-stage model	Seven-stage model	
Predeployment	Predeployment	Anticipation of departure	Deployment is becoming a reality, with no plan for memorable family events upon return from deployment; service member works increasingly long hours in preparation and is physically absent except to eat and sleep; marital conflicts may escalate; spouses shut down emotionally to avoid feelings of loss about pending separation; parents may be less attentive to child needs or preoccupied with how they will cope with parental absence; they are caught up in preparing household and personal affairs needed to have service member absent; preparation time may be a few weeks or up to a year.
		Detachment and withdrawal	
Deployment	Deployment	Emotional disorganization	Deployment occurs; service member is completely absent; remaining spouse must reorganize to fill both parental roles and may be emotionally disoriented, with feeling anger, despair, overwhelmed, abandoned and sometimes relieved that service member is finally gone; if the service member is repeatedly deployed, the spouse may feel drained; this usually lasts about a month.
	Sustainment	Recovery and stabilization	Routines are established; chores and responsibilities are learned; crises are overcome; spouse develops support system, feels confident in abilities; with repeated deployments, spouses discover that they are strong and resilient.
	Redeployment	Anticipation of return	Excitement and planning for service member's return; some frustrations as time lines or dates change; need realistic expectations of return and reunification.
Postdeployment	Postdeployment	Return adjustment and renegotiation	In the initial honeymoon period, everyone is happy; service member must reintegrate into family and resume responsibilities; spouse may relinquish gladly or resent giving up responsibility; children may have unrealistic expectations of service member parent's availability; communication is paramount.
		Reintegration and stabilization	There is continued renegotiation of roles and responsibilities; unit duties still exist—maintenance and repair of equipment; service member may be gearing up for redeployment and dealing with combat-related issues; communication remains key.

FIGURE 8.1. Cycles of deployment—family and child issues.

developmental tasks (i.e., potty training, or sleeping alone) may indicate that the child is reacting to the loss in the family. Similarly, acting out or behavioral changes in older children (i.e., sadness, depression, tantrums, substance use, somatic complaints, sleep disturbances, clinginess, and withdrawal from school or social activities) may indicate deployment-related distress in the child (Goodman et al., 2004). For all ages and developmental stages, children need consistent, open communication that is appropriate to their cognitive ability (Raveis, Siegel, & Karus, 1999).

As discussed in the previous chapters, children are more likely to experience traumatic grief if the death is unexpected. An unexpected rather than a combat-related death is more likely to occur in a military family. Children in military families often have mental images of their deployed parents' situation that bear little resemblance to reality (Hardaway, 2004). The children may have unrealistic, media-driven fears about the possibility of death for their deployed parent that are out of proportion to the actual incidence of war-related deaths (Cozza & Lieberman, 2007). As noted in the deployment cycles, despite these heightened anxieties about the safety of the absent service member, the child typically anticipates that the service member parent will return.

Unexpected death is the death that would most typically affect a child in a military family in a war situation. As of August 2008, there were 4,134 military deaths related to Operation Iraqi Freedom and 565 deaths during Operation Enduring Freedom (Department of Defense, 2008c). Militarywide, this represents 43.2% of the total deaths during this time frame (Defense Manpower Data Center, 2008b). Improvements in medical care and immediate medical attention in combat zones make it much more likely than in previous wars that the service member will be wounded and survive (Daley, 1999) (see Table 8.1). Thus, children may be forced to deal with grief and loss related to the loss of the "parent as they knew him or her" rather than the death of that parent. Moreover, because of remote assignments, training activities, and field exercises, military families and children are more frequently exposed to parental separations with unknown missions, durations, and locales (Black, 1993). Military children react to the separations, experience the related loss, and grieve in ways that are consistent with those described in Chapters 1 and 2 of this volume. However, if the service member parent dies during one of these separations, the feelings and distress that existed during the separation may be exacerbated. Further complicating the grieving process for children and surviving spouses of active duty services members who die are the unknowns surrounding war-related deaths, lifestyle changes that occur, and changes in their environment (Cozza et al., 2005; Hardaway, 2004).

TABLE 8.1. Statistics on War-Related Deaths: Global War on Terrorism (October 2001–August 2008)

	Sex		Age (years)			Active duty	Reserve/Guard	Causes of deaths		Total deaths	Wounded[a]
	Female	Males	Age < 25	25–35	≥ 35			Hostile[a]	Nonhostile[a]		
OEF	14	547	216	233	112	454	107	363	209	572	2,379
OIF	99	4,023	2,217	1,451	454	3,366	756	3,362	774	4,136	30,561
TOTALS	113	4,570	2,433	1,684	566	3,820	863	3,725	983	4,708	32,940

OEF, Operation Enduring Freedom; OIF, Operation Iraqi Freedom.
[a]Includes active duty, Reserve, and Guard. Totals differ because statistics are taken from reports that include 2 additional weeks.

MILITARY DEATHS AND DEMOGRAPHICS

As of September 2007, there were a total of 1,366,353 active duty military personnel; of these, there were 221,317 (16.2%) officers and 1,145,036 (83.8%) enlisted service members (Department of Defense, 2007a). Women comprised 196,089 (14.4%) of the forces (Department of Defense, 2007b). There were 33,550 female officers and 162,539 female enlisted active duty service members. Formerly, males primarily were deployed to war areas, but with the increased numbers of females in uniform, more females serve in combat support positions, so there is a stronger possibility that "Mom" is at risk. From 2001 to 2008 113 females have been killed in the Global War on Terrorism (Department of Defense, 2008a, 2008b). This compares to 2 female deaths in the Korean War, 8 in the Vietnam War, and 15 in the Persian Gulf War (Department of Defense, 2003).

During the Global War on Terrorism, the Defense Manpower Data Center (2008a) reports 32,940 service members wounded in action, 3,725 hostile deaths, and 983 nonhostile deaths. Of the 4,708 total deaths, 81.6% (3,840) have been active duty and 18.4% (18.4%) have been Reserve or National Guard service members. Those wounded in action have been 79.5% (26,185) active duty and 20.5% (6,755) Reserve or National Guard service members. As a caveat, Table 8.1 depicts demographic data for service members, but the total numbers may differ in some instances because the Department of Defense reports aggregated herein cover varying time periods and reflect changes pending the status of the cause of death.

CASE EXAMPLE*

Thomas and Selena live in Tacoma, Washington. Selena is a Captain in the Air Force, assigned to McChord Air Force Base (AFB). She has been in her current assignment for 14 months. Thomas is a stay-at-home dad who does some occasional freelance graphics work. The couple's decision early in Selena's military career not to have their twin boys Steve and William, age 3, and their daughter Trish, age 7, in day care or in afterschool programs has been especially important given the work schedule that Selena has recently faced. The family participates in the squadron social activities on a limited basis. As a male spouse, Thomas

---

* This is a fictitious, composite case using an existing military installation and community as the setting to provide a realistic context for assessment and treatment. Any resemblance to actual persons or situations is unintended and purely coincidental.

does not attend the spousal group meetings, because he was frequently the only male present and was not comfortable in that position. Selena's unit has been on a deployment rotation that has her gone 3 months and home 4 months. The unit has been on this schedule for 12 months and is expected to be doing this for the next 9 months at a minimum. During her deployments, Selena is especially attentive to communicating with the three children. She has made tapes of herself reading books aloud for the children to use at bedtime, phones frequently, text-messages almost daily, and the family had a webcam hooked to the computer, so they could have visual conversations whenever possible.

Thomas has family members who live in the Tacoma area. His parents are about 45 minutes away and had no connection to military family life until Thomas and Selena married. Although they were originally behind the military action in response to the 9/11 attacks on the World Trade Center, in recent years they have not been particularly supportive of the ongoing Global War on Terrorism. Selena's family is from Ohio and has a long tradition of military service. Both her father and grandfather served in the Army.

During the last deployment Trish's first-grade teacher sent home a note explaining that Trish was getting into spats with her classmates, was not completing her class work, and was disruptive in class. During the same time period, Thomas said she was hitting her brothers and woke up screaming in the night three or four times a week. Trish had always been a "daddy's girl," but she was increasingly clingy. Thomas talked to the teacher about Selena's deployment, but little changed until Selena returned home. Upon her return, Trish initially was very anxious whenever Selena was not visually present. She was clingy and difficult to put to bed. Within a month of Selena's return, these behaviors diminished, but Trish was still clingy with her mother. The twins showed little change in their behaviors and were initially most apt to seek out Thomas whenever they needed something, but they were accepting and emotionally responsive when Selena intervened or parented.

Three months after her return home, Selena was gearing up for redeployment to the rear support area working supply missions. She worked long hours and came home after the twins were asleep, with barely enough time to read a story to Trish. Selena and Thomas focused on the children and did not talk much about the upcoming separation.

Selena's unit deployed on schedule, and the family members attended only the mandatory deployment briefings because they had been through the process numerous times. Three weeks after she deployed, Selena was killed when the supply plane she was piloting had engine failure. Thomas and the children were expecting a phone call from her that day; the children cried when they had to go to bed without the call. The next day, Thomas was at home with the twins when the military notification team came to their home. Trish was at school and returned home on the bus just as the team was leaving. The next few days were a blur of activity: The squadron held a memorial service in the unit hangar, which was covered by local media; there was a church service and funeral in the National Cemetery, where Selena was buried with full military honors. Two weeks later, the casualty assistance officer suggested that Thomas see a counselor to help him in talking with the children.

INTERVENTION ISSUES AND RESOURCES

Military Identity

It is especially important for a therapist to understand the pervasiveness of the military in forming the identity and context for military service members and their families (Daley, 1999; Hardaway, 2004). For those active duty families who live on or near a military installation, military identity is reinforced by uniforms, prescribed behavior associated with rank structures (i.e., saluting and fraternization rules), housing areas, and support services (e.g., commissaries, hospitals, and base exchanges) that can only be accessed by those with a military identification card. Children may also attend schools that serve only military families on the installation or those that serve communities with a large military population.

A common experience that shapes identity for the families and children is the mobility of military life, whether in the form of deployments or relocation to a new assignment. For children, this has contributed to a unique name for their identity, too; they are frequently called "military brats." All these experiences function to reinforce the sense of belonging and identification with military life as being different and separate from the civilian community. Daley (1999) points out that as with any cultural identity, it is necessary to assess the level to which the family/child has assumed the military identity. The level of acceptance impacts the degree of loss experienced from the change in lifestyle.

Those service members who deploy as part of a National Guard or Reserve unit, or those who augment an active duty unit that deploys, face different circumstances than those active duty members assigned to a military installation. The National Guard and Reserve members may not be as imbued with the military identity, because they do not live the military life 24 hours a day, 7 days a week at work and at home (Strategic Outreach to Families of All Reservists, [SOFAR], 2008). They frequently live in remote areas, far removed from military installations, so they cannot and do not easily access the services available to active duty families (Department of Defense Task Force, 2007; National Military Family Association [NMFA], 2005). The geographical distance and lack of social identity with the military may accentuate the sense of loss and anger when a war-related death occurs, because they expect deployments with the increased war tempo, but death is not part of their expectations.

Family readiness groups, family support groups, key volunteers, and ombudsman programs form a basis for social connectivity and contribute to a sense of identity with military life (NMFA, 2005; Pincus et al., n.d.). Again, the degree to which family members associate with and identify themselves as a part of the group varies. For active duty families, the family readiness groups may be viewed as similar to other spousal groups on military installations. Spousal groups provide a ready-made friendship network, an alternative to paid employment, a means to volunteer time to help others, an informal support network to solve problems and obtain resources, and a means to access information. Family readiness groups are unit-specific support networks, loosely organized around the command structure of the unit (i.e., the commander's spouse typically takes a leadership role or designates a surrogate). There is traditionally a phone tree, so that regular communication exists between family members in the military unit. Family readiness groups are most frequently formed and activated when a military unit will be deploying and may become less active when the unit returns to the home installation. Readiness groups sponsor classes and support groups, and stage family activities and outings that both include children and are solely for the remaining spouse. Participation in the groups is voluntary, although frequently the military unit requires the service member to attend the predeployment briefings, where valuable deployment information is disseminated, thus helping to ensure that family members attend, too (NMFA, 2005). The NMFA survey regarding deployments indicates that 13% of respondents had no contact with support groups; those who did have contact with the groups reported better ability to cope during deployment.

The connectivity to the military unit is one of the primary differences between the active duty family and Reserve/Guard families. For Reserve and National Guard members, the family readiness group develops when the unit has been mobilized to deploy. For many civilian families, this is the first time they have met other such families, and they have few life experiences in common. The bond is the service member and the deploying unit, but the spouse and children may have little sense of identity with the military community. Because Reserve and Guard units form in geographic regions, there is also the possibility that the family does not have access to a family readiness group and may be isolated within its own community as well (NMFA, 2005). Community members and service providers may be completely unaware that the family has a deployed service member, and the spouse at home may not associate problems that arise as being related to the separation (Gorman & Fitzgerald, 2007).

Financial Impact

Upon the death of a service member, an immediate death gratuity is paid within 72 hours, and the designated beneficiary receives $400,000 in life insurance benefits from the Servicemen's Group Life Insurance (SGLI; NMFA, 2006). Family members also receive Dependency and Indemnity Compensation, which is a flat-rate, monthly compensation from the Department of Veterans Affairs (VA) that adjusts annually and is not taxable. Families living on military installations can remain in government housing for up to 1 year and may move from this housing at government expense. If they reside off the installation, they are authorized one relocation at government expense. The financial foundation and stability this provides is important, because in families with adequate financial resources following a parent's death, children showed fewer grief symptoms in the 2-year follow-up (Worden, 1996, as cited in Raveis et al., 1999), suggesting that the financial assistance families currently receive upon the death of the service member may in fact mitigate the distress experienced by children. Having financial resources prevents the surviving parent from having to return to or join the workforce prematurely to support the family, which allows him or her more available time to meet the children's needs. Cerel, Fristad, Verducci, Weller, and Weller (2006) suggest that this financial support and resultant increased parental presence provides stability and eliminates some of the uncertainty about life following the death of the service member, which should increase the child's resiliency and ability to cope.

Notifications

Cozza et al. (2005) has suggested that the system of notification is a potential source of disruption to activity patterns, structure, and living environments for military families. The ambiguity surrounding the initial notification of death compounds a child's sense of loss, because the surviving parent may display frustration and anger at the inaccuracies and lack of information, the inability to obtain facts about the cause or circumstances surrounding the death, and the responsiveness of the military system. Children need enough information to understand the death and to be able to grieve (Hope & Hodge, 2006). War-related deaths sometimes result in inquiry regarding the circumstances of death, or security concerns may limit the release of details.

For the surviving parent and for adult relatives, this creates a situation in which their own frustration with not knowing can lead them to minimize death-related information or to discuss information that is not appropriate for the child's developmental level or cognitive abilities (Cozza et al., 2005). The child who is left with ambiguity about the death may fill in imaginary information. The child may also lose the sense of protection and invulnerability regarding negative life events when a parent dies (Stoppelbein & Greening, 2000). Similarly, parental attempts to shelter the child from unpleasant information may contribute to inadequate parent–child communication that could help the child process the emotions associated with the death. And, as noted earlier, the child may feel personal responsibility for the death, or for failing to prevent the death, that he or she cannot express when there are poor communication patterns with the surviving parent (Raveis et al., 1999). Surviving parents have also wrestled with how to handle funeral attendance; within the military, this issue is compounded by the rituals associated with a service-connected death (NMFA, 2006). The playing of taps, the 21-gun salute, the missing man flight formation, and presentation of the U.S. flag are time-honored traditions in military funerals that may be confusing to a young child, and the adults in attendance may not be cognizant of the child's distress if they are dealing with their own emotions during the ceremonies.

The Department of Defense–assigned casualty assistance officers work with families of deceased service members from the period just after the death notification through the following year to assist family members in accessing services, from burial arrangements through their transition to civilian life (NMFA, 2006).

Other Resources

Increased recognition of the ripple effect of war-related injuries and death for service members, their families, and their communities has resulted in increased resources from the federal government within the VA treatment facilities and Vet Centers (U.S. Department of Veterans Affairs, n.d.) through TRICARE and Military OneSource, and on military installations (Department of Defense Task Force on Mental Health, 2007). In the private sector, the NMFA (n.d.) serves as an advocacy group for legislation and policy affecting military families, educates and provides information on services and resources, and works to improve military life. There is also another nonprofit organization, SOFAR, that provides free psychological services (Levin, Iskols Daynard, & Dexter,

2008). SOFAR was developed for reservists and their family members by Drs. Jaine Darwin and Kenneth Reich (Darwin & Reich, 2006; Levin et al., 2008), and includes a brochure they developed for dissemination to family members, including parents, grandparents, siblings, children, and spouses, of deploying Guard and Reserve service members (SOFAR, 2008). SOFAR focuses on all relatives of service members, which can help to reduce the incidence of transmitting unresolved grief issues between generations (Motta, Joseph, Rose, Suouzzi, & Leiderman, 1997; Stambor, 2006).

In areas of the United States that have little access to major VA or military-related resources, Military OneSource (n.d.) provides educational material about military life, resource information, Internet chat and discussion groups, toll-free nationwide referrals and appointments for services that are reimbursed through TRICARE. The Tragedy Assistance Program for Survivors (TAPS, n.d.) provides comprehensive assistance for family members who experienced the death of a service member. TAPS provides online chat groups; hosts a 24-hour, 7 day a week, support toll-free phone line; sponsors grief camps for children and family members; offers counseling services; and provides resources and support—all at no cost to the surviving family members. In isolated areas, local providers or hospice organizations that traditionally provide bereavement services may not be specific to war-related deaths, but they are available and are reimbursed through TRICARE (Tricare Management Activity, n.d.).

CASE EXAMPLE FOLLOW-UP

In the case example, circumstances in the 2 weeks following Selena's death provided constant activity, which can blunt the emotional impact of death. When the activities cease, families are frequently alone in their grief. Being approached to seek help on behalf of the children increases the likelihood that Thomas will engage in the helping process.

Thomas and Selena's family living situation is typical of many current military families who reside off the military installation and reflects issues that must be taken into account when the therapist works with family members. The family connection to military life and formation of a military identity was mitigated by Selena being the active duty service member and Thomas being the spouse. Although spousal groups are welcoming to all, they most frequently comprise female rather than male spouses, which limited Thomas's ability to identify with the group. This was compounded by his lack of prior exposure to military life, and by living in the Tacoma community rather than on McChord AFB. The voluntary nature of squadron social activities, and the couple's limited involvement in these activities, further isolated Thomas from a natural support group. Aside from an initial follow-up by the spousal group leader upon notification of Selena's death, it is unlikely that Thomas would welcome or respond to overtures of support from this source. Despite this, because Thomas has to deal with his grief, provide a stable family environment, and be available to respond to his children as they deal with the loss of their mother, it is critical that the therapist work directly with Thomas to help him cope with this emotional turmoil. Instead of looking within the active duty military community, the therapist should help Thomas identify his personal support system and prior coping skills, and encourage and provide him with information on how to access services in the future from Military OneSource, SOFAR, and TAPS.

Thomas and Selena were aware of the impact of frequent deployment on the children and had maintained as much family connection and routine as possible. The audiotapes and recorded computer conversations are invaluable resources for the children to maintain their memories of Selena and help them cope with her death. The therapist can work with Thomas on how best to incorporate their use in the family routine. The therapist can also use role playing to help Thomas anticipate and respond to questions from the children or behaviors that may arise whenever the tapes are played. Given that Trish had already been displaying clinginess and was having nightmares, Thomas needs to be made aware that these behaviors may recur and plan age-appropriate responses. Thomas can use the tapes to maintain family traditions and continue to use them within the daily routine to help stabilize the children's lives.

A positive aspect of Thomas and Selena's choice to live in Tacoma rather than on the military installation, coupled with Thomas's parents living only 45 minutes away, is that this family does not need to move to be closer to extended family. This is of great benefit to the children, because there will be less disruption to their daily routine, including their home and school environments. In this case, not relocating means the family will also remain close to the military cemetery where Selena is buried, so they can visit her gravesite easily if desired. This can help the children to make the cognitive connection between her prior deployment absences and the finality of death, which might not readily occur because of their ages—3 and 7, respectively.

The therapist can help Thomas to recognize that it is very likely that Trish and the twins, Steve and William, will regress or display behaviors similar to those that occurred when Selena deployed. The twins may not exhibit an increased number of behavioral changes, because Thomas was their primary caretaker, and at age 3, although they may ask concrete questions about their mother or death, they are not developmentally ready for long discussions (Norris-Shortle, Young, & Williams, 1993). If their grief manifests in behavioral changes, Thomas should be encouraged to bring them to a therapist for play therapy.

For Trish, age 7, school becomes a source of stability, and her teacher's knowledge of her behavior during deployments may also be a resource. The therapist should consult with the teacher and the school counselor to identify available treatment groups and behaviors that may indicate Trish needs further assistance. Trish can also be introduced to some of the TAPS resources geared toward children, and she might be the family member who serves as the bridge to services. The therapist could easily engage the grandparents to explore the TAPS resources with Trish to help them stay involved and to cope with their loss as well. The therapist must also recognize and assess the degree to which the grandparents connect with the military identity when trying to make the TAPS connection, so that barriers can be addressed as needed.

The primary work of the therapist working with Thomas and the children is to help the family grieve and adjust to the permanent loss of their mother and spouse. Thomas was able to provide a stable and nurturing family environment while Selena deployed and during her military career. This family was functioning well prior to her death, with the children displaying only minor behavioral problems related to adjustment and separation. Given their history, stability in the community, and available resources, work with this family should be of relatively short duration, and it is unlikely that this family will experience long-term "disabling grief" (Webb, 2002).

CONCLUDING COMMENTS

As occurs with any child who experiences the death of a parent, the adjustment to loss by children in military families is influenced by the reaction and actions of the surviving parent (Dunning, 2006; Lin, Sandler, Ayers, Wolchik, & Luecken, 2004). Social workers and mental health practitioners who work primarily with military populations, and those who are in practice throughout the community, must be familiar with the grieving process, the emotional cycles of deployment, resilience in military families, and the resources available to this special population group. Connection to any of the 24-hour, 7 days a week support agencies is paramount to making sure the surviving family members access the resources to which they are entitled; failure to do so adds insult to a family that has already made the ultimate sacrifice for the United States. Practitioners must also be aware and respectful of the unique nature of military life and the degree to which the family, the children, and members of their support system identify themselves as "military" or as being supportive of military families.

DISCUSSION QUESTIONS AND ROLE-PLAY EXERCISES

1. In conducting the assessment of the family system, what are some considerations that might arise from Selena being a female head of household/primary breadwinner in the view of her parents versus that of Thomas's parents?

2. What, if any, treatment issues might arise related to Selena's Air Force–related death and her Army parents in trying to engage the extended family in dealing with the death and their grief?

3. What is the impact of the local community's shift in support for war-related efforts on how Thomas and the children perceive Selena's death? How does that compare to their response to Selena's death in the few days following her death?

4. Using information from previous chapters and this case example, what types of behaviors from Steve and William, age 3, and from Trish, age 7, would suggest to you that they may need clinical intervention to deal with their loss?

5. What types of questions might Thomas anticipate from the three children as they cognitively process their mother's death?

6. As the therapist, what would you say to help Thomas "take care of himself" so that he can be available to his children?

7. Role play: Trish has been going to a bereavement group at the local counseling center, in addition to talking to the school counselor, because she continues to have sleep disturbances following Selena's death. During the last group session, she says that her daddy is really sad, and he is getting tired of coming to her room when she screams at night, so he mostly "just let's me cry." You are the therapist who must address this with Thomas. In groups of three or four, chose roles as the therapist, Thomas, and observers, to role-play this scenario.

REFERENCES

Black, W. G. (1993). Military-induced family separation: A stress reduction intervention. *Social Work, 38*(3), 273–280.

Cerel, J., Fristad, M. A., Verducci, J., Weller, R. A., & Weller, E. B. (2006).

Childhood bereavement: Pyschopathology in the 2 years postparental death. *Journal of the American Academy of Child Adolescent Psychiatry,* 45(6), 681–690.

Cozza, S. J., Chun, R. S., & Polo, J. A. (2005). Military families and children during Operation Iraqi Freedom. *Psychiatric Quarterly,* 76(4), 371–378.

Cozza, S. J., & Leiberman, A. F. (2007). The young military child: Our modern Telemachus. *Zero to Three,* 27(6), 27–33.

Daley, J. G. (1999). *Social work practice in the military.* Binghamton, NY: Haworth Press.

Darwin, J. L., & Reich, K. I. (2006). Reaching out to the families of those who serve: The SOFAR project. *Professional Psychology: Research and Practice,* 37(5), 481–484.

Defense Manpower Data Center. (2008a). Global War on Terrorism: Casualties by military service component—active, Guard, and Reserve: October 7, 2001 through August 16, 2008 (*Personnel Reports, Defense Link*). Retrieved August 20, 2008, from *siadapp.dmdc.osd.mil/index.html.*

Defense Manpower Data Center. (2008b). U.S. Active duty military deaths—1980 through 2007 (as of April 22, 2008) (*Personnel Reports, Defense Link*). Retrieved August 20, 2008, from *siadapp.dmdc.osd.mil/index.html.*

Department of Defense. (2003). Department of Defense. Active duty military deaths—race/ethnicity summary (as of March 15, 2003) (*Personnel Reports, Defense Link*). Retrieved August 1, 2008, from *siadapp.dmdc. osd.mil/index.html.*

Department of Defense. (2007a). Department of Defense active duty military personnel by rank/grade: September 30, 2007 (*Personnel Reports, Defense Link*). Retrieved August 1, 2008, from *siadapp.dmdc.osd.mil/index.html.*

Department of Defense. (2007b). Department of Defense active duty military personnel by rank/grade: September 30, 2007 (Women only) (*Personnel Reports, Defense Link*). Retrieved August 1, 2008, from *siadapp.dmdc. osd.mil/index.html.*

Department of Defense. (2008a). Operation Enduring Freedom: Military deaths October 7, 2001 through August 2, 2008 (*Personnel Reports, Defense Link*). Retrieved August 20, 2008, from *siadapp.dmdc.osd.mil/index. html.*

Department of Defense. (2008b). Operation Iraqi Freedom: Military deaths March 19, 2003 through August 2, 2008 (*Personnel Reports, Defense Link*). Retrieved August 20, 2008, from *siadapp.dmdc.osd.mil/index. html.*

Department of Defense. (2008c). Operation Iraqi Freedom (OIF). U.S. Casualty Status: Fatalities as of August 18, 2008 (*Personnel Reports, Defense Link*). Retrieved August 20, 2008, from *siadapp.dmdc.osd.mil/index.html.*

Department of Defense Task Force on Mental Health. (2007). *The Department of Defense plan to achieve the vision of the DoD Task Force on Mental Health: Report to Congress.* Retrieved January 8, 2008, from *www. ha.osd.mil/dhb/mhtf/mhtf-Report-final.pdf.*

Deployment Health and Family Readiness Library. (2006). *New emotional cycles of deployment for service members and their families.* Retrieved April 11, 2008, from *deploymenthealthlibrary.fhp.osd.mil.*

Dunning, S. (2006). As a young child's parent dies: Conceptualizing and constructing preventive interventions. *Clinical Social Work Journal, 34*(4), 499–514.

Goodman, R. F., Cohen, J., Epstein, C., Kliethermes, M., Layne, C., Macy, R., et al. (2004). Childhood traumatic grief educational materials. *National Child Traumatic Stress Network.* Retrieved December 4, 2009, from *www. nctsnet.org/nctsn_assets/pdfs/reports/childhood_traumatic_grief.pdf.*

Gorman, L. A., & Fitzgerald, H. E. (2007). Ambiguous loss, family stress, and infant attachment during times of war. *Zero to Three, 27*(6), 20–25.

Hardaway, T. (2004). Treatment of psychological trauma in children of military families. In N. B. Webb (Ed.), *Mass trauma and violence* (pp. 259–282). New York: Guilford Press.

Hope, R. M., & Hodge, D. M. (2006). Factors affecting children's adjustment to the death of a parent: The social work professional's viewpoint. *Child and Adolescent Social Work Journal, 23*(1), 107–126.

Levin, D. E., Iskols Daynard, C., & Dexter, B. A. (2008). *The "SOFAR" guide for helping children and youth cope with the deployment and return of a parent in the National Guard and other Reserve components.* Needham, MA: SOFAR: Strategic Outreach to Families of All Reservists.

Lin, K. K., Sandler, I. N., Ayers, T. S., Wolchik, S. A., & Luecken, L. J. (2004). Resilience in parentally bereaved children and adolescents seeking preventative services. *Journal of Clinical Child and Adolescent Psychology, 33*(4), 673–683.

Military OneSource. (n.d.). Retrieved August 1, 2008, from *www.militaryonesource.com.*

Motta, R. W., Joseph, J. M., Rose, R. D., Suozzi, J. M., & Leiderman, L. J. (1997). Secondary trauma: Assessing intergenerational transmission of war experiences with a modified Stroop procedure. *Journal of Clinical Psychology, 53*(8), 895–903.

Murray, J. S. (2002). Collaborative practice: Helping children cope with separation during war. *Journal for Specialists in Pediatric Nursing, 7*(3), 127–130.

National Military Family Association (NMFA). (2005). *Report on the cycles of deployment: An analysis of survey responses from April through September, 2005.* Retrieved January 15, 2008, from *www.nmfa.org/site/docserver/nmfacyclesofdeployment9.pdf?docid=5401.*

National Military Family Association (NMFA). (2006). *A survivor's guide to benefits: Taking care of our own.* Retrieved August 29, 2008, from *www. nmfa.org/site/pageserver.*

National Military Family Association (NMFA). (n.d.). Retrieved January 15, 2008, from *www.nmfa.org.*

Norris-Shortle, C., Young, P. A., & Williams, M. A. (1993). Understanding death and grief for children three and younger. *Social Work, 38*(6), 736–741.

Pincus, S. H., House, R., Christenson, J., & Adler, L. E. (n.d.). *The emotional cycle of deployment: A military family perspective* (U.S. Army HOOAH 4 Health Deployment Guide). Retrieved August 29, 2008, from *www.hooah4health.com/deployment/Familymatters/emotionalcycle.htm*.

Raveis, V. H., Siegel, K., & Karus, D. (1999). Children's psychological distress following the death of a parent. *Journal of Youth and Adolescence, 28*(2), 165–180.

Rice, K. F., & Groves, B. M. (2005). *Hope and healing; A caregiver's guide to helping young children affected by trauma.* Washington, DC: Zero to Three Press.

SOFAR: Strategic Outreach to Families of All Reservists. (2008). A program of PCFINE. Needham, MA: Psychoanalytic Couple and Family Institute of New England. Retrieved August 1, 2008, from *www.sofarusa.org*.

Stafford, E. M., & Grady, B. A. (2003). Military family support. *Pediatric Annals, 32*(2), 110–115. Retrieved August 30, 2008, from *sitemaker.umich.edu/airforce_study/files/family_support.pdf*.

Stambor, Z. (2006). War's invisible wounds. *Monitor on Psychology, 37*(1), 48–49.

Stoppelbein, L., & Greening, L. (2000). Posttraumatic stress symptoms in parentally bereaved children and adolescents. *Journal of the American Academy of Child Adolescent Pyschiatry 39*(9), 1112–1119.

Tragedy Assistance Program for Survivors (TAPS). (n.d.). Retrieved August 1, 2008, from *www.taps.org*.

TRICARE Management Activity. (n.d.). *Military health system.* Retrieved August 28, 2008, from *www.tricare.mil*.

U.S. Department of Veterans Affairs. (n.d.). *Vet Center Home.* Retrieved August 28, 2008, from *www.vetcare.va.gov*.

Webb, N. B. (Ed.). (2002). *Helping bereaved children: A handbook for practitioners* (2nd ed.). New York: Guilford Press.

PART III

DEATH IN THE SCHOOL
AND THE WIDER WORLD

CHAPTER 9

The Terminally Ill Child in School and the Sudden Death of a Teacher

ROXIA BULLOCK

As adults we have mature cognitive development that allows us to understand the concept of death as universal, irreversible, all inclusive, inevitable, and at times unpredictable for all living things (Speece & Brent, 1996). However, when a child is dying, not only the parents and family members and other caring adults but also the child has to cope and understand this unpredictable, early death. This chapter focuses on the child's physical, social, and psychological response to his or her dying. In addition, the chapter deals with the unpredictable aspect of death, even when it is anticipated. This relates to the child's reactions to the unexpected death of a teacher. The child's understanding of death at different developmental stages becomes a major consideration when dealing with children in respect to both their own death and the death of a familiar adult.

REACTION TO DEATH AT DIFFERENT DEVELOPMENTAL STAGES

Children at different developmental stages have a variety of reactions to death and dying, including crying, irritability, withdrawal, acting out, sadness, denial, play, separation anxiety, and a lack of concentration (Davies, 2004; Nagy, 1948). Factors that influence the child depend on his or her relationship with the deceased, his or her age, the circumstance and type of death (sudden or prolonged), whether it is a stigmatized death, support systems in place, previous experience with death, and the culture and religion of the family (Davies, 2004; Webb, 2003).

Children who are dying experience age-appropriate emotions, fears, and behaviors that parallel their developmental stage, beliefs, and cognitive level of understanding about death; however, in terms of medical knowledge, they are mature beyond their years (Bluebond-Langner, 2006; Easson, 1981; Webb, 2003).

Developmental Stage: 0–4 Years

The infant has a symbiotic relationship with the mother. When the mother is unavailable, either through her own grieving or death, the infant's response to this is similar to separation, with crying, whimpering, irritability, and withdrawal (Davies, 2004; Mahler, Pine, & Bergman, 1975). Exhibited physical behaviors include rocking back and forth, prolonged sleeping, and sometimes head banging. The infant prefers his or her mother's touch but can learn to be comforted by others when the family is grieving the loss of a family member.

An infant or very young child 1 or 2 years old with a diagnosed fatal illness has no cognitive understanding of death. When there is pain, the baby soon relies upon his or her instinctual responses of crying, clinging, rocking, and agitation. The infant's behavior is focused on reducing inner tension. The usual comforting and soothing of a mother's holding and feeding may at some point give way to the administration of medications to reduce the pain (Easson, 1981).

Toddlers learn to share and acquiesce to gain love and approval as they eventually come to realize they are separate individuals in the world (Mahler et al., 1975) However, toddlers continue to need the reinforcement of the mother's presence to gain mastery of the process of individuation (Bowlby, 1988; Davies, 2004; Mahler et al., 1975).

The normally developing preschool child has language and cognitive abilities to express thoughts, emotions, and physical pain. The death of a loved object for the preschooler continues to be an issue of separation, although this is often debated in the literature (Webb, 2003). Preschool children do not understand the permanence of death. Their cognitive development relies on magical thinking to explain the unknown or events that are too painful or complicated to integrate. When Sam, a 3-year-old, lost his father in a fatal car accident, he cried inconsolably when his father did not come home from work. After the initial shock, the family explained to Sam about the accident. For the next few weeks, Sam would look at the door at the usual time his father came home and ask, "Where is Daddy?" His play frequently had themes of automobile crashes and people dying, then coming to life and returning home to family. Sam also regressed and began bedwetting, thumb sucking, and having temper tantrums. Eventually, with a caring family and a short-term play therapy intervention, he returned to previously mastered developmental tasks. The regression is not unusual; however, the difficulty of regaining previously mastered tasks can have diagnostic significance.

A toddler who is dying brings his or her lack of understanding of the permanence of death to the dying process (Easson, 1981). The preschool child uses primitive emotions to express feelings: He or she reflects the surrounding mood and emotions. The child is unaware of the significance of death but may mirror the emotions that the family is overtly or covertly expressing. When the preschool child is sick and hospitalized, he or she is afraid of an unfamiliar place and separation from family. Already in pain, the child has pain inflicted upon him or her with needles and tests. Preschoolers live in a concrete world and believe there is a cause for everything. They may think they are being punished for doing something wrong. Preschoolers may withhold their anger toward much loved and needed parents, then take it out on hospital staff, who in turn may respond in kind, reinforcing negative beliefs. Parents must constantly reassure children that they have not been "bad" and help them understand that the hospitalization is to help them feel better (Easson, 1981). If the child asks whether he or she is dying, which is unlikely but possible due to previous experiences of death, the child needs to have things explained in age-appropriate language: "We are doing all we can do to help you get better."

Developmental Stage: 5–8 Years

The early latency-age child has begun to move away from the family into the school setting and peer relationships. Gender and family roles have become more established. The child is included in cultural rituals. There is more independence in his or her daily activities. This child is more aware of time, including the past, the present, and the future. He or she understands birth, growth, living, and dying (Easson, 1981). The child works toward mastery of tasks, emotions, and fears. This child has usually been exposed to loss or death in some manner, either through loss of a grandparent or a pet, or through watching television cartoons, movies, or news reports. He or she is aware of being alive and fears death or not being (Easson, 1981). The child is still in the realm of concrete thinking; there is a reason for everything (Davies, 2004). If the child does something wrong, he or she will be punished. If the child becomes sick or hospitalized, it must be because he or she did something wrong and needs to be punished (Easson, 1981). Although aware of death, the child continues to use magical thinking in the early years of this developmental stage. Death is personified by monsters and strange-looking people (Nagy, 1948). As the child approaches age 9 to 10 years, he or she becomes aware that death is irreversible. He or she holds on to concrete and understandable beliefs (e.g., old people die and bad people die) but wants to keep fears of youth dying at bay. When a schoolmate dies, the child's fears may surface and cause anxiety about his or her own existence. The child tries hard to ignore and shut out these feelings.

When a child becomes sick and is hospitalized, he or she understands a diagnosis and prognosis. The child looks to his or her parents for the strength that is lacking within him- or herself. The parents need to reassure the child that he or she is not being sent away as punishment for doing something bad. The child is scared, lonely, and saddened by the separation that hospitalization necessitates and tries hard to be brave and control fears, which may be expressed as anger and frustration at the medical team. The child needs his or her parents, relatives, and schoolmates to visit and to provide comfort (Easson, 1981). He or she soon becomes savvy to the hospital routine. If the hospital specializes in a specific disease, then the child soon learns the language and innuendos about the severity of the illness and its ultimate result, death. Frequent visits by parents and removal to another room or a position close to the door are often interpreted as death being close. The child watches this and learns (Easson, 1981). Denial is a defense mechanisms used by the child and his or her family, and other children in the hospital.

Developmental Stage: 9–12 Years

Moving from concrete thinking to the beginnings of abstract thinking is one of the hallmarks of the later latency developmental stage (Davies, 2004). This age group also has developed language capable of expressing thoughts and emotions (Davies, 2004). School and peers have become a large part of these children's lives. Belonging to a peer group means exhibiting behavior that is acceptable to that group, and these preteens soon learn the behavior and culture of the group. Self-regulation is expected of this age group. Anything that makes this preteen different creates angst and anxiety about not being part of the group. Illness and death are seen as different and possibly as punishment. There is also a macabre fascination with death and a curious, gruesome interest in its details.

Death in the family or his or her own illness makes this child feel different at a time when being like everyone else signifies inclusion in the peer group (Webb, 2003). Because this group understands the finality of death, defense mechanisms, such as denial, avoidance, and compensation, are available at this developmental stage. On the other hand, the need for control can be used to support treatment, by having the child participate in his or her own treatment. The child is capable of taking his or her own medications when appropriate. This awareness may cause anxiety when, in a hospital setting, this child is aware of the rotation of beds or removal of a child who will soon die. This is part of the hospital culture that this young patient picks up on quickly (Easson, 1981). A child is aware of what is happening when he or she is dying and needs his parents' support and caring. He or she needs to be told the truth in age-appropriate language. Research has shown that parents who recognize their child's awareness of his or her own death do not regret having talked to their child about death (Kreicbergs, Valdimarsdottier, Onelov, Jenter, & Strineck, 2004). Parents also need to give hope that remission or cure is a possibility. When medical procedures are explained in advance, the young patient is usually more cooperative (Easson, 1981). He or she has the emotional ability to face dying, and to ask for support and comfort from those around him. The child needs to mourn the separation. He or she may feel sad and angry, because he knows what he or she is leaving behind (Easson, 1981).

A family that is not honest, or that does not talk of death creates a greater burden for the child in several ways: the child feels that he or she has to take care of family members, because they cannot tolerate the child's death; it leaves the child feeling alone in his or her grief; the child may feel angry at the parents, then feel guilty for feeling angry (Bearison, 2006, Alexander, 1995). Openness of parents, relatives, peers, and religious counselors, and family support are necessary for this child to navigate the process of dying. At times, this process, and how to cope with it, spills over into the school system in times of remission when the child returns to the school setting.

SCHOOL AND THE DYING CHILD

The law provides education for all children. When a child is diagnosed with a life-threatening illness, school continues to be a part of his or her life. However, school attendance can often be interrupted by hospitalizations, treatments, clinical appointments, and sick days. The school system must deal with accommodating the needs of chronically ill and dying children. School remains important to children who are terminally ill, because education is a normal part of a child's life. School provides a routine that gives children a purpose in life, a distraction from the illness, a feeling of normality and of belonging to a peer group, a sense of accomplishment in working to fulfill their potential, and a chance for parents to see their children participating in the normal development of childhood (Wood, 2006).

How does the school accommodate the needs of a child who is frequently absent due to illness, falling behind academically, suffering physical discomfort, and/or enduring physical or mental limitations, behavioral problems, or learning disabilities? There are two Acts that accommodate these eligible children: Section 504 of the Rehabilitation Act of 1973 and the Individuals with Disabilities Education Act of 1990 (Rothstein, 1995).

The 504 policy and procedures states: "No otherwise qualified handicapped individual in the United States . . . shall, solely by reason of his handicap, be excluded from the participation in, be denied the benefit of, or be subjected to discrimination under any program or activity receiving federal financial assistance" (Rothstein, 1995, p. 27).

How does a concerned parent obtain a Section 504 assessment for his or her child? If a parent or teacher considers a child to have a disability (neurological, respiratory, speech, hearing, vision, etc.) that impairs a major life activity, the 504 Coordinator is notified in writing by the teacher or parent, and an assessment to determine eligibility is arranged. However, if the student compensates in some way (medication, equipment, corrective devices) and is able to participate equally with his or her nondisabled peers, then the child is not considered eligible for 504 accommodations (Rothstein, 1995).

Using the appropriate form supplied by the school, a parent can initiate a 504 request for his or her child. If school staff initiate the request, they contact the 504 Coordinator, who then must notify the parent within 5 days in writing and send forms to be completed by the parents and/or health care provider(s). To determine whether a child is eligible for 504, the team must answer three questions (Rothstein, 1995): Does the student have a physical or mental impairment? Is a major life activity affected by the physical or mental impairment? Is the major life activity substantially impaired?

After parental notification and forms are completed, the following steps are instituted:

- The team determines whether an assessment is appropriate and if so, requests an assessment.
- The team does an assessment.
- The team notifies the parents of the results of the assessment and informs them of their rights, including the right to appeal, if they disagree.
- The modifications and/or accommodations are put in place.

The Individuals with Disabilities Education Act (IDEA) includes the educational and psychological evaluations of a child. The evaluations are included under the auspices of the Committee of Special Education in the local school district. The process often begins with a teacher or guidance counselor/social worker discussing with parents that their child is not performing on grade level, and/or that standardized test scores are substantially below grade level. Another area that may initiate the request for an evaluation is behavior problems. An evaluation is recommended to determine whether there may be a learning disability or some other reason for the academic and/or behavior problems. The parents then send a written request for an evaluation to the Committee on Special Education in their school district. The parents are interviewed for a social history by a social worker. Then the child is evaluated by a school psychologist. The parent, social worker, psychologist, teacher, and child, if age appropriate, have a conference, and the results of the evaluation are presented. If the child is found to be eligible, services are implemented. The services are provided at the child's public school and guided by an individualized education plan (IEP) (see *schools.nyc.gov*).

Difficulties may emerge in the school setting for a child who is terminally ill and taking medication and treatments that may alter his or her appearance. The child may be teased, bullied, or shunned. Although difficult, it can be helpful for the child to educate classmates about his or her condition. This reduces fears and opens communication. In addition, the teacher needs to become educated and in turn educate the children. The guidance counselor and/or social worker can initiate communication with the medical team to become informed about this particular disease (Openshaw, 2008; Webb, 2009).

The social worker or guidance counselor uses different therapeutic techniques to help the chronically ill or dying child to adjust to the school environment. Individual counseling can help the child discuss or play out his/her fears and anxieties. Family counseling can help the school and family work cooperatively both educationally and medically (Webb, 2009). The parents and school nurse can help educate school professionals so they can better serve the child. Group counseling can be effective with children who have illness conditions or mixed with those who do not so as to promote interaction, understanding, and empathy (Clifford, 1991). Group counseling is intended to be supportive and reduce the feelings of being alone with this illness.

CASE EXAMPLE: DEATH OF A STUDENT

Mrs. Perez, a fourth-grade teacher in a mainstream classroom in an elementary public school in a large metropolitan city, has been somewhat reluctant to seek out the services of the social worker for fear of seeming incompetent. However, the school social worker had helped her with Luis, an acting-out child with attention-deficit/hyperactivity disorder, and now she needs help again. In November, John, a 10-year-old student of Hispanic and German ethnicity, had been absent 8 days this school year and was beginning to act out. She had a meeting with his parents, Mr. and Mrs. Fein, who informed her that John had been diagnosed with leukemia in the second grade and had been in remission for 1 year and was doing well. Recently John had been showing symptoms of nosebleeds, vomiting, fatigue, bone pain, and fever. They were distraught. His recent doctor's appointment and tests confirmed that the leukemia was back; he had relapsed. This explained his absences. Mrs. Perez, completely unprepared for such news, was shaken. She has an 11-year-old son and can empathize. How could she teach and help John? His parents explained the diagnosis and the next steps of treatment, and gave Mrs. Perez a list of days and possibly weeks he was expected to be absent. His parents asked for schoolwork to help John keep up with his studies. Having been through this in the second grade, they were just recovering from the exhaustive ordeal. Now it was happening again. They were angry, anxious, and afraid. After the parents left, Mrs. Perez asked to see the social worker to request help.

The social worker did not know John. She called Mr. and Mrs. Fein, introduced herself, and asked permission to meet with John about his health concerns and his behavior when he returned to school. The social worker explained how she would respect their feelings about what to say about the disease. They were concerned about how to tell John about the risks involved with a relapse. There was discussion about how it is important to give hope yet at the same time be honest (Kreicbergs et al., 2004). An appointment was set for the following week to discuss John's developmental and health history and current medical condition. His parents were appreciative of the call and any help the school could provide.

The Social Worker's First Meeting with John's Parents

The following week, the social worker met Mr. and Mrs. Fein. They were eager for any help with John. The boy's recent behavior included answering the teacher back in a rude way, not doing homework, not passing in class work, and having confrontations with other students. This was uncharacteristic of John. Until the diagnosis of cancer in the second grade, John had been a good student, receiving A's and B's. He had good behavior and was respectful. He was well liked by his peers, who appreciated his athletic ability. His recent participation in sports activities provided the key to diagnosing his leukemia this time around.

He began having headaches, fatigue, frequent bruising, and bleeding more than previously when involved in contact play. He was diagnosed with acute lymphocytic leukemia (ALL). His parents were devastated. They were bewildered with this relapse, because John had been healthy and was returning to the typical activities of a child his age. When he was 7 years old and received the diagnosis of leukemia, they were shocked. Their lives became consumed with tests, hospitalizations, and clinic visits. John was subjected to many blood tests, and finally a bone marrow test confirmed the diagnosis (Siegel & Newton, 1994). He began chemotherapy immediately. He had terrible side effects but was a trouper through it all. He even had a catheter for the drugs. This went on for a year; then, amazingly, he went into remission. He was administered postinduction therapy after the remission to destroy any lingering cancer cells in his body (Siegel & Newton, 1994). His parents hoped he would make the 5-year mark and be considered cured. They were distraught to hear this recent news. They felt as if they were back at square one. It was quite likely that this time they would be looking for a bone marrow transplant. Finding a donor would be another difficult process.

The social worker asked for signed releases for permission to contact John's doctor and other medical team members (Openshaw, 2008). She hoped his team could help her support John and his parents. The team included a hospital social worker, whom the parents liked and found helpful. The school social worker needed to learn about this disease so she could be knowledgeable. John had a younger sister, Maria, who was in the first grade, and the social worker asked, to meet with her when appropriate. Well siblings of chronically or terminally ill children have concerns that need to be addressed (Bluebond-Langner, 1996).

The First Meeting with John

Three weeks later John returned to school and the social worker met with him.

Content	Analysis
SW: Hi, John. How are you today?	
J: OK, tired. You are the person who talks to kids with problems. Luis came to you.	Nothing gets past the gossip of the students.
SW: Yes.	
J: I behave. Well, most of the time. Why am I here?	He has a charming sense of humor. This question caught me

SW: Your teacher told me you have been absent for a long time and before that there were some homework problems. I do talk to students about problems, but I listen to students who talk to me.

J: My friend said you play games. I have been absent. I was in the hospital. (*John is quiet, fighting back tears.*) I was sick before in the second grade and it is back. You talked to my parents?

SW: Yes, they told me how brave you are. You had some chemotherapy in the hospital 2 weeks ago. How did that go?

J: Awful, I was pretty sick. I take medicine now. I'll do better in school. Can we play a game?

SW: Sure. Your choice. (*John picks Battleship.*) If you need help with schoolwork, let me know.

J: (*John wins the game.*) If you practice, you will get better.

SW: Maybe you can help me. How about if we meet next week?

J: OK.

off guard. I could have asked him why he thought I called him to my office, but I went for straightforward honesty. It is the kind of relationship I want to establish with him.

I am thinking ahead to discussions of his cancer. I need to establish honesty. I give him some quiet time. He may not be ready to talk about this to a stranger. I need to build a trusting relationship. In reality, he knows why I sent for him.

I pushed the cancer issue a little and left it up to him.

He was brave, but he had told me enough for now.

The symbolism of the "battle" was evident.

I had to laugh.

Usually I have children draw, but I really wanted to give John some sense of control, given that he was in a situation over which he had little or no control.

He returned to class.

The Next 3 Months

John's relapse seemed worse than his first experience with leukemia. The chemotherapy did not work as well, and his parents and the doctors were discussing a bone marrow transplant. John was in and out of school. The school social worker was given permission to talk to the hospital social worker when needed. John met with the social worker weekly, or as often as he needed, when he was in school. He seemed relaxed in her office as he played and talked openly. He liked to draw and engaged easily when drawing. He had lost his hair from the chemotherapy and had a bloated look due to drugs. Through the Department of Education, the social worker arranged for a certified teacher to tutor John at home when there were long hospital or home stays due to reactions to treatments. John, although a smart child, was falling behind in his academics and his skills due to absences. There was a meeting and discussion with his parents and teacher about initiating a Section 504 for John. The team coordinator sent the necessary papers to his parents, and John was found to be eligible for services, including nurse visitations as needed, counseling visits as needed, a tutoring service, and classroom modifications where appropriate (Rothstein, 1995).

John was physically tired and frustrated. He did not feel that his parents were being honest with him about the cancer, and he wanted more information. John was 10 years old and knew that certain diseases were fatal, and cancer was one of them. He knew how to use the Internet and did so. He had survived leukemia once, but this time was different. He felt sicker than before. He talked about the "culture" of the hospital ward and how kids knew things adults tried to hide from them (e.g., José being taken from the room before he died, and Sally recently going home and not returning although John knew she was not cured).

The social worker spoke to Mr. and Mrs. Fein about John's frustration and desire for more information about his cancer. They agreed to try to be more open and honest, although this was very difficult for them. They gave the social worker full permission to have any conversations with John regarding the boy's concerns about death.

4 Months after the First Meeting

Content	Analysis
J: Hi, Pete is a jerk. He thinks he is so "all that." He was making fun of my head.	John has lost his hair. Will he be willing to tell his class about leukemia and educate them? I present the idea to him.
SW: What did you say?	Is he angry at Pete or at the cancer for making him look different than the other kids?
J: I told him to go "*#!" himself. Sorry.	
SW: Sounds like you stood up for yourself. It must be hard to look different and to have no	

control over what the
medications are doing to your
body. I have an idea for you
to think about. Would you
be willing to tell your class
about leukemia, so they would
understand better what you are
going through and hopefully
be more understanding and not
say "dumb" things?

J: You mean stand up and talk
about it? Maybe, it would
make Pete look like a jerk. I
don't know. I am embarrassed
sometimes about how I look,
and I am not sure I want them
to ask me a lot of questions.
What if I don't know the
answer?

I distracted John from his real
feelings, and he is not going to let
me do it. Good for him.
He is wondering about the
possibility of his not getting
better, of his own death.

SW: You don't have to know all
the answers because you will be
talking about your experience,
and who knows that better
than you? I'll help and set it up
with your teacher and if you
want me to be there I'll stay in
the classroom while you talk.

I have promised his parents
that they will be the ones to
have this conversation about his
deteriorating health. I have to call
them.

J: What if they ask me . . .
(quiet) . . . you know, can you
die from leukemia.

SW: Then you tell them,
sometimes, but that 80% of
children get better and are
cured.

He is so brave. He has put into
words his fear of dying and I was
honest but able to give him hope.

J: Maybe. But it still sucks. I just
want this to be over but what
if . . . ? (quiet) Remember I told
you about José in the hospital,
he died. They don't want you
to know, but we all know. He
went home and didn't come
back.

SW: They try to keep secrets from you.

J: What a joke.

SW: How does that make you feel?

J: How do you think? Mad. Scared. (*in a little voice*) I don't want to be sick anymore.

He is angry at everyone who is not making him better. He is doing his part by putting up with terrible meds, so why is he still sick? John is 10, and he still uses cause-and-effect thinking. He takes meds. He should get better.

SW: It doesn't seem fair, you are doing your part by taking your meds, and the cancer is not playing fair.

I reflect back his feelings.

J: (*quiet*) They are still looking for a bone marrow match, but they haven't found one. My sister is not a match. I was hoping, but it is not her fault.

He is moving back and forth between the wishful thinking of a child and the mature understanding that it is not his sister's fault. It would be easy to blame someone and distance himself from the anger.

SW: No, it is not her fault. They have banks of donors. Maybe a match will come up.

I try to give him hope.

J: Maybe. Do we have time for a game?

SW: Yes.

I can tell he is not convinced, so again we see the child needing to move away from the intensity of the emotions. Again he chooses Battleship. Could destroying my ships be a metaphor for his wish to destroy the cancer? I listen carefully as we play.

The Social Worker's Second Meeting with John's Parents

This meeting was emotional. After the social worker met with John, he was admitted to the hospital. He was very sick. Mr. and Mrs. Fein shared with difficulty that John's condition was deteriorating, and that the search for a bone marrow match, so far, was not successful. His white blood cell count was very high, and he was becoming weaker (Siegel & Newton, 1994). They had many decisions to make about his care. The doctors were encouraging them to prepare for his death, but they felt paralyzed to do this. How could they tell John that he was dying? How much longer could he stay in the hospital? Should they bring him home or place him in a hospice facility? The social worker and parents discussed the need to be honest with John, because he probably knew (Kübler-Ross, 1983). Children who are dying pick up on adult behaviors and emotions. When the child feels that the adult cannot tell the truth, he or she begins to protect the parent by withdrawing and withholding his or her own anxious and fearful feelings (Easson, 1981). This becomes a burden and increases the child's anger, fear, and anxiety. The child may direct these feelings at others, outside of the family, to protect the family (Easson, 1981). Both parents agreed that in the end they wanted to keep John at home for as long as possible. They began to make preparations to accommodate his needs. They did not want to give up and still hoped for a bone marrow transplant, but time was running out. John's mother repeated several times that he had recovered before and maybe he would do so again. Both parents turned to their church and religious faith for comfort and understanding, and to find a purpose in their son's life, illness, and possible death. The social worker and parents discussed John's classmates visiting him and/or sending cards. They agreed that this would be a good idea.

1 Month Later

The school social worker received a telephone call from Mr. Fein that John had died quietly at home 2 days earlier, with his family around him. He asked that the social worker take care of informing the school. She agreed and asked about funeral arrangements, and Mr. Fein gave her the information. She asked whether he would mind if school staff and some students attended the funeral. He thought that would be nice.

The social worker met with the principal and wrote a memo to all the staff. The social worker met with the principal, guidance counselor, and Mrs. Perez and the other fourth-grade teachers to discuss how they would tell the students. They agreed to read a memo to ensure that the message was delivered uniformly. This would also help the teachers control their emotional feelings. The guidance counselor and social worker would be present in the classroom at that time to talk to the children and answer any questions. They would also be looking for high-risk students who might recently have had a relative die, have a sick family member, or be an especially vulnerable child. They would set up a special meeting with those children and their parents to provide support through this time. They also composed a letter to inform families of the children in these classes of the event and to explain some of the signs of grief their children might display, and how to comfort their children. They included the guidance office telephone number for those parents who felt they needed help at this time (Stevenson, 2002).

Mrs. Perez was upset when she heard the news, but she was able to tell the children and answer questions. What would she do with John's desk and the belongings he had in school? She did not want to eliminate them, like he had never existed. Two days later, she decided to have a "farewell" for John in her class. She had the students sit around John's desk and tell memorable stories about him as they packed his things in a nicely decorated box to return to his parents, with a sympathy note from the class. Each class member, if he or she wanted to, said a final goodbye to John. Again, this gave Mrs. Perez and the social worker a chance to observe the children for any high-risk behaviors. There were some tears but, all in all, she felt it was a lovely ritual and formal goodbye.

CASE EXAMPLE: SUDDEN DEATH OF A TEACHER

Other than home and family, school is the place children spend the most time, develop social relationships and skills, and engage in intellectually stimulating lessons. Involvement with adults outside of the family and developing both emotional and working attachments is part of this milieu. When adult school personnel die, it is an emotional experience for not only the teachers and staff but also for the students in that teacher's class, as well as students who have forged a close relationship with that teacher. The school's role has been documented by several authors in terms of how to handle the sudden or prolonged death of an administrator, teacher, counselor, staff person, or student (Bullock, 2007; Stevenson, 2002; Dudley, 1995; Doster & McElroy, 1993; Hickey, 1993). Children at different developmental stages have both predictable and individualized reactions to the death of a person who touched their lives in some way. We can anticipate age-specific symptoms of children. Then there are the unique emotional reactions of each individual, depending on his or her relationship with the deceased, previous death experience, support systems, proximity to the death situation, psychological problems, developmental deficiencies, and religious and cultural beliefs (Webb, 2002).

Certain death situations are understandable and acceptable within the child's cognitive conceptions, such as the death of an elderly person or someone dying from a disease. No matter how sad these events are, with time these deaths are incorporated into the child's life experience and developmental maturation. Some specific deaths are stigmatized (e.g., suicide, AIDS, drug overdose, and homicide) (Doka, 1989). Other deaths are difficult to accept, such as the death of a child, the death of an adolescent due to high-risk behavior, and the sudden death of a person in an accident. The sudden, unexpected death of a young beloved teacher and how a school responds is the theme of this section. The case has been disguised to protect confidentiality.

Mr. Pratt was a second-grade teacher in a large metropolitan elementary school. He had been a member of the staff for 5 years. This school was his first assignment as a teacher. The administration and teachers were impressed with his natural talent, organizational skills, teaching skills, and genuine interest in the children. He especially had a gift for working successfully with difficult students. Mr. Pratt was single and lived close to his parents. His older sister also lived in the area. He came from a close-knit family. His professional life was focused on motivating the children, and learning and implementing new and innovative teaching techniques. He was also involved in school-related extracurricular activities, including the Homework Helper Club, Lunchtime Chat Groups, and Parent Workshops (teaching parents how to help their children with homework). He was becoming well known in his school's community.

In late August, just before the new school year was to begin, the principal received a call early Sunday morning from Mr. Pratt's sister. Mr. Pratt had been killed instantly in a car accident. It had rained heavily Saturday night, and he had been on his way home from visiting friends. His car was hit by a speeding drunk driver. The other car had been occupied by three teenagers who had been out drinking. The teenager driving the car was also killed. The two teenage passengers were in critical condition.

The principal was shocked that such a promising life had been cut short. She called her crisis team, which consisted of the assistant principal, the math teacher, the guidance counselor, the social worker, and the parent coordinator (Dudley, 1995). This would be an especially delicate situation. The students of Mr. Pratt's new class would be expecting him. In fact, certain parents had specifically requested Mr. Pratt as their child's teacher. His former students would also be expecting to see him. The principal arranged an appointment for early Monday morning to meet and set up a plan for breaking the news to the teachers and staff. The children would be informed when they returned to school the following week. She asked the crisis team members not to say anything until the meeting. She had arranged to call Mr. Pratt's sister on Monday morning to gather more details, in order to convey accurate information (Bullock, 2007; Dudley, 1995; Doster & McElroy, 1993). The principal would arrange for her crisis team to join her to attend the funeral on Tuesday. That Sunday, the principal had personalized the generic announcement form created by the crisis team to send to parents when the children resumed school Wednesday of the following week.

Monday morning turned out to be more difficult than the principal had anticipated. The news media had reported the accident. They focused more on the teenager's death, but Mr. Pratt's name was mentioned. Some of the children and their parents had heard the news. Many parents called the school to verify the news of Mr. Pratt's death. The secretary was given specific instructions about what to say. She provided the factual information on which the family had agreed. The principal would respect the family members' wishes about funeral attendance and calls.

The crisis team meeting had been scheduled for 8:00 A.M. Monday morning. The priority was preparation of the announcement letter to parents per the details Mr. Pratt's sister would provide. Then the secretary would make copies for each student in the school to take home (see Figure 9.1). The principal provided the agenda, then the team would take over and prepare the details of informing the school population and handling the grief that would follow. The first order of business would be to inform the school staff at a 7:30 A.M. meeting on the first

---

Dear Parents,

The summer is coming to an end and the school year is about to begin. I hope you all had a wonderful summer break. We are happily anticipating the return of the children to our school community. The children will return Wednesday September ____, 2008.

However, it is with great sadness that I am informing you that Mr. Pratt was killed in a severe car accident on August ____, 2008. We will miss him and his devotion to the children.

We will address this event on the first day that the children return to school. We have chosen to do this because many of you and your children already know about this event due to news coverage. We also plan to have parent meetings not only to discuss the usual school agenda but also to give you some information about how to discuss this event with your child. The meetings will be scheduled according to grades, because children react to death according to their age. The parent meetings are as follows in the auditorium:

9/____/08 Wednesday evening 5:00 P.M. to 6:30 P.M. PreK through second grade
9/____/08 Thursday evening 5:00 P.M. to 6:30 P.M. third grade through fifth grade
9/____/08 Friday evening 5:00 P.M. to 6:30 P.M. sixth grade through eighth grade

I look forward to meeting with all of you.

Sincerely,

_____
Principal

FIGURE 9.1. Announcement letter to parents.

day back to school, which would be that Thursday. The team would be careful to share the facts of the accident. They would allow time for questions and processing of emotions. They would model the process the teachers would use with the children. Many teachers knew of the accident, yet they were shocked to hear the news become real. Many cried and all were given information about union counseling services. The team empathetically explained that the teachers would need to tell the students and allow time to listen to students' concerns and sadness. Each teacher was given a written statement to read, so that all would be giving the same information. This helped the teachers focus on the event and the children, and control their own emotions in an appropriate way. Teachers were encouraged to share appropriate feelings, such as "I will miss Mr. Pratt also." The team members would be available in each room to help, and one of them would read the prepared statement if any teacher felt he or she could not perform this task. The team explained to the teachers that this was a situational type of crisis that carried with it shock, suddenness, randomness, and disbelief (James & Gilliland, 2005). The social worker explained how the developmental stages of the children would govern their reactions to this death. The teachers were also instructed to observe any high-risk students and give their names to the social worker or the guidance counselor for follow-up. "High risk" would include any students who had experienced a death in the past year, those particularly close to Mr. Pratt, those with psychological problems, and students in his class (Dudley, 1995).

That Mr. Pratt died over the summer presented the school with a unique situation both for the students and the administration. The death of Mr. Pratt would be a loss for the students who had known him personally, especially last year's students, who would be expecting him to help them transition to their new teacher and new grade. It is not unusual for younger children to have some difficulty transitioning from one grade to another. These students feel the loss of a teacher to whom they have become accustomed and may feel jealous that his new students have displaced them (Davies, 2004). Returning to school and engaging with last year's teacher can help the children understand the process of moving on and developing a caring relationship with the new teacher. This process was prematurely interrupted by Mr. Pratt's death. Younger children do not yet understand the permanence of death and might expect Mr. Pratt to return. Second graders, Mr. Pratt's grade, are on the cusp of understanding this irreversibility of death. The stress of beginning a new school year can pull children back into earlier beliefs that the dead person will magically return. This age group has probably experienced death with pets, grandparents, or television characters, but depending on a child's maturity and other factors, he or she might expect Mr. Pratt to return to the classroom. Children of this age may feel responsible if they have had any angry thoughts about Mr. Pratt and/ or guilty about their teacher's death. The new teacher would observe students for possible high-risk behaviors of acting out or withdrawing. Another potentially high risk would be any child who knew any of the teenagers in the other car.

The social worker and the guidance counselor opened their offices for students to visit as needed to discuss feelings about the death of Mr. Pratt. In addition, they both set class schedules for such meetings. They also set up early morning appointments the first week for parents who wanted to stop by and talk.

The beginning of the school year was also an appropriate time to have parent meetings. Three meetings according to the breakdown of grades (pre-K–2; 3–5; 6–8) would allow the social worker and guidance counselor an opportunity to explain some of the age-appropriate reactions to death, and how parents might comfort and talk to their children about Mr. Pratt's tragic death. There would be time set aside for parents to ask questions.

Parents who had more than one child in different classes would be encouraged to attend different meetings. Parents were asked to prepare their children by telling them about the death of Mr. Pratt as noted in the letter sent out on the first day. They were reassured that the school would also inform the children in an appropriate and sensitive way. If the parents had any questions or reservations about this process, they were encouraged to ask questions. Mr. Pratt's second-grade class was of particular concern. The principal asked the guidance counselor and social worker to work with the new teacher to help the children cope. A retired teacher agreed to return for the full school year to provide consistency for the children. Fortunately, this experienced teacher could move into the position easily.

On the first day of school, after the children settled into their new classes, they were told of Mr. Pratt's death. They were given time to ask questions and to share feelings and concerns about what would happen to them and their work.

Groups

When an event influences a large number of people, including children, forming groups is an efficient way to provide support through the crisis; it is a technique that allows all to know that they are not alone. Groups are an appropriate modality for a school setting (Maden, 2000; Stevenson, 2002). It is important to screen each child before the group begins to ensure that each member is appropriate for group counseling. The group needs to have a purpose, a common theme that connects each member in the group; in this case, the theme was bereavement. Often groups are homogeneous in gender depending on age and theme. However, in this situation, it was determined to be appropriate for the groups to have both boys and girls (Clifford, 1991, Brown, 2004). It would also be a good opportunity to screen for any students who might need a referral for further counseling.

The guidance counselor and the social worker were concerned about Mr. Pratt's second-grade class. They decided to create several groups for all who were interested. All of the children wanted to participate. All the parents gave permission. Groups can accommodate a variety of sizes, but six to eight members is a good number (Clifford, 1991, Brown, 2004). There were 28 students in his class; therefore, two groups of six and two groups of eight were created.

The groups were scheduled to meet at the end of lunchtime and include recess time once a week for 10 weeks. The guidance counselor and the social worker would co-lead the groups Monday through Thursday. The guidance counselor and the social worker agreed on a bereavement theme with supportive activities for each week. Drawings and other types of artwork would comprise some of the activities (DiLeo, 1973; Landreth, 2002; Malchiodi, 1998). This gave structure to the group and at the same time allowed flexibility for the children to express feelings they were experiencing at that time. The first session laid out the purpose of the group; group rules and confidentiality, discussion of how the children were feeling and thinking about the death of Mr. Pratt, any concerns, and anything else they wanted to discuss. The children all knew one other, so there were no formal introductions except to acknowledge who was in a particular group.

After each session, the guidance counselor and the social worker processed the group to discuss children's reactions and identify any potentially high-risk students. Processing is beneficial for the group facilitators to discuss their own feelings and thoughts about the students in the group, as well as how they interacted with the students and with each other (Ryan & Cunningham, 2007).

CONCLUSION

The modern school system emphasizes its traditional responsibilities of education but also includes areas of students' lives that impact education, such as the death of a student and/or a teacher. The school community now includes parents/guardians in many aspects of the school environment, such as permission to evaluate for academic or emotional disabilities, support of Section 504 assessment and accommodations, and dealing with death within the community. Chronically or terminally ill children can continue to attend school in times of health or remission. This helps the children stay connected to peers, teachers, and the school environment. This connection allows the children a feeling of purpose, a sense of normality, and a distraction from their disease. Life experiences, such as trauma and death, are a part of life. Some of these difficult events enter children's lives unexpectedly and inevitably become part of the school environment. Schools must be prepared to help their students deal with these painful life passages.

DISCUSSION QUESTIONS AND ROLE-PLAY EXERCISES

1. Discuss, in debate format, how involved the school should be with the family of a terminally ill child. One group is supportive of school involvement and the other group is not, preferring to leave the dying process entirely to the family.

2. Discuss the possible impact on the social worker of dealing with the death of a child. What might be some vicarious traumatization to the social worker, and how can this be handled to avoid burnout?

3. Role play: Role-play with your class how you might set up an environment and activities to have closure about the death of a student in a second- or (any-grade) class. How would you change it for different grade levels?

REFERENCES

Alexander, P. (1995). The child and life-threatening illness. In K. Doka (Ed.), *Children mourning mourning children* (pp. 45–46). Washington, DC: Hospice Foundation of America.

Bearison, D. J. (2006). *When treatment fails: How medicine cares for dying children.* New York: Oxford University Press.

Bluebond-Langner, M. (1996). *In the shadow of illness.* Princeton, NJ: Princeton University Press.

Bluebond-Langner, M. (2006). Children's view of death. In A. Goldman, R. Hain, & S. Liben, (Eds.). *Oxford textbook of palliative care for children* (pp. 85–94). Oxford, UK: Oxford University Press.

Bowlby, J. (1988). *A secure base: Parent–child attachment and healthy human development.* London: Basic Books.

Brown, N. W. (2004). *Psychoeducational groups.* New York: Routledge.

Bullock, R. (2007). The crisis of deaths in schools. In N. B. Webb (Ed.), *Play therapy with children in crisis* (3rd ed., pp. 270–293). New York: Guilford Press.

Clifford, M. W. (1991). A model for group therapy with latency-age boys. *Group, 15*(2), 116–124.

Davies, D. (2004). *Child development: A practitioner's guide* (2nd ed.). New York: Guilford Press.

DiLeo, J. H. (1973). *Children's drawings as diagnostic aids.* New York: Brunner/Mazel.

Doka, K. (1989). *Disenfranchised grief: Recognizing hidden sorrow.* Lexington, MA: Lexington Press.

Doster, G. P., & McElroy, C. Q. (1993). Sudden death of a teacher: Multilevel intervention in an elementary school. In N. B. Webb (Ed.), *Helping bereaved children* (pp. 212–238). New York: Guilford Press.

Dudley, J. (1995). *When grief visits school: Organizing a successful response.* Minneapolis, MN: Educational Media Corporation.

Easson, W. M. (1981). *The dying child: The management of the child or adolescent who is dying.* Springfield, IL: Thomas.

Hickey, L. O. (1993). Death of a counselor: A bereavement group for junior high school students. In N. B. Webb (Ed.), *Helping bereaved children* (pp. 239–266). New York: Guilford Press.

James, R. K., & Gilliland, B. E. (2005). *Crisis intervention strategies* (5th ed.). Belmont, CA: Brooks/Cole.

Kreicbergs, U., Valdimarsdottier, U., Onelov, E., Jenter, J., & Strineck, G., (2004). Talking about death with children who have severe malignant disease. *New England Journal of Medicine, 351*(12), 1175–1186.

Kübler-Ross, E. (1983). *On children and death.* New York: Macmillan.

Landreth, G. (2002). *Play therapy: The art of the relationship* (2nd ed.). New York: Brunner/Routledge.

Maden, C. (2000). Child-centered play therapy with disruptive school students. In H. G. Kaduson (Ed.), *Short-term therapy with children* (pp. 53–68). New York: Guilford Press.

Mahler, M., Pine, F., & Bergman, A. (1975). *The psychological birth of the human infant.* London: Hutchinsons.

Malchiodi, C. A. (1998). *Understanding children's drawing.* New York: Guilford Press.

Nagy, M. (1948). The child's theories concerning death. *Journal of Genetic Psychology, 73,* 3–27.

Openshaw, L. (2008). *Social work in schools: Principles and practice.* New York: Guilford Press.

Rothstein, L. F. (1995). *Special education law* (2nd ed.). New York: Longman.

Ryan, K., & Cunningham, M. (2007). Helping the helpers: Guidelines to prevent vicarious traumatization of play therapist working with traumatized children. In N. B. Webb (Ed.), *Play therapy with children in crisis: Individual, group, and family treatment* (pp. 443–460). New York: Guilford Press.

Siegel, D. S., & Newton, D. E. (1994). *Leukemia.* New York: A Venture Book.

Speece, M. W., & Brent, S. B. (1996). The development of children's understanding of death. In C. A. Corr & D. M. Corr (Eds.), *Handbook of childhood death and bereavement* (pp. 29–50). New York: Springer.

Stevenson, R. G. (2002). Sudden death in schools. In N. B. Webb (Ed.), *Helping bereaved children* (2nd ed., pp. 194–213). New York: Guilford Press.

Webb, N. B. (Ed.). (2002). *Helping bereaved children: A handbook for practitioners* (2nd ed.). New York: Guilford Press.

Webb, N. B. (Ed.). (2003). *Social work practice with children*. New York: Guilford Press.

Webb, N. B. (Ed.). (2009). *Helping children and adolescents with chronic and serious medical conditions: A strengths-based approach*. Hoboken, NJ: Wiley.

Wood, I. (2006). School. In A. Goldman, R. Hain, & S. Liben (Eds.), *Oxford textbook of palliative care for children* (pp. 128–140). Oxford, UK: Oxford University Press.

CHAPTER 10

Violent, Traumatic Death in Schools and Community Responses

PATTI HOMAN ANEWALT

CASE EXAMPLE

When 16-year-old Kevin Haines attended school on Friday, May 11, 2007, he did not know it would be his last day in school, much less the last day of his life. His older sister Maggie had arrived home from college the night before. By Saturday morning Kevin and his parents had been brutally murdered in their home. Upon waking up to "sounds of struggle and the smell of blood" (Kelly, Crable, & Robinson, 2008), Maggie ran to her parents' bedroom, where her mother's last words instructed her to go to the neighbor's house for help.

In the days and weeks that followed, with the killer still at large, the high school, the school district, and the entire community were in crisis. Hospice grief counselors supplemented the elementary, middle, and high school counselors and psychologists from the district that first Monday following the murders. Faculty met before school to review plans for the day and to identify key concerns. The high school staff lounge was designated as a place to support faculty members who needed to talk. Two counselors followed Kevin's class schedule. Staffed with school and community counselors, the gym became the central location where students could go to talk with someone. School psychologists, counselors, and a social worker identified at-risk students and faculty to determine

190

where additional support was needed. Administration personnel cooperated with local police, while continually assessing priorities and areas of concern. At the end of that first day, faculty again gathered to receive administrative updates, to support one another, and to prepare for the next day. Local pastors provided a community prayer service, and hundreds of students and parents attended. On that Monday after the murders, school staff and students pinpointed by police were interviewed to gather information about the family (which continued intermittently until school let out in June).

School personnel advocated to the College Testing Board for students who felt unable to focus on scholastic aptitude tests (SATs), and the students were allowed to postpone the test. An informational session about coping with the stress of the unsolved murders was held in the high school auditorium the following Monday. A panel of a school psychologists, counselors, and local police fielded myriad parental concerns.

Ironically, the funeral for Kevin and his parents was held on his parent's wedding anniversary. Recognizing that the killer could be present, close family and friends entered the church after everyone else was seated. With the church packed to capacity, including over 150 students, the police were a heavy presence. More than 75 students remained after the service to talk with counselors, including 16-year-old Alec Kreider, one of the last to leave (Berkebile-Kane, personal communication, June 4, 2008). Five weeks later, Alec threatened suicide and was admitted to an inpatient psychiatric facility, where he confessed to a therapist and then to his father that he was the one who had murdered the family (Kelly et al., 2008). Police arrested Kreider after his father accompanied him to the local police station. Questioned about his motive during the trial a year later, Kreider denied having an explanation for committing the murders.

The ripple effects in the community were significant in the 5 weeks between the time of the murders and Alec's confession. Until Alec was apprehended, children, teens, and adults throughout the county were afraid to be alone. Kevin's parents were locally employed and active in their church. Kevin's mother Lisa had taught preschool for over 10 years. Current and past children she had taught, as well as their parents, were deeply affected. There was an ongoing focus in the media, criticism of the police, and heightened anxiety throughout the community. Children and teens were afraid to be home alone after school, and many children slept with their parents. Home security businesses quickly developed long waiting lists as people purchased dead bolts, alarm systems, and infrared cameras for their homes.

What would the response be if this occurred in your community? Would your schools feel prepared and equipped to respond? Are school resources and agreements in place so that school personnel work collaboratively with others in the community to address the myriad problems that would arise? Previous chapters have established how children experience death in numerous ways. Though not an every day occurrence at the local level, *all* school districts throughout the country have many students at any given time grieving significant losses. "Americans have been exposed to increased levels of mass violence during the past decade" (National Institute of Mental Health, 2002, p. 1). Constant media coverage of war, terrorism, and community violence has resulted in more exposure to sudden and violent death than that in previous generations. It is not a matter of *if*, it is a matter of *when* the next school crisis will occur. The Amish shooting in October 2006, in a rural Pennsylvania village, confirms that "no school is immune" (Dwyer, Osher, & Warger, 1998, p. 1) and everyone can be impacted. The tragedy in Columbine High School in 1999 and the September 11, 2001, terrorist attack long before the Amish schoolhouse shooting illustrates how pervasive the ripple effects can be. The impact lingers and spreads at individual, community, national, and even international levels.

Most schools now have a crisis plan, as well as an identified crisis response team, but enough time usually elapses between crises to leave teams feeling less than fully prepared. This chapter outlines four components of school crisis response: *preparing* for sudden or violent incidents; *assessing* the impact; *responding* to the crisis, with the goal of mitigating the impact on all who are affected; and *collaborating* with community resources in the days, weeks, and months that follow school-based violence or sudden death. Many school districts and crisis teams focus most of their planning on the immediate response to a school crisis. With an emphasis on preparation, this chapter addresses key considerations and interventions in "temporal sequence" (Vernberg & Vogel, 1993, p. 485).

RESPONSES THAT AFFECT CHILDREN

Parent/Adult Reactions

Most studies of children who are traumatized and affected by sudden death stress the important role that adults, particularly parents, play in the emotional well-being of the children (Cohen, Mannarino, Greenberg, Padlo, & Shipley, 2002; Coates, Schechter, & First, 2003; Galante & Foa, 1986; Smilde-van den Doel, Smit, & Wolleswinkel-vanden Bosch, 2006; Webb, 2007). Children only cope as effectively as do the adults around them. The best way to support students affected by crisis and loss is to work with the parents and adults closest to the children. Informing, including, and involving parents and key adults are critical. Most parents need guidance on how to talk with and remain connected to their children in times of crisis. Coates, Schechter, and First (2003), working with children in New York City after September 11, 2001, were unable to separate out the children's reactions from the way the entire family responded to the attack. In the case example at the beginning of this chapter, many parents were uncomfortable discussing the circumstances surrounding the (stabbing) death of the Haines family. Stemming from their own feelings of vulnerability, they unintentionally projected their anxiety onto their children, and everyone was afraid to be home alone.

Within hours of the Amish schoolhouse shooting, Amish parents congregating at the local firehouse had many questions about what to say and how to talk to their children about what happened in the schoolhouse that morning. Psychologists and counselors met with over 50 Amish parents to field their questions and help them understand how best to support and talk to their children. When traumatic death impacts a school, parents often seek other influential adults to address their reactions and best meet their children's needs. After the Amish shooting, teachers in the neighboring Amish schools were afraid to return to their own schools. As teachers expressed their concerns to counselors, they were able to identify what they needed to feel safe enough to resume classes. How adults respond and interpret the significance of the event directly influences children's ability to cope. Children pick up on the intensity of the emotions, even when the adults around them provide no information. Regardless of how horrific the actual incidents are, children's imaginations often fabricate something worse than what occurred. Informing, supporting, and reassuring students are key components in any response to sudden death in schools.

Community Reactions

Drawing from Webb's (1991) preference for the word "crisis" rather than "trauma" in certain circumstances, it is important to recognize that everyone reacts differently to extreme stress. Not everyone is necessarily traumatized. "Trauma" refers to the psychological wound that can occur, and it is best understood from the perspective of the person experiencing the crisis. When a tragedy affects a school, if the community is unable to heal, then those who are traumatized will also be unable to heal. Trauma is best understood on two levels—how it is experienced by the individual, and how it is experienced by a community (Myers, 1996). After the Amish schoolhouse tragedy, several communitywide sessions were attended by both Amish and "English" (the Amish word for non-Amish). Time and again, they gathered, intuitively needing to acknowledge how their entire community was affected. By coming together as a group, people could heal individually as well. This chapter outlines suggestions for addressing not only the immediate crisis-related issues but also the longer-term aspects of grief for individuals, as well as the entire school community.

PREPARATION IN THE SCHOOL

The Role of the School

The most significant environment outside a child's immediate family is the school. Consuming most of a student's weekday hours, school provides the primary source of social relationships and activities. It is a safe, familiar environment. School personnel play an important role in helping students cope with their grief (Doka, 2008). "Unique effects were found for support from teachers and classmates . . . lending credence to the position that socially supportive relationships within the classroom are important for children's psychological well-being after a major disaster" (Vernberg, Silverman, LaGreca, & Prinstein, 1996, p. 245). Following the September 11, 2001, terrorist attacks, many experts felt that New York City schools were some of the most effective environments for providing follow-up services to students (Gould, Munfakh, Kleinman, Lubell, & Provenzano, 2004). The importance of this role should not be underestimated.

Preparation before a crisis is essential to ensure effective and sensitive handling of a crisis situation. An intentional focus on prevention, education, and clear lines of communication is an important component of school preparation. Well-organized crisis response teams that meet regularly and have resources on hand are better prepared when the next school crisis occurs. No matter *how* prepared school personnel try to be, all crises include unexpected aspects. No school administration can plan for or feel completely confident in responding to the situation described at the beginning of this chapter.

Education and Prevention

Preparation before a tragedy occurs involves an emphasis on education. Although it is impossible to prevent all tragedies, schools decrease the likelihood of a crisis by being proactive. Numerous studies (e.g., Slovak, 2002) identify the relationship between household guns and suicide or homicide. Schools that stress the importance of eliminating access to firearms can prevent many potential tragedies. Educating students about signs of potential violence in the form of either suicide or homicide is crit-ical. Helping students understand how and when to report anything sus-picious to an adult is another component of preventive education. Schools must identify an easy, confidential process in which students may make someone else aware of something they observed that may be of concern.

Several areas need attention when it comes to educating others about suicide prevention. Having studied school violence for many years, Cornell (2007) emphasizes the importance of a good relation-ship that fosters strong communication and trust, so that students will make faculty aware when a potentially violent or threatening situation exists. With suicide as the leading cause of death for adolescents, having in place a protocol for addressing the effects of a suicide is an equally important preventive action (Doka, 2008). Physicians and medical facil-ity personnel also need to take these threats seriously. It is frustrating for caring school personnel when they ask parents to take their child to the emergency room or to their doctor, only to have the child turned away by both. This undermines faculty members' assessment of the serious-ness of the situation, because they then lose credibility with parents and students about coming to them for help (Berkebile-Kane, personal com-munication, June 4, 2008).

Offering death education in the schools, whether in preparation for possible suicides or tragedies, provides students with a level of familiar-ity and knowledge that prepares them to cope more effectively when a death occurs (Stevenson, 2008). Similarly, school districts that provide in-school services on issues of grief, loss, sudden death, and traumatic responses familiarize school personnel with what to expect when a cri-sis occurs. Even well-trained crisis response teams feel challenged as the extensive ripple effects occur in the days and weeks that follow a crisis. Most school districts are woefully unprepared when it comes to dealing with the aftermath of a situation such as what happened at Columbine High School (Lattanzi Licht, 2008) or the example cited at the beginning of this chapter. Because affected students feel more comfortable turning to a teacher they trust than to a little-known counselor (Gould et al., 2004), teachers, as well as counselors and administrators, need training on what to expect and how best to support students affected by a crisis.

Education and Communication

A proactive preventive stance that emphasizes resilience rather than weakness, and well-being rather than pathology, encourages a response to crisis that draws from the perspective of being a survivor rather than a victim. Schools that foster good communication and a strong relationship between home and school provide a firm foundation on which to draw when a school tragedy occurs. Similarly, when schools keep parents informed and help families understand how to maintain healthy, strong parental relationships with their children, they can draw upon this strength when school-based violence or sudden death occurs. Numerous studies emphasize the correlation between resilience in coping with a crisis and a strong relationship between parents and children (Christ & Christ, 2006; Cohen et al., 2002; Lin, Sandler, Ayers, Wolchik, & Leucken, 2004).

In preparing for a school crisis, the communication plan is critically important. Clear chains of command in communication, specific protocols, and an approach that conveys competence, expertise, and honesty significantly impacts the success of the response (Reynolds, 2004). Communication within the school community, as well as beyond, to all outside organizations with which the school interfaces ensures a collaborative focus and avoids the problem that can sometimes arise with territorial issues that are more competitive than collaborative in nature. Those responding to the Virginia Tech shooting realized, in retrospect, that they should have planned for a more centralized system of communication in their response plans (Kennedy, 2007).

The Department of Homeland Security developed the National Incident Management System (NIMS), which provides a uniform, consistent approach to any type of crisis. NIMS compliance is another way to ensure effective communication (Federal Emergency Management Agency, 2008). Familiarity with and training in the NIMS system ensures that school personnel share the same language, concepts, priorities, and processes with police and emergency medical personnel who are trained in this system of communication and structure.

Determining School Readiness

The very nature of school-based violence and sudden death means that an incident will take place when least expected. Schools should identify which crises will most likely occur, what their procedure will be, and who will respond. Each school must develop a crisis plan that meets the unique needs of its particular community. All staff should be aware of the plan and have a clear understanding of their role in its implementation. The self-evaluation tool (Figure 10.1) is one way schools can determine their level of readiness.

Crisis Response Teams

The crisis response team should include a wide variety of individuals. It is important to include school personnel who work closely with students,

There are two kinds of schools—those that have faced the crisis of a death, and those that are going to do so. Preparation for handling deaths in the school community is essential before the crisis happens, because it ensures effective and sensitive handling of the situation when it occurs. To respond effectively, the school must have a plan. Staff must be aware of the plan and have a clear understanding of their role in implementing that plan. This self-evaluation tool may be a helpful way to determine how prepared your school really is.

Rate how prepared your school is on each of the components using the following scale. Note what you would like to improve, add, or change in each area.

1 = Excellent; 2 = Good; 3 = Fair; 4 = Poor; NA = Not Applicable

School Crisis Response Components	Rating	Ways to improve
District Readiness:		
Our district takes a proactive, preventive approach to planning for crisis response.		
District policy guidelines clarify what is treated as a crisis and what responses are needed.		
Our district has a procedure in place to commemorate a death.		
School Readiness:		
Administration has a strong/positive commitment to planning for and addressing issues of crisis and death in our school.		
All school personnel (not just crisis response team members) have had training in grief, loss, and crisis response.		
Materials and resources are prepared and ready to distribute in the event of illness or loss in the school.		
Our phone chain is updated every 6 months to ensure names and phone numbers are current.		
Our crisis response team meets regularly.		

(cont.)

FIGURE 10.1. Are You Prepared?: A self-evaluation tool.

School Crisis Response Components	Rating	Ways to improve
School Readiness *(cont.)*:		
Our crisis response training includes information about age-specific student responses and possible intervention strategies.		
The size of our counseling staff is adequate to address the needs of our school.		
Crisis Plan Components:		
Addresses student, faculty, and parent needs for the *first few* hours, days, and week after the incident.		
Considers *ongoing* needs and issues for the weeks and months that follow an incident or death.		
Specifically addresses the needs of students before, during, and after funerals.		
Includes ways to communicate effectively with the media.		
Includes a variety of notification procedures (announcements and notices to students and faculty; student assembly, faculty, and parent meetings).		
Identifies ways to enlist assistance in the community (other schools or community agencies) if needed.		
Clarifies the role of nonteaching staff (custodian, office and cafeteria staff, aides, bus drivers).		
Addresses the needs of parents who may be calling or coming to the school.		
Includes high-risk students' needs.		
Includes library staff (for reading or audiovisual material and resources) to address students, faculty and classroom needs following a death.		
Plans for location and staffing of "counseling areas" for additional support.		
Includes a variety of notification procedures (announcements and notices to students and faculty; student assembly, faculty, and parent meetings).		
Has a system in place to support crisis response team members.		

FIGURE 10.1. *(cont.)*

such as teachers, counselors, psychologists, social workers, and aides, in addition to the administrators, security and custodial staff, office staff, district personnel, counselors from other schools, and community mental health resources (e.g., hospice grief counselors or crisis hotline staff). Crisis response teams should meet regularly to review their roles and role-play potential scenarios. By discussing previous and potential incidents they will feel more prepared for the next crisis. Team members must be aware of their own unique beliefs, values, and areas of both strength and vulnerability, because the knowledge and skills set that accompany an individual team member's awareness will influence how effectively he or she responds.

Crisis response team members trained on the differences between normal and traumatic grief reactions must assess and address all who are impacted (Goodman & Brown, 2008). Human beings strive to know and to understand; therefore, whenever a tragedy occurs, existential issues arise, and the question "Why?" often surfaces. Training and skills building topics for crisis response team members should include the following:

- Current theories of grief
- Current theories of trauma
- *How* to be a calm, nonanxious presence in times of crisis
- Ways to involve community resources
- Self-awareness
- Stress, self-care, and coping strategies
- Team building
- Scenarios to role-play (individual support, central locations to provide support—referred to by some as "safe rooms," and group interventions)

When a school experiences an unexpected death, the impact is felt throughout the faculty and student body. The crisis response team monitors and assesses this impact as the response unfolds, while outside resources provide an objective perspective of the situation. Community mental health agency representatives are excellent consultative resources and additions to the team (Kerr, Brent, McKain, & McCommons, 2003; Lovre, 2007). The involvement of hospice grief counselors in the example at the beginning of this chapter illustrates how to utilize these supplemental community resources. Establishing reciprocal arrangements with other districts is another way to supplement the team. As part of the standard protocol, these reinforcements can be immediately implemented.

Each school response team must be clear about its primary areas of focus. The U.S. Department of Education (2002) suggests that *readiness, response,* and *recovery* are three key components on which to concentrate. *"Themes of relationships, community* and *responsiveness"* (Lattanzi Licht, 2008, p. 336) are three alternative priorities to consider. Osofsky (1995) emphasized *individual resources, a safe environment,* and *identifying a supportive individual* in that environment to be the most important factors when addressing the impact of violence on pre-school- through elementary-school-age children. The elements of *"balance, communication, connectedness* and *support"* suggest four other areas a school could consider for its focus on crisis prevention, intervention, and response (Consortium to Prevent School Violence, 2008, p. 1).

Resources

Looking for or developing resources amid the shock and confusion of a crisis contributes to the feeling of being overwhelmed and out of control. Schools can establish a shared file server or intranet to make handouts available for all school faculty long *before* a crisis occurs. Separate handouts for students, parents of students, and faculty can address normal reactions in times of unexpected crisis and suggest ways to cope, as well as ways to support others. Having a template of a letter to send home to parents, prepared long before a school crisis occurs, is an additional resource that is helpful (see Figure 10.2 for a sample).

WHEN AN INCIDENT OCCURS: ASSESSING THE IMPACT

From the moment an incident occurs, the crisis response team must continually assess the impact on students, faculty, parents, and the community at large. The model of responses to trauma and bereavement in Figure 10.3 illustrates how reactions and needs change over time in the minutes, hours, days, weeks, and even years that follow a crisis event. Schools must tailor their intervention(s) to the specific phase of recovery (Myers, 1996). Thoughtful and intentional implementation of the crisis plan, usually initiated by someone the school principal designates, such as the school social worker or psychologist, begins with an assessment of the magnitude of the event. Although ultimately responsible for the response effort, administrators and superintendents often rely heavily on the head of the crisis response team to coordinate all the specific plans. In the example at the outset of this chapter, the principal met with the crisis response team and hospice grief counselors at 6:30 A.M. and 3 P.M.

WHAT: Parent letter and information packet to send home with students

WHEN: Sent on school letterhead after the death of a student or teacher

WHY: Conveys continued concern for students, provides direction and resources for families

Dear Parent,

We are saddened by recent deaths that have touched our lives and the lives of our students. As a school community, we express our condolences to the families and friends of _____.

As school staff we encourage you to listen carefully to your child. Answer questions openly and honestly as they occur, and let your child know that even as adults we don't have all the answers concerning questions about death. When children, regardless of the age, are affected by a loss, it is not uncommon for them to struggle with fears, experience poor concentration, nightmares, physical complaints, eating or sleeping difficulties, regressive behaviors, crying or irritability. Monitor your child and know that accepting his/her feelings and validating whatever they may be feeling is important.

Enclosed is some information you may find helpful in the coming weeks and months. If you have any questions or concerns about how your child may be affected by the recent death(s) in our school (list a community resource and phone number they can access, such as a hospice bereavement program that might be part of your crisis response team).

Counselors will be available at the school to talk with students who are struggling. Our counselors and teachers are also available to provide support and answer any questions you may have. Please feel free to call me also at _____ if you have any concerns.

Sincerely,

School Principal

FIGURE 10.2. Sample elementary school letter, an opportunity for outreach after the death of a student or teacher.

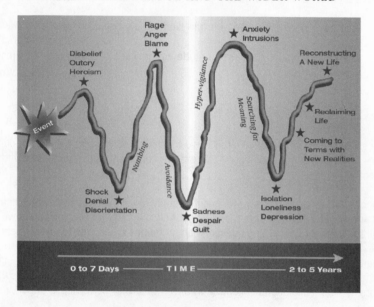

FIGURE 10.3. Model of psychological responses to trauma and traumatic bereavement. From U.S. Department of Health and Human Services (2004).

that first day of school. Similar to death(s) when tragedy occurs on a larger scale, particularly if there is no forewarning, reality can become distorted. Suddenly nothing feels safe or certain. Adults need to help children understand and maintain a realistic context for the specific situation. After every school shooting, schools throughout the country review and tighten their security measures. This can at times exacerbate the feeling of vulnerability. Children and adults need to be reminded that schools *usually are* safe environments. "Fewer than one percent of all violent deaths of children occur on school grounds, indeed a child is far more likely to be killed in the community or at home" (Dwyer et al., 1998, p. 1). Everyone, including the media, quickly focuses on school safety when a school tragedy takes place, despite the fact that violent crime occurs more commonly in communities than in schools (Cornell, 2007). Adults and children become more aware that a school shooting is a *possibility* once one has occurred, but they need to be reminded that this does not increase the *probability* that it will occur again.

Also akin to the overall grief process, the trajectory for recovery after school-based violence or sudden death is always longer than what is comfortable for most individuals. Despite the desire for routines to "return to normal," the process is not linear. This adjustment process includes many ups and downs, often with changes occurring when least expected. When something triggers a reminder, such as an anniversary, the grief reactions usually take students, as well as adults, by surprise. Eventually these grief bursts lessen in frequency and intensity, but when experienced, many people wonder whether their reactions are normal. The ability of each student to revisit the incident varies, depending on his or her personality and opportunities to acknowledge the impact it has had on his or her life. Children develop their own "rhythm" (Nader, 1997) in adjusting to the incident, and counselors and psychologists actively monitor this impact, allowing them to adjust overt time in their own unique ways. Sensitivity to the unique needs of the individuals who are mentally challenged or emotionally disturbed must also be an integral part of assessing who is affected.

Even in times of disaster, most experiences represent normal grief reactions to an abnormal situation (Myers, Zunin, & Zunin, 1990). However, supporting others who are affected by sudden or violent death requires a great deal of flexibility. Needs change over time as the circumstances change; it is a *process* of adjustment. Frequently, when working with traumatically bereaved children after September 11, 2001, the interventions were adapted as needs changed over time (Goodman & Brown, 2008).

Immediate Interventions

How schools respond, particularly in the first few minutes and hours following the incident, has the potential either to exacerbate or to ameliorate the crisis at hand. Regardless of a school administrator's personal reactions, appearing calm and in control establishes a reassuring atmosphere for the school and the community. Being direct and intentional in decision making and clearly communicating the next steps are more likely to ensure that others will embrace and follow these plans. Students need simple, developmentally appropriate information. School personnel must be mindful of what they discuss within earshot of students. By the time a mother picked up her daughter for early dismissal from kindergarten after a school lockdown due to a murder–suicide in Iowa City, the daughter knew many of the details, because she had spent the day listening to the teachers whisper to each other (Sanders, personal communication, June 8, 2008). Adults, as well as students, need reassurance that they are experiencing common reactions. Whenever possible, it is important to emphasize how unlikely it is that the situation would occur again, unless, of course, that is not the case. One of the challenges in the example at the beginning of this chapter was the difficulty in providing this reassurance in the days and weeks following the tragedy.

Keeping in mind Maslow's (1954) hierarchy of needs, the initial interventions are basic and readily apparent. Physical and emotional safety is the greatest priority. In the evening after a murder–suicide occurred in a middle school cafeteria, the mother of an elementary school student shared her concerns about her son, who felt safer at school than at home. The mother could not understand why he would feel safer at school, where the shooting took place, until the son explained that the school doors were kept locked, unlike the doors in their home. Although basic, individual needs vary greatly, thereby explaining the need for a wide range of interventions. Designating someone to keep a running log of what takes place, plans implemented, and who is doing what helps those in charge stay on top of the countless details that they must monitor and track.

In the first few hours of response to a school crisis, there is "a high level of activity with a low level of efficiency" (Myers, 1996, p. 2). Emotions are magnified; everyone wants to "do something" in response to feeling helpless and overwhelmed. This only contributes to the chaos and confusion. When schools provide a clear delineation of plans, and roles within that plan, there is structure and a sense of order in what otherwise is very chaotic. Simultaneously, accompanying the reactions of shock, denial, disbelief, and disorientation experienced by the entire school is the challenge of handling "spontaneous volunteers." Whether well-meaning members of the community or opportunistic individuals, the offer of additional support presents a challenge for crisis response teams. Schools need to identify who will assess the training, skills level, and experience of these volunteers. Particularly if short staffed and needing additional help, this assessment will determine whether, how, and where to utilize them appropriately. When a tragedy occurs, the response to feeling helpless is the desire to help, ironically, so people can feel better, not necessarily because their help is needed. Gathering a list of volunteer names and phone numbers, and explaining that someone will contact them when additional needs are identified is an effective way to handle spontaneous volunteers.

Designating a location where people can bring cards, flowers, and mementos is an additional way schools can address this natural need to "do" something. Particularly when those who have died were known well by school faculty or students, it is wise intentionally to identify a specific location. After the Challenger exploded, the Concord High School library was designated for this purpose. Mementos from all over the world, as well as messages from those more directly touched by the life of Christa McAuliffe, were placed on display throughout the library.

A crisis management briefing (CMB; Everly & Mitchell, 2002), called by some schools an "informational briefing" (U.S. Department of Health and Human Services, 2004), is an effective way for schools to assess and address needs proactively in the first day or two after a traumatic incident. CMBs provide the opportunity to convey how the school is handling the situation, to assess who is most significantly impacted, and to offer a forum for parents to air concerns, feel heard, and be supported. This helps to dispel rumors and reduce anxiety, and to provide information on resources available. Following a school shooting, almost 700 people attended two CMBs (Seebold, 2003), a clear illustration that the school accurately identified and addressed this need. Timing is critical, and soon after an incident is usually the best time to provide informational sessions, because people tend to be more receptive to support soon after the crisis. After two high school teens died in a car accident, many parents asked the school to coordinate some type of group meeting. When the meeting was finally arranged a week later, few attended— the opportunity had passed. Needs change as the days and weeks unfold after an incident. Monitoring and addressing needs, at the right time, is the "art" of crisis response.

Early Interventions: The First Week

Even in a well-prepared school with an organized crisis response team, the initial response to a crisis can feel like "the day that won't end" for those involved in addressing the needs. This, then, leads to what usually feels like "the week that won't end." Critical aspects of intervention in the week that follows a tragic event include continually assessing, reprioritizing plans, and being flexible. Webb's tripartite approach for assessing the child (see Chapter 2, this volume) also provides an excellent framework for understanding the impact of the crisis on affected adults.

Nonverbal clues provide valuable information about what interventions to provide. One elementary school relocated classes to another building after a minor fire in the boys' bathroom. For days, many kindergarten boys repeatedly drew pictures of the school burning and played "firemen" at recess. It was not until the teacher asked a fireman to talk to the class about the fire safety features in the school that these behaviors began to subside.

In the first few days after an incident, many students (and adults) have trouble focusing, feel disoriented, and need reassurance about plans in place to address needs. This is the ideal time to disseminate information and education that fosters resilience and recovery. The most common areas of focus include what to expect behaviorally, cognitively, emotionally, and physically; how to cope with stress, grief, trauma, and loss; normal versus abnormal grief; and concerns to watch for (National Institute of Mental Health, 2002). Interventions are most effective when they complement the innate resilient responses and strengths of affected individuals.

Educationally focused support groups and time to talk within the classroom provide a safe place for students to realize they are not unique in their reactions and anxieties about an incident. School-based groups allow students to talk about their individual reactions to the crisis, clarify misperceptions, and learn basic strategies about coping with stress, crisis, and loss (Vernberg & Vogel, 1993). When offered soon after the incident, groups provide students the opportunity to express and address their experiences rather than suppress them and only increase students' stress levels over time. When a student killed the principal and himself in the crowded cafeteria of a middle school (Seebold, 2003), students and parents attended individual counseling and support group sessions the day after the incident. Many of the 250 students in the cafeteria at the time of the shooting felt guilty, because they either froze or ran out of the cafeteria as soon as it happened. Parents were distressed, because many of the teachers who were on duty in the cafeteria also fled when the first gunshot went off. By providing opportunities to express what troubled them, parents and students were able to move beyond the experience rather than dwelling on or becoming consumed by their concerns.

Ongoing Interventions

Specific interventions are found in Part IV of this book. The magnitude of the incident influences how long a school should continue to offer opportunities to process the event, but the adjustment always takes longer than most people expect. More than 2 years had passed before the administrative personnel at Columbine High School felt they had returned to a "normal" routine (Ochberg, 2000). Following September 11, 2001, students in New York City had "somewhat metabolized" (Coates, Rosenthal, & Schechter, 2003, p. 34) the worst aspects of the trauma, but for several weeks they continued to re-create the World Trade Center scenario in their drawings. Flashbacks, nightmares, and other posttraumatic stress reactions may continue or become evident as individuals gain more distance from the incident.

Psychologists and counselors who recognize the differences between trauma and grief play an important role in identifying who might need more support. There is a distinct correlation between the degree of exposure to an incident and its impact on the child. Clearly, children who have been previously traumatized are at greater risk (Doka, 2008; Godeau et al., 2005). Comparing students' behavior after an incident to how they had acted previously is one way to determine who might benefit from additional intervention. When this is the case, specialized training is necessary (Cohen et al., 2002). Schools may not have the resources to provide the treatment for traumatized children, but, at a minimum, they must be able to identify the more significantly affected children and make referrals. The brief screening tool (Figure 10.4) is a helpful assessment resource. Although most children did not need psychotherapeutic intervention after the Oklahoma City bombing, there was less stigma when students were screened and treated in the schools (Allen, Tucker, & Pfefferbaum, 2006). If unaddressed, students may become "stuck" on the traumatic aspects and never fully grieve (Cohen & Mannarino, 2006). Because of the stigma still associated with seeking mental health support, schools play an important role in monitoring the impact of an event on students and faculty, and "normalizing" anxiety responses.

Particularly with adolescents, music is a helpful way to encourage mourning after significant loss. Whether through individual or group support, encouraging students to bring in and share songs that speak to their emotions provides a vehicle for healing. Choosing a specific song to play at a memorial service, commemorative event, or end-of-year graduation illustrates how music can be a source of comfort and connection between students.

Unique to this generation of students, the advent of the Internet brings with it an additional avenue for commemoration and support. Although it is "Public," in the sense that others read the postings, and interactive in nature, it also affords a sense of privacy, because one's identity is hidden. Websites such as *www.remembered-forever.org* provide opportunities to leave tributes and condolences, and to post photos, videos and audio clips. Termed "e-mourning" (Larson, personal communication, June 13, 2008), such places on the Internet to post memories and correspond with others who are also bereaved present a new avenue of support in the 21st century. Monitoring these websites and the postings on Facebook, MySpace, or a funeral home website helps school personnel and parents learn more about how students are impacted when an incident or death has occurred. It is important to note, however, that many schools prohibit faculty access to those areas of the Internet while on school property, so concerned school personnel must do this at home on their own time.

Another aspect of ongoing interventions is the role environment and cultural influences in grief and mourning play out. Although trauma is experienced throughout the world, sensitivity to cultural influences and their role in the grief and mourning process is an important consideration when determining appropriate interventions. Referencing the Amish girls who were tragically murdered in the schoolhouse shooting, the front page article of the Amish community newspaper ("Thank you, 2006") spoke of the healing qualities of the Amish faith and asked for

When a traumatic incident occurs, its impact can affect children in a variety of ways. The following tool was developed after September 11, 2001, because many children and adolescents exhibited one or more of the following signs and symptoms of posttraumatic stress. Although not all affected youth require treatment, there are times when it is wise to contact a mental health professional. Reasons to be concerned would be if academic or social functioning becomes impaired or if a child or adolescent is experiencing several symptoms, particularly if some time has gone by since the traumatic event occurred.

Infants up to age 6
____ Separation anxiety
____ Psychomotor agitation
____ Regressive behaviors (thumb-sucking, bedwetting, fear of the darkness)
____ Persistent and repetitive trauma-related play
____ Irritability and low frustration tolerance
____ Disruptive or aggressive behavior
____ Nightmares, sleep problems

Children 6 to 11 years of age
____ Regressive behaviors
____ Irritability and low frustration tolerance
____ Disruptive or aggressive behavior
____ Problems with peers
____ Nightmares, sleep problems
____ Extreme withdrawal
____ Extreme fearfulness
____ Inability to concentrate
____ Refusal to attend school
____ Academic decline
____ Physical complaints (headaches, stomachaches without a medical basis)
____ Sadness, feeling hopeless about the future
____ Emotional numbing or flatness

Adolescents 12 to 17 years of age
____ Nightmares, sleep problems
____ Withdrawal and isolation
____ Inability to concentrate
____ School avoidance
____ Academic decline
____ Physical complaints without a medical basis
____ Sadness, feeling hopeless about the future
____ Suicidal thoughts
____ Emotional numbing or flatness
____ Flashbacks
____ Avoidance of reminders of the traumatic events
____ First-time or increased use of alcohol or drugs
____ Problems with peers
____ Antisocial behavior

FIGURE 10.4. Children's Reactions to a Traumatic Event: A brief screening tool. Reprinted with permission from *Contemporary Pediatrics, 19*(9), September 2002, p. 49. *Contemporary Pediatrics* is a copyrighted publication of Advanstar Communications Inc. All rights reserved.

blessings on all who had responded to the Amish in their time of need. This note of appreciation provides an illustration of how grief is influenced by the cultural context.

The ways culture can influence the mourning process are also found in research. Several studies compare African Americans' openly expressive emotions after a loss and the more constrained reaction of most Asian Americans (Corr, Nabe, & Corr, 2003). Related to environmental considerations, turf issues and gang factors are more commonly related to violence in a city school than in more rural school districts. Sensitivity to culture, local traditions, and environment should not be overlooked when considering the most appropriate interventions.

Certain days of the year, particularly the anniversary of a tragedy, can be stressful times when grief reactions resurface and anxiety increases. Some want to avoid any reminders, while others embrace opportunities to commemorate and acknowledge all that has occurred. It is helpful when schools offer suggestions for private ways to remember, times to reflect and reminisce, and activities in the form of public rituals. This can provide the opportunity to acknowledge the resilience and compassion experienced in such a difficult time in the past, serving as another marker toward healing. It is important to realize that every time something happens in regard to the event in the months that follow, it is not necessary to set up a crisis response. For instance, a year after the Haines family murders, described earlier, when Alec Kreider was under trial, the videotaped plea of sole survivor Maggie Haines to the judge made many specific details of the murders public. Some administrators, although they had not been involved in the original crisis response, put out the message that if students needed help, they could go to the school. Several members of the crisis response team who were involved felt incorrectly that this was unnecessary and only served to exacerbate an already stressful situation. The crisis response team that is involved at the outset of an incident should continue to be involved in assessing and coordinating needs in the weeks, months, and even years following a significant event.

Community Collaboration

Given the limited resources in all school districts, many sources emphasize the value of utilizing community resources to strengthen and enhance the quality of the response to a school tragedy (Coates et al., 2003; Kerr et al., 2003; Myers, 1996; U.S. Department of Education, 2007). The U.S. Department of Education (2002) emphasizes the importance of collaboration between community agencies and schools "based on recognition that schools cannot do all of this work, in many cases being overburdened with demands that should be addressed in other community systems" (p. 11). Developing an infrastructure of collaboration with community mental health agencies ensures an objective, outside perspective and is a necessary supplement to school mental health resources, particularly in large-scale incidents. Also, as time passes and schools settle back into a noncrisis routine, community resources can address the ongoing needs of those who are still affected in the aftermath of the crisis. When students and faculty lost family members on September 11, 2001, Capital Hospice's Point of Hope Grief Counseling Center in the Washington, DC, area conferred with school officials about services they could offer (McMahon, 2005). Over the next 12 months, they provided a wide range of support services to affected families, in this way relieving DC area school district personnel from feeling obligated to address needs that were mainly psychologically rather than educationally focused.

After the Amish school shooting in Lancaster County, Pennsylvania, grant funding enabled the local Victim Witness Program to offer psychotherapy for first responders. Affected Amish family members received services from another local counseling agency. Schools that collaborate with community resource personnel before a crisis occurs find the transitions to be smoother in the weeks and months following a significant school incident.

CONCLUSIONS

One hears in the news about terrorist attacks, natural disasters, casualties from war, local homicides, and accidents nearly every given day. There is a fine line between being able to balance a realistic view of today's world and dwelling on the potential ways that tragedy can affect anyone at a personal level. Vulnerability and uncertainty intensify when there is school-related violence or a sudden death. The initial focus of the school is to restore a sense of safety and security. Schools that have made prevention and preparation a priority utilize relationships they have established both within the larger community and the school itself. In a potentially vulnerable position of criticism from parents as a result of fear, anxiety, and blame, schools that proactively foster a strong relationship with parents can then draw from this foundation when a crisis occurs. In noncrisis times, the best-case scenario is the school that offers preventive educational forums for parents and students, encouraging communication and sensitivity to students' needs in all realms—emotionally, behaviorally, psychologically, socially, and spiritually.

All eyes turn toward the school administration and the crisis response team for guidance when the unexpected occurs. Ironically, those most knowledgeable, skilled, and trained to respond recognize that the individuals most affected will inform them about what they need, when, and where they need it. In a crisis, these relationships are further strengthened, capitalizing on the innate resilience of the human spirit and the strength gained from this sense of belonging to a larger community. Crises provide a unique opportunity to strengthen the community as individuals reach out and deepen their connections, learning from and supporting one another. School personnel who prepare in advance and, when a crisis occurs, intentionally assess and respond, utilizing all the resources available to them in their community, experience the privilege of witnessing what Rachel Naomi Remen (1994) suggests: "Perhaps every 'victim' is really a survivor who does not know it yet" (p. 28).

DISCUSSION QUESTIONS

1. Consider yourself the counselor at the high school in the case example presented at the beginning of the chapter. Would you feel comfortable advising parents about how to talk with and support their children? What about this situation would be difficult for you, and how would you address that?

2. Identify one area of prevention that should be addressed in your community, and talk about why you think this is important.

3. What community resources can you involve to strengthen the crisis response team in your school?

4. Consider a significant or traumatic loss that you have experienced in your personal life. What was most difficult part of that for you? What helped you eventually to be able to move forward and put that experience behind you?

REFERENCES

Allen, J., Tucker, P., & Pfefferbaum, B. (2006). Community outreach following a terrorist act: Violent death and the Oklahoma City experience. In E. Rynearson (Ed.), *Violent death resilience and intervention beyond the crisis* (pp. 311–334). New York: Routledge/Taylor & Francis.

Children's reaction to 9/11: A brief screening tool. (2002). *Contemporary Pediatrics, 19,* 49.

Christ, G., & Christ, A. (2006). Current approaches to helping children cope with a parent's terminal illness. *CA: A Cancer Journal for Clinicians, 56,* 197–212.

Coates, S., Rosenthal, J., & Schecter, D. (Eds.). (2003). *September 11 trauma and human bonds.* Hillsdale, NJ: Analytic Press.

Coates, S., Schecter, D., & First, E. (2003). Brief interventions with traumatized children and families after September 11. In S. Coates, J. Rosenthal, & D. Schecter (Eds.), *September 11 trauma and human bonds*. Hillsdale, NJ: Analytic Press.

Cohen, J., & Mannarino, A. (2006). Treating childhood traumatic grief. In E. Rynearson (Ed.), *Violent death resilience and intervention beyond the crisis* (pp. 255–273). New York: Routledge/Taylor & Francis.

Cohen, J., Mannarino, A., Greenberg, T., Padlo, S., & Shipley, C. (2002). Childhood traumatic grief concepts and controversies. *Trauma, Violence, and Abuse, 3*(4), 307–327.

Consortium to Prevent School Violence. (2008). School shooting position statement. Retrieved May 1, 2008, from *www.ncsvprp.org*.

Cornell, D. (2007). Virginia Tech: What can we do? *Monitor on Psychology, 38*(6), 1–3.

Corr, C., Nabe, C., & Corr, C. (2003). *Death and dying, life and living* (4th ed.). Belmont, CA: Wadsworth/Thompson Learning.

Doka, K. (2008, February 14). Resiliency in the face of trauma—study examines impact on 9/11 children. *Hospice Foundation of America's Hospice and Caregiving Blog*. Retrieved February 19, 2008, from *www.hospice-foundation.org/blog/2008/02/resiliency-in-face-of-trauma-study.html*.

Dwyer, K., Osher, D., & Warger, C. (1998). *Early warning, timely response: A guide to safe schools*. Washington, DC: U.S. Department of Education.

Everly, G., & Mitchell, J. (2002). *Critical incident stress management: Advanced group crisis intervention: A workbook* (2nd ed.). Baltimore: International Critical Incident Stress Foundation, Inc.

Federal Emergency Management Agency. (2008). National Incident Management System FAQs. Retrieved June 18, 2008, from *www.fema.gov/emergency/nims/faq/compliance.shtm*.

Galante, R., & Foa, O. (1986). An epidemiological study of psychic trauma and treatment effectiveness for children after a natural disaster. *Journal of the American Academy of Child Psychiatry, 25*, 357–363.

Godeau, E., Vignes, C., Navarro, F., Iachan, R., Ross, J., Pasquier, C., et al. (2005). Effects of a large-scale industrial disaster on rates of symptoms consistent with posttraumatic stress disorders among schoolchildren in Toulouse. *Archives of Pediatric and Adolescent Medicine, 159*, 579–584.

Goodman, R., & Brown, E. (2008). Service and science in times of crisis: Developing, planning, and implementing a clinical research program for children traumatically bereaved after 9/11. *Death Studies, 32*, 154–180.

Gould, M., Munfakh, J., Kleinman, M., Lubell, K., & Provenzano, D. (2004). Impact of the September 11th terrorist attacks on teenagers' mental health. *Applied Developmental Science, 8*(3), 158–169.

Kelly, J., Crable, A., & Robinson, R. (2008, June 17). Kreider: Life in jail. *Lancaster New Era Newspaper*, pp. 1, A6.

Kennedy, A. (2007, June). We are Virginia Tech: How counselors responded to the grief and trauma on campus after the startling events of April 16. *Counseling Today*, pp. 1, 46–48.

Kerr, M., Brent, D., McKain, B., & McCommons, P. (2003). *Postvention stan-

dards manual, a guide for a school's response in the aftermath of a sudden death (4th ed.). Pittsburgh: Western Psychiatric Institute and Clinic of UPMC Presbyterian Shadyside Services for Teens at Risk.

Lattanzi Licht, M. (2008). When tragedy strikes: Response and prevention. In K. Doka & A. Tucci (Eds.), *Living with grief children and adolescents* (pp. 335–349). Washington, DC: Hospice Foundation of America.

Lin, K., Sandler, I., Ayers, T., Wolchik, S., & Luecken, L. (2004). Resilience in parentally bereaved children and adolescents seeking preventative services. *Journal of Clinical Child and Adolescent Psychology, 33*(4), 673-683.

Lovre, C. (2007, April 25–28). *Crisis response in the school setting, five day team training.* Crisis Management Institute presentation for IU13 in Lancaster, PA.

Maslow, A. H. (1954). *Motivation and personality.* New York: HarperCollins.

McMahon, R. (2005, September). Retrospectives from members who made a difference in the aftermath of 9/11, reflections. *Insights,* pp. 38–39.

Myers, D. (1996). *Disaster response and recovery: A handbook for mental health professionals.* Menlo Park, CA: National Center for Posttraumatic Stress Disorder.

Myers, D., Zunin, H. S., & Zunin, L. M. (1990). Grief: The art of coping with tragedy. *Today's Supervisor, 7*(11), 14–15.

Nader, K. (1997). Treating traumatic grief in systems. In C. Figley, B. Bride & N. Mazza (Eds.), *Death and trauma: The traumatology of grieving* (pp. 159–192). Washington, DC: Taylor & Francis.

National Institute of Mental Health. (2002). *Mental health and mass violence: Evidence-based early psychological intervention for victims/survivors of mass violence: A workshop to reach consensus on best practices.* NIH Publication No. 02-5138. Washington, DC: U.S. Government Printing Office.

Ochberg, F. (2000). Bound by a trauma called Columbine. Retrieved March 15, 2008, from *www.giftfromwithin.org/html.columbin.html.*

Osofsy, J. (1995). The effects of exposure to violence of young children. *The American Psychologist, 50*(9), 782–788.

Remen, R. (1994). *Kitchen table wisdom: Stories that heal.* New York: Berkley.

Reynolds, B. (2004). *Crisis and emergency risk communication: By leaders for leaders.* Atlanta, GA: Centers for Disease Control and Prevention.

Seebold, A. (2003). Responding to a murder/suicide at a rural junior high school. *International Journal of Emergency Mental Health, 5*(3), 153–159.

Slovak, K. (2002). Gun violence and children: Factors related to exposure and trauma. *Health and Social Work, 27*(2), 104–112.

Smilde-van den Doel, O., Smitt, C., & Wolleswinkel-vanden Bosch, J. (2006). School performance and social-emotional behavior of primary schoolchildren before and after a disaster. *Pediatrics, 118*(5), 1311–1320.

Stevenson, R. (2008). Helping students cope with grief. In K. Doka & A. Tucci (Eds.), *Living with grief children and adolescents* (pp. 317–333). Washington, DC: Hospice Foundation of America.

Thank you. (2006, October, 16). *Die Botschaft, 32*(16), p. 1.

U.S. Department of Education. (2002). *The 3 Rs to dealing with trauma in* schools: Readiness, response, and recovery [Broadcast materials]. Retrieved June 17, 2008, from www.walcoff.com/prevention/broadmat.html.

U.S. Department of Education. (2007). Practical information on crisis planning: A guide for schools and communities. Retrieved June 17, 2008, from www.ed.gov/admins/lead/safety/emergencyplan/crisisplanning.pdf.

U.S. Department of Health and Human Services. (2004). Mental health response to mass violence and terrorism: A training manual (DHHS Pub. No. SMA 3959). Rockville, MD: Center for Mental Health Services, Substance Abuse and Mental Health Services Administration.

Vernberg, E., Silverman, W., La Greca, A., & Prinstein, M. (1996). Prediction and post-traumatic stress symptoms in children after Hurricane Andrew. Journal of Abnormal Psychology, 105(2), 237–248.

Vernberg, E., & Vogel, J. (1993). Task Force Report Part 2: Interventions with children after disasters. Journal of Clinical Child Psychology, 22(4), 485–498.

Webb, N. B. (Ed.). (1991). Play therapy with children in crisis. New York: Guilford Press.

Webb, N. B. (Ed.). (2007). Play therapy with children in crisis (3rd ed.). New York: Guilford Press.

CHAPTER 11

Children's and Adolescents' Exposure to the Mass Violence of War and Terrorism

Role of the Media

KATHLEEN NADER

Evidence suggests that people with direct exposure to and/or perceived life threat from a mass violent event are those who most commonly report posttraumatic stress disorder (PTSD) and other posttrauma symptoms (Bosgieter, Rasmussen, Cook, Kofford, & Caldarella, 2006; Marshall & Galea, 2004; Nader, 2008). In addition to direct exposures, prolonged and/or repeated TV watching of traumatic events, or disturbing images related to these events, has been linked in youth to PTSD and other symptoms, such as anxiety, depression, grief, social distrust, trauma-specific fears, conduct disturbances, and altered information processing (Aber, Gershoff, Ware, & Kotler, 2004; Bosgieter et al., 2006; Nader, Pynoos, Fairbanks, Al-Ajeel, & Al-Asfour, 1993; Pfefferbaum, Gurwitch, Robertson, Brandt, & Pfefferbaum 2003; Wang et al., 2006).

Media depictions of fictional and actual violence influence youth in a variety of ways. Repeated exposure to TV, movie, and video game violence has been linked to aggression, including mass killings. The journalists and others who interview youth and publish their interviews via TV or printed media following mass traumatic events may either help or exacerbate youth's posttrauma reactions. TV, newspaper, and other media can assist by providing useful information and helping to gather resources and other information. Youth watch TV displays of traumatic events for a number of reasons. Differences in these reasons may be important to treatment. Studies have confirmed for a variety of events the symptomatic impact of viewing violent and other traumatic events on TV. Youth of all ages may have symptoms after media exposure. Media exposure has been linked to increased symptoms for youth directly exposed to a traumatic event and for those with only media exposures.

THE INFLUENCE OF ELECTRONIC MEDIA ON YOUTH

Youth are clearly influenced by the electronic media that they watch. Their mimicry of clothing choices, ways of speaking, attempted personas, behavioral choices, and more demonstrate that influence. Youth compare themselves to media figures and characters when making self-assessments (e.g., body image; Beullens, Eggermont, & Van den Bulck, 2008). For fictional or truth-based TV and theater movies, presentations with repeated themes that elicit intense emotions and/or that are fun to mimic are likely to have the strongest influence. In the past, youth living in violent neighborhoods were exposed to images and experiences from which children in safe neighborhoods were protected. Now youth are exposed to such images through TV, movies, and video games. Huesmann (2007) refers to them as "virtual" bad neighborhoods.

The effects of watching "media violence"—intentional injury or irritation of a person by another person or character—have been well documented (Huesmann, 2007; Bushman & Huesmann, 2006). For children and adults, well-designed research has repeatedly shown that watching violence on electronic media increases the risk of behaving aggressively right after viewing and years later. Even after researchers controlled for early aggressiveness, early habitual exposure to media violence in middle-childhood predicted increased aggressiveness 1, 3, 10, 15, and 22 years later (Huesmann, 2007). Long-term effects have been greater for children than for adults, perhaps because children more readily encode new beliefs, scripts, and schemas through observational learning (Bushman & Huesmann, 2006).

Media can have a positive or a negative effect on youth. Across studies, violent media, including TV, movies, video games, music, and comic books, have been linked to aggressive thoughts and behaviors, angry feelings, arousal levels, and helping behavior. Well-known rampage killers, such as the Virginia Tech shooter (33 dead, 15 injured) and Columbine High School shooters (23 dead, 24 wounded), among others, were influenced by violent movies and/or violent video games (Nader, in press).

JOURNALISTS AND OTHER MEDIA INTERVIEWERS

Media personnel are often among the first to have contact with those who are traumatized after catastrophic events. Media presentations may assist the recovery of those exposed to traumatic events by, for example, encouraging preparedness, eliciting aid, providing needed information, or mobilizing action. In contrast, insensitive, ill-timed and/or untrained actions of media professionals can produce long-term difficulties for individuals with traumatic exposure (Nader, 1993, 2008). Because traumatized children and adolescents become vulnerable in a number of ways, it is important to examine media actions that are potentially harmful to them and those that can be of assistance. Teichroeb (2006) has provided some guidelines for journalists interviewing children. As she points out, "Journalists have a responsibility to report the truth with compassion and sensitivity" (p. 2) (see also Ocberg, 1995/2008).

Exacerbating Problems

Understanding a traumatized youth's state of mind, issues of closure, and the aftereffects of interviewing are crucial to effective and harmless interviews (Nader, 1997, 2008). Children may appear to be OK when they are not (Teichroeb, 2006). A variety of harmful effects, including worsened symptoms, suicides and suicide attempts, murder, severe depressions, and acute psychotic episodes, have followed interviews by untrained or poorly trained, unskilled, or culturally uninformed interviewers (Mayou, Ehlers, & Hobbs, 2000; Nader, 1997; Raphael & Wilson, 2001; Ruzek & Watson, 2001; Swiss & Giller, 1993).

Following traumatic exposure, children may have a diminished capacity to cope with both external intrusions and internal psychological intrusions (Nader, 1993). In the immediate aftermath of events, symptoms may be exacerbated by, for example, the intrusion of a stranger or being delayed from having contact with caregivers and/or from needed interventions. Parents may be too disconcerted to provide a child protection from intrusion (Teichrobe, 2006). Reduced stress tolerance, ongoing attempts to contend with peritraumatic experiences (those that occurred during the trauma), intrusive mental imagery, and other traumatic reactions may render external intrusions, such as the influx of reporters and cameras or the questions of a single interviewer, distressing, frightening, and additionally intrusive (Nader, 1993). The passage of time does not guarantee that ill effects from interviews will not occur.

Feeling Betrayed

Children may feel betrayed because of the content of news releases or because an interviewer was misleading (Nader, 1993). They may feel abandoned after a great focus of attention, followed by withdrawal of attention. Children may be pleased with the attention, only to feel embarrassed later. Some children have been teased by peers or have been horrified, for example, that they were shown on TV in their pajamas (Libow, 1992) or in an emotional or victimized state (see case of Jordan, Box 11.1a). Youth may feel humiliated by the portrayal of themselves, for example, as part of a rejected culture. No matter how right or wrong a group is, its youth may be innocent victims of world or community opinion. For example, Jabr (2004) complained that despite their mal-nourishment, exposure to continuous war attacks, deaths in large numbers, and anxiety and other symptoms, Palestinian children are stereotyped as violent and portrayed as unloved by their families.

Reinforcing the Perpetrators

Guaranteed media attention is sometimes a component in acts of public violence. School rampage shooters (e.g., Columbine and Virginia Tech) expected and planned for extensive media coverage. Terrorists count on publicity to further their causes and to instill fear in their targets. Ways to ensure freedom of the press without encouraging increased violence and traumatic exposure are needed.

Helping after War or Terrorism

Media often assist intervention efforts (Nader, 2008; Fang & Chen, 2004). Local newspapers, radio, and TV can prepare and educate a populace after mass traumas. Media may provide parent and other posttrauma education, basic information that relieves distress, preparation for varied courses of response, and possible coping methods. Local media can announce intervention programs and the scheduling of assessment and treatment events. They can educate parents about how to recognize traumatic reactions in their children (Teichroeb, 2006). They can interview families that are successfully putting their lives back together, in order to inspire hope and healing in a manner that does not diminish those who continue to suffer. After events such as terrorism and other mass violence, the media can assist initial and anniversary memorialization of those who died. Perhaps because of the nature of terrorist attacks, people, and the media stories about them, events can have some positive effects. After 9/11, many youth reported greater close-

BOX 11.1. Case Examples

a. Jordan, a third grader, was afraid to return to school after recovering from a drive-by gang shooting. His peers had seen the story on TV, and he was afraid they would think of him as a victim and think he was strange because of his eye patch. When he returned, Jordan's classmates were reluctant to be near him, as though victimization and injury were contagious.

b. *Eight-year-old Kimberly* heard an explosion and crashing noises but was quickly knocked unconscious. She did not remember what had happened to her. Kimberly spent weeks in the hospital recovering from her injuries. When she was released, repairs had been made and there was no evidence of the event. She had no visual memory of the devastation until she saw the media coverage on the anniversary of the event.

c. *Shawn, a 15-year-old Californian*, watched the events of 9/11 repeatedly. He said that he kept hoping it would turn out to be a hoax—"You know, like *War of the Worlds*, when my grandfather was a child." Everyone was really scared when they turned on the radio and heard that space ships were attacking. Shawn said, "I just couldn't believe it was really happening and kept hoping it would end a different way."

d. *A man who was in a massacre as a preadolescent* described how, from adolescence to adulthood, he read every book he could find and watched every TV show or documentary he could that described mass killers. His desire to understand included the possibility that he could prevent future victimization by understanding who would do such things and why they might do it.

e. *Nine-year-old Joshua* moved out of New York City to upstate New York just prior to the 9/11 attacks on the World Trade Center. Most of his school peers did not have significant reactions, unless they had family members directly affected in the disaster. Joshua did not know anyone who was killed or injured in the disaster, or anyone involved in rescue or recovery. His traumatic response to the disaster occurred after watching news coverage of the event. Having previously lived in New York City, combined with repeatedly seeing the news coverage, seemed to contribute to his traumatic response. He was preoccupied with the event, drew pictures of the Twin Towers, and talked about what happened for weeks after watching. He was afraid to go back to New York City or the area surrounding it, where he still had relatives. He exhibited regressive behavior, fear of sleeping alone, a need to talk about the event repeatedly, and reenactment of the event in his play. A strained relationship between his parents contributed to his distress and reactions.

ness to others, increased appreciation and gratitude, more altruistic and caring acts, increased interest in world events, elevated patriotism, and enhanced security and alertness (Phillips, Prince, & Schiebelhut, 2004; Whalen, Henker, King, Jamner, & Levine, 2004; Mapp & Koch, 2004).

MEDIA EXPOSURE TO WAR AND TERRORISM

Media exposure can affect youth whether or not they are exposed directly to war or terrorism (Nader, 2008; Nader et al., 1993; Pfefferbaum, Seale, et al., 2003; Schuster et al., 2001). Media exposure may be a part of multiple types of exposure or a youth's only exposure to an event.

Issues Affecting Comparisons of Findings for Media Exposure

Manner of assessment and failure to assess important variables may influence findings (Nader, 2008). Although Bleich, Gelkopf, and Solomon (2003) found no significant differences between adults actually injured in a terrorist attack and those who were not directly exposed, they theorize that this could be because the respondents understated their reactions in telephone interviews, or because a major national trauma is not limited to those who experience it directly. Studies do not assess all possible symptoms, nor do they study exactly the same sets of symptoms and variables. Time since assessment often differs across studies. Failure to assess or control for mediating and moderating variables may affect findings. Such failures may be part of why some findings (e.g., relative to gender) have been mixed. Exposure to an event and to the media often increases with age (Bosgeiter et al., 2006; Schuster et al., 2001; Thabet, Abed, & Vostanis, 2004). Youths' abilities to understand the meaning of death and the long-term implications of events also vary by age (Table 11.1; Webb, Chapter 1, this volume). Specific symptoms may be more pronounced at some ages because of developmental issues. The source of information matters to findings. Children often report more symptoms for themselves than parents report for them (Lengua, Long, Smith, & Meltzoff, 2005; Phillips et al., 2004). Differences may exist in what is displayed during and after events. Images of mutilated and bloody bodies were displayed repeatedly on TV and in photos in war-torn Kuwait (Nader et al., 1993), the Gaza strip (Thabet et al., 2004), and Croatia. In Kuwait, a room was dedicated to torture instruments and images.

(text resumes on p. 227)

TABLE 11.1. Age and Reactions to Media Displays of Terrorism or War

Age group Understanding of media images	Study (authors)	Age range/ time	Event-related media viewing and symptoms or findings
Toddler–preschool (2–6 or 7) • Difficulty understanding —Replays are the same event. —The permanence of death or impact of numerous deaths. —Fictional vs. nonfictional events. • May recall or dream distressing images.	9/11— Terrorism, National Survey (Schuster et al., 2001)	Young children/ 3–5 days after	• Protection from viewing was more likely for younger children. • Number of hours of viewing was related to number of symptoms.
	Gaza Strip— War (Wang et al., 2006)	1–4/ ongoing	• Type of exposure was related to variations in response. • Media exposure was linked to increased externalizing, oppositional defiance, aggressive behavior, and emotional reactivity.
Middle childhood (6 or 7–11 or 12) • Understand the permanence of death. • Understand that one event is replayed repeatedly. • May be drawn to media watching in order to cope with arousal or the event and symptoms, out of curiosity, or to help process the event/deaths.	Gulf War, Kuwait (Nader et al., 1993) (*see also* "Adolescence")	7–12/4 mo after	• Total exposure score (12 types of exposure) was linked to severity of PTS, PTS criteria, and grief. • Media exposure added significantly to PTS scores. • Increased PTS symptoms occurred for both directly exposed and only media exposed. • TV watching and worrying about someone during the event was associated with higher PTS.
	Gaza Strip— war (Thabet et al., 2002)	9–15/ ongoing	• PTSD was predicted only by exposure to bombardment; trauma-specific fears were higher for direct exposure; anxiety was related to media exposure. • Anxiety symptoms/disorders were higher in areas with no direct bombing (media exposed).
	Gaza Strip— war (Thabet et al., 2004)	9–15/ September 2000, ongoing	• Trauma and depression scores were significantly related to the number of traumatic exposures (media was one of the exposures). • TV viewing and symptoms increased with age.

(cont.)

TABLE 11.1. *(cont.)*

Age group Understanding of media images	Study (authors)	Age range/ time	Event-related media viewing and symptoms or findings
Middle childhood *(cont.)*	OKC bombing— terrorism (Pfefferbaum, Moore, et al., 1999)	Grades 6–12/ 7 wk after	• Hearing and/or feeling the explosion, knowing an injured or deceased victim, and TV exposure correlated with PTS and difficulty calming after TV. • TV viewing was a stronger predictor of PTS than hearing and/or feeling the explosion, gender, or knowing an injured or deceased victim. • Youth knowing victims had sig. higher PTS; hearing/feeling the bomb was a better predictor of persistence than TV exposure for this group. • Girls had more symptoms and were more likely to have difficulty calming down after watching TV.
	OKC— terrorism (Pfefferbaum, Nixon, et al., 1999)	Middle school and high school/ 7 wk after	• Local TV coverage was continuous after bombing. • Bereaved youth had higher PTS and arousal scores, greater worry about family at the time of the explosion, and more difficulty calming down after bomb-related TV viewing. • Youth who lost an immediate family member had the highest PTS scores. • Retrospective report of arousal during the blast was highly predictive of PTS.
	OKC— terrorism, 100 mi. away (Pfefferbaum, Seale, et al., 2003)	Sixth graders/ 2 yr after	• PTS reactions increased with increased exposure to both print and broadcast media. • PTS reactions were contingent upon emotional reactions to media coverage.
	9/11— terrorism, Washington, DC (Phillips et al., 2004)	5–12/ 3 mo after	• TV coverage was continuous across the nation. • Symptoms increased with TV watching; intrusive thoughts, hyperarousal, and nightmares;

(cont.)

TABLE 11.1. *(cont.)*

Age group Understanding of media images	Study (authors)	Age range/ time	Event-related media viewing and symptoms or findings
Middle childhood *(cont.)*			shaken sense of safety, sleep disturbance, increased fatigue, cessation of thoughts of future, more easily irritated, and increased startle response. • Media-exposed youth's fears for safety increased with activities such as attending memorials, patriotic gestures, and donating to charities.
	9/11— terrorism, Washington state (Lengua et al., 2005)	9–13/1 mo and 6 mo after	• Increased media exposure was related to increased child-reported worry and upset. • Youth reported PTS symptoms comparable to those of youth directly exposed to traumas (more reexperiencing and less PTS than for an earthquake). • Youth reported more symptoms for themselves than parents reported for them. • Youth and parents initially reported a drop in youth's symptoms. • Strong emotions during TV viewing were related to more symptoms. • Previous symptoms, worrying about someone during the event, or knowing someone who died was linked to increased symptoms. • More externalizing reported for boys before and after attacks; more upset reported by girls. • Protective factors: high self-esteem and social competence.
	9/11— terrorism, NYC (Hoven et al., 2005)	Fourth to fifth graders/ 6 mo after	• All disorders increased with increased exposures. • 28.6% of all youth (grades 4–12) had one or more of six probable anxiety and depressive disorders—most prevalent were PTSD, probable separation anxiety, and agoraphobia.

(cont.)

TABLE 11.1. *(cont.)*

Age group Understanding of media images	Study (authors)	Age range/ time	Event-related media viewing and symptoms or findings
Middle childhood *(cont.)*			• Girls had more anxiety and depressive disorders; boys and older youth had more conduct disorders. • Younger children (fourth to fifth graders) had more direct and family but less TV exposures, and more symptoms. • Risk factors: two or more direct exposures, family exposure, high media exposure, and previous traumas (two or more); female gender, low maternal education, and mh service use.
	9/11— terrorism, Washington state (Lengua et al., 2006)	9–13/ 1 mo after	• Coping styles and tendency to threat appraisal style remained consistent pre- and postattack. • Stress load, inactive coping style, and threat appraisal predicted PTS. • Preattack symptoms and 9/11 threat appraisal predicted functional impairment. • Coping style and appraisal style contributed before and after 9/11 and independently to post-9/11 PTS, over and above preattack symptoms; they mediated the effects of preattack stress load.
	9/11— terrorism, London (Holmes et al., 2007)	10–11/ 2 and 6 mo after	• Significant minority of assessed media-exposed youths had PTS symptoms. • Combined intrusive imagery and experiencing threat predicted persistence of symptoms. • Without the combination of intrusive imagery and threat, symptoms, but not functional impairment, declined over time.

(cont.)

TABLE 11.1. *(cont.)*

Age group Understanding of media images	Study (authors)	Age range/ time	Event-related media viewing and symptoms or findings
Adolescence (13–17) • Understand the reality of thousands of deaths. • To varying degrees, understand the meaning and/or greater impact of the event. • May be drawn to media watching in order to cope with or to increase arousal, cope with or process the event or symptoms, honor the dead.	Gulf War, Kuwait (Nader et al., 1993)	13–18/ 4 mo after	• Increased exposures related to higher PTS and grief. • When exposure was divided into three subcomponents, witnessing was the best predictor of PTS. • TV related to increased PTS symptoms for directly exposed and for the few only media-exposed youth. • Older children tended to have greater exposures and higher PTS total scores. • Highest mean score was for *hurting others*; the adolescent who killed had the highest PTS score.
	9/11— terrorism, NYC (Aber et al., 2004)	6–14 for preattack data 12–20/ 4 mo to 2 yr after	• Exposures and reactions varied: direct 9/11 exposure—depression and PTSD; media exposure—anxiety and PTSD (not conduct disturbance); family exposure—social mistrust. Exposure to NYC violence (witnessing/victimization)—PTSD, anxiety, depression, conduct disturbances, hostile attribution bias, social mistrust. • Witnessed violence and violent victimization, and 9/11 exposure increased with age; family exposure decreased with age. • Nonwhite youth were more likely exposed to community violence; white youth (and girls) more likely exposed to 9/11.
	9/11— terrorism, national sample (Gil-Rivas et al., 2004)	Mean age: 15.27 yr/ 2 wk and 1 yr after	• Female gender and mh problem history were associated with acute stress reactions. • One year later, no gender differences; higher levels of PTS and functional impairment were associated with parent–youth conflict.

(cont.)

TABLE 11.1. *(cont.)*

Age group Understanding of media images	Study (authors)	Age range/ time	Event-related media viewing and symptoms or findings
			• History of mh disorders and learning disabilities more likely to report acute stress symptoms and symptoms at 1 yr after 9/11; learning disabilities and mh disorders were associated with more distress when parental support was low.
			• Over and above distress, parent–youth conflict was related to functional impairment.
			• Protective factors: parental positive affect and sense of self-efficacy; higher levels of father support.
	9/11— terrorism, California (Whalen et al., 2004)	14–18/1–3 yr before and 2–5 mo after	• Media exposures, increased rules, less travel.
			• Negative affect when reminded; reported only low to moderate levels of most PTS symptoms; higher levels of difficulty paying attention and enjoying things as much were related to media exposure.
			• State and trait anxiety contributed to distress.
			• Benefits: greater interpersonal closeness; togetherness; increased appreciation and gestures of caring, increased security measures, patriotism, learning world events.
			• Optimism was protective.
	9/11— terrorism, NYC (Hoven et al., 2005)	6th–12th graders/ 6 mo after	• 28.6% of youth had one or more of six probable anxiety and depressive disorders.
			• All disorders increased with increased exposures as were, more weakly, conduct disorder and alcohol abuse (see "risk factors," Hoven et al., 2005, above).
			• Girls had more anxiety and depressive disorders; boys had more conduct disorders.
			• Older youth had greater proximity to events; more prior traumas, more conduct disorders.

Although people were shown jumping from the Twin Towers in New York City, actual bloody, mutilated bodies were not shown across the United States.

Reasons That Youth Watch

Youth view traumatic TV images for a number of reasons, such as access, coping needs, processing issues, and grief (Nader, 2008). Some researchers have suggested that hyperaroused youth may be drawn to media coverage to reduce or to sustain their heightened arousal (Pfefferbaum et al., 2001; Pfefferbaum, Seale, et al., 2003). Some youth may happen upon traumatic images, view them in unsupervised periods, or be shown images by others. An 11-year-old girl who first saw the devastation of a bombing on TV a year later, for example, began to reexperience the images (see case of Kimberly, Box 11.1b). Some youth watch to overcome disbelief (see case of Shawn, Box 11.1c).

Viewing TV during or after war or terrorism has served as a coping mechanism for adults and youth (Bleich et al., 2003; Nader, 1997). Following 19 months of terrorism, Israeli and Arab–Israeli adults' most prevalent methods of coping were gathering information about friends and family and watching or listening to TV and radio reports (Bleich et al., 2003). During the Gulf War that ended in 1991, Kuwaiti youth inside the country watched, for example, to learn the proximity of the enemy and the safety of home. Youth outside of the country watched to learn about the progress of the war and the status of relatives who remained in Kuwait (Nader et al., 1993). Early during the ongoing Iraq War, TV and radio communications were cut off in Iraq. No access made it more difficult to know how near or from what direction the threat would come, whether loved ones were threatened, whether the war was over, or whether and when needed resources (e.g., food and water) would be available (Nader, 2008).

War survivors have expressed the need for others in the world to see and for survivors themselves to remember what the enemy has done to them. In 1992, in Croatia, and 1991, after the Gulf War, families reported watching gruesome video, TV, and photographed war images over and over again, as though unable to stop. At an international conference, a Bosnian psychiatrist showed pictures of war horrors to others. She expressed a need for people to understand the horrors imposed on them by the Serbians. Kuwaiti families watched such images while "glued to the TV," and they passed around photos of bloody, mutilated bodies during mealtimes. One Kuwaiti mother of six explained, "We must watch. These bodies are our dead. We must never forget what they [the enemy] have done to us."

A need to understand or to regain some sense of control may be a part of being drawn to media depictions of traumas. For example, an intense need to understand why an event happened, and/or why it happened to oneself, is common after a traumatic experience. To process a traumatic experience and the "Why?" of it, youth may watch repeatedly and/or read about a variety of traumatic events (see Box 11.1d).

THE RELATIONSHIP BETWEEN MEDIA WATCHING AND SYMPTOMS

Researchers have documented PTSD and other trauma-related symptoms following media exposure at varying distances away from events and after a variety of events (Bosgieter et al., 2006; Terr et al., 1999). Bosgieter et al. (2006) found a significant relationship between the parent-reported anxiety symptoms of a small group of children and their TV watching of three events: 9/11, hurricane Katrina, and the Indonesian tsunami. Following the September 11, 2001, terrorist attacks on the New York City World Trade Center, the Pentagon, and air flights, Schuster et al. (2001) found that parents across the United States who reported that their children were stressed were likely to restrict the children's TV watching. For youth whose TV watching was not restricted, the number of their parent-reported stress symptoms was associated with the number of hours of 9/11-related TV watching. One study, in which youth with the most direct exposures (fourth to fifth graders) had the least media exposure, did not find a media effect. For these New York fourth to twelfth graders exposed to the 9/11 attacks, Hoven et al. (2005) found a strong effect between family exposure and anxiety, and depressive disorders.

During or after events, specific media images, such as people falling to their deaths (Ahern, Galea, Resnick, & Vlahov, 2004) or bloody and/or mutilated bodies (Nader et al., 1993; Thabet et al., 2004), may induce arousal, trauma, and other anxiety symptoms, especially with repeated viewing. Both positive (e.g., heroics or helping efforts) and negative images of the 9/11 attacks were associated with PTSD symptoms among children outside of the New York area (Gershoff & Aber, 2004; Saylor, Cowart, Livpovsky, Jackson, & Finch, 2003). The effects of distressing media images on youth are influenced by multiple variables (Nader, 2008). A youth's early and ongoing attachments and support systems impact whether a youth is stress reactive or stress resilient, for example (Ford, 2009; Nader, 2008; Yates, Egeland, & Sroufe, 2003). Personal and developmental differences may affect a youth's reactions to watching (Aber et al., 2004; Pfefferbaum, Gurwitch, et al., 2003; Table 11.1).

A young child, for example, may think that each showing is a different event or a movie. An adolescent will understand the repeated showing of one event and the implications of the event.

For media and direct exposures, it appears that anything that increases the emotional impact of the experience or decreases effective coping may contribute to reactions. A youth's proximity to the event, previous traumas, current traumatic exposures, reactions during viewing, and/or relationship to those experiencing the trauma may make a difference in reactions to media images. Researchers have observed that experiences such as watching the events on TV at a safe distance while knowing a friend or relative is endangered (Nader et al., 1993), ineffective coping (Silver, Holman, McIntosh, Poulin, & Gil-Rivas, 2002), watching from the affected area along with other exposures, lack of social support, and strong emotions (Ahern et al., 2004; Pfefferbaum, Seale, et al., 2003) have contributed to increased reactions. For currently and previously traumatized youth, media images of a new event may serve as traumatic reminders or as confirmation of an unsafe world.

Exposure Variables

Research shows that exposure is an important variable in relation to the severity of a youth's traumatic reactions (Fletcher, 2003; Nader, 2008). Exposure includes subjective exposure (e.g., intensity of emotional response, perception of danger), as well as actual proximity to the event and/or its dangers (Lengua et al., 2005; Nader et al., 1993). After the explosion of the Challenger space vehicle, Terr et al. (1999) found that youth who lived in closer proximity to the teacher who was killed had greater average reactions than those thousands of miles away. The impact of proximity in combination with media exposure may vary with other factors that increase emotional impact, child-specific factors, environmental circumstances, and the extent to which events a long distance away engender a sense of life threat or a confirmation of the lack of safety (Box 11.1e).

Directly Exposed Youths

Media exposure to war or terrorism can increase symptoms in youth directly exposed to the events. With exposure to mutilated bodies and wounded people on TV as one of a list of wartime exposures, Thabet, Abed, and Vostanis (2004) found that trauma and depression scores were significantly related to the *number of exposures*. For youth who remained in Kuwait during the Gulf War (Nader et al., 1993), total exposure score (especially hurting another) was associated with posttraumatic stress (PTS) and grief scores. After researchers controlled for the effects of each of the 12 types of exposure (e.g., Threat to Significant Other—knowing a captured, injured, or deceased person; Witnessing— seeing injured or dead bodies on the ground, mutilated bodies on TV, death or injury while it was happening; Life Threat—felt threatened with injury, death, or was injured; Hurt Someone Else), witnessing muti- lated bodies on TV was the strongest predictor of PTS. For New York City (NYC) adults, Ahern et al. (2004) found that age, race/ethnicity, social support, previous traumatic events, seeing the attacks in person, a peritraumatic event panic attack, death of a friend or relative in the attacks, and participation in rescue efforts were all associated with both TV viewing and probable PTSD. After researchers adjusted for the other variables, individuals who watched the most 9/11-related TV were still 66% more likely to have probable PTSD than those who viewed the least TV.

Highly exposed youth may watch more and have more difficulty recovering from watching event-related TV. Children who heard or felt the explosion, or knew direct victims of the Oklahoma City bombing (OKC; Pfefferbaum, Moore, et al., 1999), and bereaved children (Pfef- ferbaum, Nixon, et al., 1999) reported more bomb-related TV view- ing than did unexposed or nonbereaved youth. Difficulty calming down after viewing bomb-related events correlated significantly with relation- ship to the deceased.

Youth Not Directly Exposed

Youth with only media exposures have had PTS and other symptoms (Nader et al., 1993). For 119 sixth-grade students, Pfefferbaum, Seale, et al. (2003) found that even with no direct exposure to the terrorist bombings in OKC, PTS reactions increased with increased exposure to both print and broadcast media when youth had moderate or intense reactions to media coverage. Youth in Washington state (Lengua et al., 2005), California (Whalen et al., 2004), and London (Holmes, Creswell, & O'Connor, 2007) reported PTS symptoms in response to 9/11. Hol- mes et al. found that for youth in London assessed 2 and 6 months after 9/11, although total PTS significantly decreased between the two times (14.5% initially; 9.2% at 6 months), impairment in the ability to func- tion normally did not decrease.

Constructive efforts of media-exposed youth may increase some symptoms. For kindergarten to sixth graders in Washington, DC, 3 months after 9/11 (Phillips et al., 2004), self-reported negative reactions were significantly influenced only by the degree of their exposure to TV news related to the attacks. In contrast to parents' reports, engaging in constructive activities, such as patriotic gestures or volunteer efforts, was associated with increased child-reported feelings of threatened safety.

Parent–youth relationships are important to reactions. One year after 9/11 (Gil-Rivas, Holman, & Silver, 2004), after researchers adjusted for acute stress symptoms, prior mental health problems, and learning disabilities, parent–adolescent conflict was significantly associated with higher levels of adolescent PTS symptoms. Parent–adolescent conflict was the only variable associated with higher levels of functional impairment. In addition, youth with prior mental health disorders or learning disabilities who reported lower levels of parental support also reported higher levels of distress 1 year later. Parental distress or trauma was not associated with youth distress, PTS, or functional impairment.

More study is needed to determine qualitative and quantitative differences between reactions of directly exposed versus only media-exposed youth. Whalen et al. (2004) found that California adolescents' postevent negative emotional reactions and PTS symptoms were present when youth were reminded of 9/11 but were comparable to previous levels of symptoms when they were not reminded. For these media-exposed youth, PTS symptoms were generally at a medium level except for high ratings for fears of recurrence, difficulty paying attention, and not enjoying things as much. In London, functional impairment persisted even when PTS did not for youth who did react to 9/11.

Comparisons by Exposure Levels

More studies are needed to understand variations in response by type of exposure, age, and event type. Wang et al. (2006) assessed 95 Israeli children, ages 1–4. Parents reported that directly terrorism-exposed children had significantly increased risk of externalizing, internalizing, and total problems. Preschool children who daily watched 5 minutes or more of TV with terrorism content showed increased risk of externalizing, emotional reactivity, aggressive behavior, and oppositional defiance. Preschoolers with nonterrorism-related traumas had increased risk of anxiety/depression, affective problems, and anxiety. For NYC adolescents assessed before (ages 6–14) and after (ages 12–20) 9/11 (Aber et al., 2004), direct exposure was associated with increased depression and PTSD. Media exposure was related to more anxiety and PTSD but fewer conduct disturbances. Family exposure was associated with social mistrust. When researchers accounted for prior levels of symptoms, hostile bias, and exposure to other violence (witnessing and victimization), only the association between media exposure to 9/11 and adolescent PTS symptoms remained: Symptoms increased with increases in reported media exposure. On the other hand, youth's exposures to intrafamilial or community violence in NYC were associated with all assessed mental health outcomes (PTSD, depression, conduct disturbances, anxiety), hostile attribution biases, and social mistrust. For 9- to 12-year-olds, Thabet, Abed, and Vostanis (2002) found that Palestinian children's exposures to bombardment and home demolition (B&HD) were the strongest predictors of PTS reactions and predicted higher fear scores as well. Children exposed through the media reported more anticipatory anxiety and cognitive distress than children who were directly exposed. Anxiety symptoms and disorders were consistently higher in children living in parts of the Gaza Strip not directly affected by B&HD than in those directly exposed. Lengua et al. (2005) compared 9/11 media-exposed Washington state youth to youth exposed to the Northridge, California earthquake. Although the earthquake sample reported more total PTS symptoms, the Washington youth reported more reexperiencing symptoms.

Peritraumatic Emotions

Controlling for peritraumatic panic attacks (i.e., those occurring during exposure to the event) accounted for a large proportion of the reduction in association between TV viewing and probable PTSD for adults after 9/11 (Ahern et al., 2004). Pfefferbaum, Stuber, Galea, and Fairbrother (2006) confirmed the association between peritraumatic panic attacks and probable or subthreshold PTSD for adolescents with an average of 2 hours of TV watching and a variety of other exposures. Pfefferbaum, Seale, et al. (2003) and Lengua et al., (2005) found that strong emotions during watching increased reactions to televized terrorism. For London youth, Holmes et al. (2007) reported that mean PTS scores (but not necessarily functional impairment) were significantly higher if children reported that they felt scared, endangered, helpless, sick, or that the world was a more dangerous place. After controlling for second-month symptoms, peritraumatic feelings of endangerment was the only variable to predict symptoms at 6 months.

Worry about others or knowing someone who died during an event increases emotional proximity to events (Lengua et al., 2005; Nader et al., 1993). Youth watching from a distance during war or terrorism have reported increased or high levels of symptoms when worried about others, or when they knew someone who died. Individual U.S. children, whose family members are/were in Iraq as a part of the current ongoing war, have told of increased (sometimes unbearable) worries, anxiety, and fears related to news reports of faulty armor, dead soldiers, bombings, and other horrors in Iraq.

Gender

In relationship to media exposure, researchers have found no gender effects on PTS scores (Nader et al., 1993; Phillips et al., 2004; Thabet et al., 2004; Whalen et al., 2004), initial but not prolonged gender effects (Gil-Rivas et al., 2004), or gender effects that may or may not be explained (Hoven et al., 2005; Pfefferbaum, Moore, et al., 1999; Lengua et al., 2005). As in other types of trauma exposure, Lengua et al. found that boys exhibited higher levels of externalizing symptoms and girls reported greater levels of upset by the 9/11 attacks. This may reflect girls' greater readiness to admit emotional upset or a gender difference in manner of expressing distress. Boys in this study had greater levels of externalizing problems before 9/11.

Youth Characteristics and Symptoms

For media exposed youth, preexisting symptoms (e.g., anxiety) and emotionality have been associated with increased traumatic reactions (Lengua et al., 2005; Whalen et al., 2004). State and trait anxiety have made independent contributions to the prediction of distress for adolescents (Whalen et al., 2004). When they assessed temperamental traits (fear, irritability, poor attention regulation, low inhibitory control, impulsivity), Lengua et al. (2005) found a trend for children with lower levels of inhibitory control (self-regulation) to have more PTS symptoms. Problems with self-regulation may be particularly evident for young children who are only beginning to develop it (Table 11.1). Lengua et al. found more avoidance symptoms and more upset in African American youth. They exhibited higher levels of anxiety, depression, and conduct disturbances both pre- and postattack.

In Washington State, Lengua, Long, and Meltzoff (2006) found that youth whose appraisal style was to perceive threat from stressors and who used inactive coping before 9/11 tended to do the same after 9/11. Youth who viewed stressors as challenges and felt they had the resources to deal with them tended to appraise 9/11 more positively and had lower symptoms. Post-9/11 threat-style and inactive coping were associated with more PTS symptoms. Preattack stress level predicted 9/11 threat appraisal and avoidant coping, which predicted PTS. Although PTS symptoms were related to greater functional impairment, only preattack symptomatology, measured by the Child Behavior Checklist, and 9/11 threat appraisal predicted functional impairment.

Protective Factors

A few studies have examined protective factors related to media exposure. After 9/11, effective coping was associated with fewer symptoms for adults (Silver et al., 2002) and youth (Lengua et al., 2006). Gil-Rivas et al. (2004) found that the strongest contributors to adolescents' positive affect 1 year after the 9/11 attacks were parents' self-reported positive affect and parenting self-efficacy. Perceived support from fathers, but not from mothers, was linked to higher levels of youths' positive affect. Adolescent optimism (Whalen et al., 2004) or positive appraisal style (Lengua et al., 2006) and preattack self-esteem, social competence, and a trend for inhibitory control (Lengua et al., 2005) have served as protective factors (lower PTS levels).

Media Images as Reminders

For youth exposed to a traumatic event, media images may serve as reminders of the experience and instigate physiological and/or psychological symptoms (Nader, 2008; Pfefferbaum, Gurwitch, et al., 2003). Anniversary or later replays of the event may remind and again elicit the full range or a subset of symptoms. Media depictions of events may also serve as reminders for youth exposed to other violent events, such as mass shootings (Nader, 2008). Some child trauma therapists reported calls after 9/11 from clients who had years ago completed treatment. A young man who was shot during a mass shooting at a restaurant in California, in which many died and were injured, began to reexperience trauma symptoms (especially arousal symptoms) after seeing the 9/11 attacks on TV. A woman who, at age 7, was exposed to a school shooting had increased symptoms with each news report of killings. The first experience, soon after the sniper attack, was news of people dying after eating poisoned watermelons in the northern part of her state. Each new event confirmed that the world is unsafe and frightening.

CONCLUDING COMMENTS

Exposure to war and terroristic events can provoke serious negative reactions, including symptoms of PTS (Phillips et al., 2004). Although more study is needed to assess the differences in intensity and nature of reactions across studies, extensive media viewing of such events is clearly associated with problematic reactions for youth from all age groups and from varying locations. Pfefferbaum, Gurwitch, et al. (2003) recommend that after children's exposure to media coverage of potentially traumatic events, adults may need to discuss the event with children, reassure children about their safety, assist them in processing emotions, suggest and practice coping strategies, and/or redirect their attention. Increased visible efforts to ensure safety, among other supportive behaviors, may also be of help to previously and currently traumatized youth. Mental health professionals need to assist parents in understanding reactions to traumatic events and the impact of TV watching, in processing their own reactions, and in understanding the influence of their reactions and behaviors on the children. Phillips et al. (2004) suggest that, for young children, media exposure to disastrous events should be limited. Youth of all ages should be protected from graphic images of death and injury (Nader et al., 1993). For children who seek knowledge of the events, adults should enable them to become informed while assisting them to cope. Engaging in community or patriotic efforts after events may be a part of moral training for youth. Parents must be cognizant of its potential stressful impact on children, and the need for their support and assistance after these gestures as well. Findings also suggest the need to provide initial interventions for all youth who might be affected either directly or through the media, and to focus more long-term interventions on youth who exhibit more serious and prolonged reactions (Phillips et al., 2004).

DISCUSSION QUESTIONS

1. In what ways does watching media violence affect youth of different ages?
2. How do journalists help or hurt the healing process for youth? What is the role of parents in permitting or discouraging media exposure?
3. What are the differences in response related to exposure variables?

ACKNOWLEDGMENT

My sincere thanks to Christine Mello for her input.

REFERENCES

Aber, J. L., Gershoff, E. T., Ware, A., & Kotler, J. A. (2004). Estimating the effects of September 11th and other forms of violence on the mental health and social development of New York City's youth: A matter of context. *Applied Developmental Science, 8*(3), 111–129.

Ahern, J., Galea, S., Resnick, H., & Vlahov, D. (2004). TV images and probable posttraumatic stress disorder after September 11: The role of background characteristics, event exposures, and perievent panic. *Journal of Nervous and Mental Disease, 192*(3), 217–226.

Beullens, K., Eggermont, S., & Van den Bulck, J. (2008, May). *TV viewing, adolescent females' body dissatisfaction and the concern that boys expect girls to be attractive.* Paper presented at the annual meeting of the International Communication Association, Sheraton New York, New York, NY. Retrieved July 11, 2008, from *www.allacademic.com/meta/p14081_ index.html*.

Bleich, A., Gelkopf, M., & Solomon, Z. (2003). Exposure to terrorism, stress-related mental health symptoms, and coping behaviors among a nationally represented sample in Israel. *Journal of the American Medical Association, 290*(5), 612–620.

Bosgieter, B., Rasmussen, T., Cook, L., Kofford, J., & Caldarella, P. (2006, April 20–22). *Media exposure to traumatic events and its relationship to childhood anxiety.* Paper presented at the Rocky Mountain Psychological Association annual meeting, Park City, UT.

Bushman, B., & Huesmann, L. (2006). Short-term and long-term effects of violent media on aggression in children and adults. *Archives of Pediatric Adolescent Medicine, 160,* 348–352.

Fang, L., & Chen, T. (2004). Community outreach and education to deal with cultural resistance to mental health services. In N. B. Webb (Ed.), *Mass trauma, stress, and loss: Helping children and families cope* (pp. 234–255). New York: Guilford Press.

Fletcher, K. E. (2003). Childhood posttraumatic stress disorder. In E. J. Mash & R. A. Barkley (Eds.), *Child psychopathology* (2nd ed., pp. 330–371). New York: Guilford Press.

Ford, J. D. (2009). Neurobiological and developmental research: Clinical implications. In C. Courtois & J. D. Ford (Eds.), *Treating complex traumatic stress disorders: An evidence-based guide* (pp. 31–58). New York: Guilford Press.

Gershoff, E., & Aber, J. (2004). Assessing the impact of September 11th, 2001, on children, youth, and parents: Methodological challenges to research on terrorism and other nonnormative events. *Applied Developmental Science, 8*(3), 106–110.

Gil-Rivas, V., Holman, E., & Silver, R. (2004). Adolescent vulnerability following the September 11th terrorist attacks: A study of parents and their children. *Applied Developmental Science, 8*(3), 130–142.

Holmes, E., Creswell, C., & O'Connor, T. (2007). Posttraumatic stress symptoms in London school children following September 11, 2001: An exploratory investigation of peritraumatic reactions and intrusive imagery. *Journal of Behavior Therapy and Experimental Psychiatry, 38,* 474–490.

Hoven, C. W., Duarte, C. S., Lucas, C. P., Wu, P., Mandell, D. J., Goodwin, R. D., et al. (2005). Psychopathology among New York City public school children 6 months after September 11. *Archives of General Psychiatry, 62,* 545–552.

Huesmann, R. L. (2007). The impact of electronic media violence: Scientific theory and research. *Journal of Adolescent Health, 41,* S6–S13.

Jabr, S. (2004). The children of Palestine: A generation of hope and despair. *Washington Report on Middle East Affairs,* 23(10), 18–76.

Lengua, L., Long, A., & Meltzoff, A. (2006). Pre-attack stress load, appraisals, and coping in children's responses to the 9/11 terrorist attacks. *Journal of Child Psychology and Psychiatry, 47*(12), 1219–1227.

Lengua, L., Long, A., Smith, K., & Meltzoff, A. (2005). Pre-attack symptomatology and temperament as predictors of children's responses to the September 11 terrorist attacks. *Journal of Child Psychology and Psychiatry, 46*(6), 631–645.

Libow, J. (1992). Traumatized children and the news media. *American Journal of Orthopsychiatry, 62*(3), 379–386.

Mapp, I., & Koch, D. (2004). Creating a group mural to promote healing following a mass trauma. In N. B. Webb (Ed.), *Mass trauma and violence* (pp. 100–119). New York: Guilford Press.

Marshall, R., & Galea, S. (2004). Science for the community: Assessing mental health after 9/11. *Journal of Clinical Psychology, 65*(1), 37–43.

Mayou, R. A., Ehlers, A., & Hobbs, M. (2000). Psychological debriefing for road traffic accident victims: Three-year follow-up of a randomized controlled trial. *British Journal of Psychiatry, 176,* 589–593.

Nader, K. (1993, October 4). *Violence and the media: Impact on traumatized children.* Conference presentation, Violence and the Media: Helping Victims of Trauma, Virginia Mason Medical Center, Seattle, WA.

Nader, K. (1997). Assessing traumatic experiences in children. In J. Wilson & T. Keane (Eds.), *Assessing psychological trauma and PTSD* (pp. 291–348). New York: Guilford Press.

Nader, K. (2008). *Understanding and assessing trauma in children and adolescents: Measures, methods, and youth in context.* New York: Routledge.

Nader, K. (Ed.). (in press). *School rampage shootings and other youth disturbances: Early preventive interventions.* New York: Routledge.

Nader, K., Pynoos, R. S., Fairbanks, L. A., Al-Ajeel, M., & Al-Asfour, A. (1993). A preliminary study of PTSD and grief among the children of Kuwait following the Gulf Crisis. *British Journal of Clinical Psychology, 32,* 407–416.

Ochberg, F. (2008). PTSD 101 for journalists. Retrieved May 4, 2008, from *www.giftfromwithin.org/html/ptsd101.html.* (Original work published 1995)

Pfefferbaum, B., Moore, V., McDonald, N., Maynard, B., Gurwitch, R., & Nixon, S. (1999). The role of exposure in postraumatic stress in youths following the 1995 bombing. *Journal of the Oklahoma State Medical Association, 92*(4), 164–167.

Pfefferbaum, B., Nixon, S., Tivis, R., Doughty, D., Pynoos, R., Gurwitch, R., et al. (2001). Television exposure in children after terrorist attacks. *Psychiatry, 64*(3), 202–211.

Pfefferbaum, B., Nixon, S., Tucker, P. M., Tivis, R., Moore, V., Gurwitch, R., et al. (1999). Posttraumatic stress responses in bereaved children after the

Oklahoma City bombing. *Journal of the American Academy of Child and Adolescent Psychiatry, 38*(11), 1372–1379.

Pfefferbaum, B., Seale, T., Brandt, E., Pfefferbaum, R., Doughty, D., & Rainwater, S. (2003). Media exposure in children one hundred miles from a terrorist bombing. *Annals of Clinical Psychiatry, 15*(1), 1–8.

Pfefferbaum, B., Stuber, J., Galea, S., & Fairbrother, G. (2006). Panic reactions to terrorist attacks and problable posttrauamtic stress disorder in adolescents. *Journal of Traumatic Stress, 19*(2), 217–228.

Pfefferbaum, R., Gurwitch, R., Robertson, M., Brandt, E., & Pfefferbaum, B. (2003). Terrorism, the media, and distress in youth. *Prevention Researcher, 10*(2), 14–16.

Phillips, D., Prince, S., & Schiebelhut, L. (2004). Elementary school children's responses 3 months after the September 11 terrorist attacks: A study in Washington, DC. *American Journal of Orthopsychiatry, 74*(4), 509–528.

Raphael, B., & Wilson, J. (Eds.). (2001). *Psychological debriefing: Theory, practice and evidence.* Cambridge, UK: Cambridge University Press.

Ruzek, J., & Watson, P. (2001). Early intervention to prevent PTSD and other trauma-related problems. *PTSD Research Quarterly, 12*(4), 1–7.

Saylor, C., Cowart, B., Livpovsky, J., Jackson, C., & Finch, A. (2003). Media exposure to September 11: Elementary school students' experiences and posttrauma symptoms. *American Behavioral Scientist, 46*, 1622–1642.

Schuster, M. A., Stein, B. D., Jaycox, L. H., Collins, R. L., Marshall, G. N., Elliott, M. N., et al. (2001). A national survey of stress reaction after the September 11, 2001 terrorist attacks. *New England Journal of Medicine, 345*(20), 1507–1512.

Silver, R. C., Holman, E. A., McIntosh, D. N., Poulin, M., & Gil-Rivas, V. (2002). Nationwide longitudinal study of psychological responses to September 11. *Journal of the American Medical Association, 288*, 1235–1244.

Swiss, S., & Giller, J. E. (1993). Rape as a crime of war: A medical perspective. *Journal of the American Medical Association, 270*(5), 612–615.

Teichroeb, R. (2006). Covering children and trauma: A guide for journalism professionals (Washington State University, Dart Center for Journalism and Trauma). Retrieved July 5, 2008 from *www.dartcenter.org.*

Terr, L., Bloch, D., Michel, B., Shi, H., Reinhardt, J., & Metayer, S. (1999). Children's symptoms in the wake of Challenger: A field study of distant-traumatic effects and an outline of related conditions. *American Journal of Psychiatry, 156*, 1536–1544.

Thabet, A., Abed, Y., & Vostanis, P. (2002). Emotional problems in Palestinian children living in a war zone: A cross-sectional study. *Lancet, 359*(9320), 1801–1804.

Thabet, A., Abed, Y., & Vostanis, P. (2004). Comorbidity of PTSD and depression among refugee children during war conflict. *Journal of Child Psychology and Psychiatry, 45*(3), 533–542.

Wang, Y., Nomura, Y., Pat-Horenczyk, R., Doppelt, O., Abramovitz, R., Brom, D., et al. (2006). Association of Direct Exposure to Terrorism, Media Exposure to Terrorism, and Other Trauma with Emotional and Behavioral

Problems in Preschool Children. *Annals of the New York Academy of Sciences, 1094*, 363–368.

Whalen, C., Henker, B., King, P., Jamner, L., & Levine, L. (2004). Adolescents react to the events of September 11, 2001: Focused versus ambient impact. *Journal of Abnormal Child Psychology, 32*(1), 1–11.

Yates, T. M., Egeland, B., & Sroufe, A. (2003). Rethinking resilience: A developmental process perspective. In S. S. Luthar (Ed.), *Resilience and vulnerability: Adaptation in the context of childhood adversities* (pp. 243–266). New York: Cambridge University Press.

CHAPTER 12

Deaths Connected
to Natural Disasters

JENNIFER BAGGERLY
ALISON SALLOUM

PREVALENCE OF NATURAL DISASTERS

The enormous prevalence and increasing rate of natural disasters com-
pels mental health clinicians to be prepared to provide help to bereaved
children who survive these deadly events. Consider the following statistics: In 2007, 414 natural disasters affected over 211 million people
worldwide, killed 16,847 people, and caused over $74.9 billion in eco-
nomic damages (Scheuren, le Polain, Below, Guha-Sapir, & Ponserre,
2008). In 2005, Hurricane Katrina caused 1,833 fatalities and about
$110 billion in damage in the United States (Abramson, Redlener, Steh-
ling-Ariza, & Fuller, 2007; Knabb, Rhome, & Brown, 2005). Unfortunately, the rate of natural disasters, especially storms and floods, appears
to be increasing. "In recent decades, the number of reported hydrologi-
cal disasters has increased 7.4% per year" (Scheuren, et al., 2008, p. 11).
In 2007, 44 floods were declared as federal disasters in the United States
compared to only 28 in 1997 (Federal Emergency Management Agency,
2008). Other natural disasters, such as fires, have caused thousands of
deaths per year. In 2006, 412,500 U.S. families experienced house fires
that resulted in 2,620 deaths and 12,925 injuries (U.S. Fire Administration, 2007).

IMPACT OF NATURAL DISASTERS ON CHILDREN

Natural disasters can cause short and long-term physical and mental health problems in children that impede their growth and development (Silverman & La Greca, 2002; La Greca, 2008). One study revealing the short-term impact found that 3 months after Hurricane Andrew, 56% of 1,086 third-, fourth-, and fifth-grade children reported moderate to very severe symptoms (Vernberg, La Greca, Silverman, & Prinstein, 1996). Another study demonstrating the long-term impact found that 2 years after Hurricane Katrina, between 46,582 and 64,934 children had an educational, health, or mental health problem that put them at risk for long-term poor outcomes (Abramson et al., 2007). More specifically, this study also found that 31.5% of parents reported that since Hurricane Katrina their child experienced clinically diagnosed depression, anxiety, or a behavior disorder.

Research has identified numerous physiological, emotional, behavioral, and cognitive symptoms in children who have experienced a natural disaster (Silverman & La Greca, 2002; Speier, 2000). Common physiological responses to natural disasters can be categorized along two continua. In a dissociative response, children may have decreases in their heart rates, blood pressure, and awareness of pain (Perry, Pollard, Blakely, Baker, & Vigilante, 1995). Yet, in the arousal response, children may have increases in their heart rate, blood pressure, cortisol, and adrenaline, as well as suppressed immune functioning (Perry et al., 1995; Silverman & La Greca, 2002). Other commonly reported physiological symptoms in children include headaches, stomachaches, chest pains, sleeplessness, hypervigilance, and inattentiveness (American Academy of Pediatrics, n.d.).

Typical emotional, behavioral, and cognitive symptoms in preschool- and elementary-age school-children include fear, anxiety, depression, irritability, crying, withdrawal, nightmares, regression, bedwetting, clinginess, school refusal, aggression, and play reenactments (Silverman & La Greca, 2002; Speier, 2000). For adolescents, expected symptoms include withdrawal, depression, antisocial behavior (e.g., stealing), high-risk behavior, alcohol and drug use, as well as school problems (Speier, 2000).

For most children, these symptoms usually resolve within a short time (Speier, 2000). However, some children may have ongoing problems that result in acute stress disorder (less than 30 days), posttraumatic stress disorder (PTSD) (over 30 days), other anxiety disorders, or depression (LaGreca, 2008; Speier, 2000). PTSD symptoms include (1) reexperiencing the traumatic event through intrusive thoughts, dreams, and play reenactments; (2) avoidance of trauma reminders and numbing feelings; and (3) hyperarousal, such as sleeplessness, irritability, and exaggerated startle response (La Greca, 2008). "In community studies, approximately 24% to 39% of children and adolescents exposed to destructive natural disasters have been found to meet criteria for a PTSD diagnosis in the first few weeks or months following the event" (La Greca, 2008, p. 124).

After natural disasters, some children also experience traumatic grief. Absolute horror combined with an incomprehensible death of someone known to the child only begins to describe "childhood traumatic grief" (CTG). More formally, CTG has been defined as "a condition in which both unresolved grief (i.e., yearning and searching for the deceased and difficulty in accepting the death) and PTSD symptoms are present" (Cohen, Mannarino, & Deblinger, 2006, p. 17). Children who have had a loved one killed during natural disasters are very susceptible to PTSD (La Greca, 2008).

RISK AND RESILIENCY FACTORS

Mental health clinicians can help to triage children who have survived natural disasters by being aware of not only possible symptoms, as described earlier, but also risk and resiliency factors. Several researchers have identified the following four categories of risk and resiliency factors that predict more severe symptoms after natural disasters:

1. Preexisting characteristics
2. Levels of trauma exposure
3. Social support
4. Coping style

First, preexisting characteristics, such as prior trauma, female gender, ethnic/racial minority, younger age, and preexisting anxiety, predict higher rates of PTSD (La Greca, 2008; Vernberg et al., 1996). Second, high levels of trauma exposure, particularly intensity, duration, and perception of life threat, predict higher rates of PTSD (La Greca, 2008; Vernberg et al., 1996). Researchers who corroborated these risk factors (Weems, Pina, & Costa, 2007) found that predisaster trait anxiety and negative affect predicted posttraumatic stress in youth after Hurricane Katrina. Likewise, LaGreca, Silverman, and Wasserstein (1998) previously found that children's predisaster anxiety, inattention, academic skills, and high trauma exposure predicted posttraumatic symptoms 3 months after Hurricane Andrew. They also found that predisaster anxiety, exposure, and African American ethnicity 7 months after the Hurricane Andrew predicted posttraumatic stress symptoms. However, differences in distress postdisaster between and within racial/ethnic groups may be better accounted for by differences in culture, acculturation, and socioeconomic status (Jones, Frary, Cunningham, Weddle, & Kaiser, 2001).

The third risk and resiliency factor category that predicts PTSD is social support from parents, peers, and teachers (Vernberg et al., 1996). Parents have been acknowledged as the single, most important component for children's recovery after a disaster, because they provide nurturance and a sense of safety (Vernberg et al., 1996; Webb, 2004). In addition, Hurricane Katrina researchers Abramson, Stehling-Ariza, Garfield, and Redlener (2008) recommend that children be reconnected quickly with social supports, such as religious events, formal education, and recreational activities.

The fourth risk and resiliency factor category is coping style, in which positive coping predicts lower rates of PTSD, while negative coping (e.g., anger and blaming) predicts higher rates of PTSD (La Greca, 2008; Vernberg et al., 1996). Coping strategies of talking, staying informed, and praying were found to predict less psychological stress in people displaced after Hurricane Katrina according to a survey by Spence, Lachlan, and Burke (2007). Methods for enhancing children's cognitive, physical, emotional, behavioral, and spiritual coping strategies and social supports are explained in Baggerly and Exum (2008) and Baggerly (2007).

PSYCHOLOGICAL INTERVENTIONS

A range of psychological interventions for children after natural disasters has been summarized by La Greca (2008). For the immediate impact phase, she describes critical incident stress debriefing and psychological first aid. For the short-term recovery phase, she recommends school-based cognitive-behavioral therapy and community-based "stress and coping" interventions, such as her workbook entitled *After the Storm*. For the long-term recovery phase, she includes multimodality trauma treatment, brief trauma/grief-focused psychotherapy, school-based psychosocial intervention, and eye movement desensitization and reprocessing (EMDR).

Cohen et al. (2006) recommend trauma-focused cognitive-behavioral therapy (TF-CBT) for treating CTG. This treatment consists of individual child and parent sessions, and joint parent–child sessions. Their trauma-focused components include psychoeducation, parenting skills, relaxation, affective expression and modulation, cognitive coping and processing, trauma narrative, *in vivo* mastery, conjoint child–parent sessions, and enhancing future safety. Their grief-focused components include grief psychoeducation, grieving the loss and resolving ambivalent feelings about the deceased, preserving positive memories, and redefining the relationship with the deceased and committing to present relationships. A newer, empirically supported approach to CTG that combines many of these recommendations into a group format for children is described below.

GRIEF AND TRAUMA INTERVENTION FOR CHILDREN

Grief and trauma intervention (GTI) is a time-limited group psychotherapy model for children who are experiencing high levels of traumatic stress due to disaster, violence and/or death (Salloum, 2006). Although used most recently with younger children, GTI may also be used with adolescents (e.g., Salloum, 2004). The foundation of the GTI includes developmentally specific methods, an ecological perspective, and culturally relevant approaches. The theoretical ordering of themes addressed occurs within three overlapping phases: (1) resilience and safety; (2) restorative retelling; (3) and reconnecting (Herman, 1997; Rynearson, 2001). Techniques from cognitive-behavioral therapy and narrative therapy are combined to address loss and trauma.

A specific process of drawing, discussing, writing, and witnessing (DDWW) is used to elicit, explore, and expand children's narratives of loss and traumatic events to understand the meaning of the event(s) to the children, while also serving as a type of narrative exposure to traumatic aspects of the event(s). A child is asked to draw a picture of a particular topic (Pynoos & Eth, 1984) pertaining to the specified themes. Afterward, the drawing is discussed, with a clinician-guided exploration of the child's thoughts and feelings. Restorative questions help place the child within or close to the story as opposed to having the child recount the story as an observer (Rynearson, 2001). The clinician then "plays secretary" (Stacey & Loptson, 1995) and writes the child's story about the drawing in the child's book (*My Story*). Last, the clinician, parent, and/or group members serve as "outside witnesses" (White & Epston, 1990) to the child's story while empathetically responding. GTI includes 10 child group sessions, one parent session, and one individual child session, with additional family and individual sessions as needed.

GTI was first developed and evaluated with children, ages 7–12, who had had someone close to them murdered (Salloum, 2008). Although results were promising, revisions to strengthen the effect were made, and the intervention was tested with children experiencing losses and at least moderate posttraumatic stress after Hurricane Katrina (Salloum & Overstreet, 2008). In this study, 56 children (ages 7–12) were randomly assigned to receive the GTI in a group setting or individually. GTI was provided in school and in afterschool programs. Results of the intervention with children after Hurricane Katrina suggest that children in both treatment modalities experienced significant decreases in posttraumatic stress, depression, traumatic grief, and global distress, and the effect sizes from pretest to posttest were $d = 1.16$, $d = 0.53$, $d = 0.73$, and $d = 0.51$, respectively (Salloum & Overstreet, 2008). Additional studies on GTI are underway, and GTI may be adapted to address cultural differences and different developmental ages.

APPLICATION OF GRIEF AND TRAUMA INTERVENTION

Assessment

Often survivors of natural disasters speak of their lives in terms of "before" the disaster and "after" the disaster. Assessment needs to include prior (before the disaster) and current biological–psychological–social–spiritual–cultural information, and the strengths of the child, including child and family social supports, coping efforts, and protective factors.

Strengths and resources of the child may include factors such as the child's parent providing emotional support to the child; open and age-appropriate communication within the family; child and family members sharing positive memories of the deceased; child and family members having a positive outlook for the future (optimism and hope); the child engaging in activities that interest him or her; the child having a positive peer support network; the child doing well academically; the child and family having a safe and adequate living environment; and the child and family engaging in active coping strategies to recover from the disaster (Rosenfeld, Caye, Ayalon, & Lahad, 2005; Silverman & LaGreca, 2002).

The assessment also needs to include asking direct questions of the child and family about disaster-specific matters related to proximity exposure, threat, loss, changes, and unique events during and after the disaster that impact the child and family (see Figure 12.1). These questions may be posed in a yes-or-no format to the child, then followed up by further exploration when applicable. If the child is highly anxious, it may be best to teach relaxation skills, such as deep-breathing exercises, before asking these questions, or to let the child know that he or she does not need to explain any details at this time. It is important to help the

Type of question	Sample questions	Yes	No
Proximity exposure	1. Were you close to the (name disaster) when it happened?	___	___
	2. Did you see (name the major destruction caused by the disaster, such as the burned buildings, the rubble, destroyed homes, the water)?	___	___
	3. Did you read or see the news about (name the disaster)?	___	___
	4. Do you continue to see the destruction caused by (disaster)?	___	___
Threat related	1. Were you separated from (name who the child would have been with at the time of the disaster, such as family, a teacher, a coach) during the disaster?	___	___
	2. Were you scared that you or someone you knew might get hurt or die due to (disaster)?	___	___
	3. Did you or someone you know get hurt or injured?	___	___
	4. Is someone close to you missing since (the disaster)?	___	___
	5. Did someone you know die? If yes, did you witness the person getting hurt or dying? (See note below.)	___	___
	6. Did you think that you were going to die?	___	___
	7. Did you think that someone close to you was going to die?	___	___
	8. Are you still scared that you or someone you know is going to be hurt or die due to the (the disaster)?	___	___
	9. Do you think that it (the disaster) is going to happen again?	___	___
Losses and changes	1. Did you lose your toys in (the disaster)?	___	___
	2. Did you lose your pet in the (name disaster)?	___	___
	3. Did you lose your clothes in the (name disaster)?	___	___
	4. Did you lose friends due to (the disaster)?	___	___
	5. Did you go to a new school because of (the disaster)?	___	___
	6. Have the things you used to do for fun changed?	___	___

(cont.)

FIGURE 12.1. Examples of disaster-specific questions with a yes-or-no response format.

Type of question	Sample questions	Yes	No
Losses and changes *(cont.)*	7. Did your house get damaged?		
	8. Did you move to a new place to live after (the disaster) and/or death?	___	___
	9. Did you move to a new neighborhood after (the disaster) and/or death?	___	___
	10. Have there been major changes in your family since (the disaster) or death?	___	___
	11. Has your daily routine changed since (the disaster) and/or death?	___	___
Unique events during and after the disaster	1. Did you have time to prepare for (the disaster)?	___	___
	2. Do you think you or someone else could have stopped (name the person who got injured or died) from getting injured or dying?	___	___
	3. Did you see (name the disaster-specific element, such as flood waters or fire)?	___	___
	4. Did you smell, taste or touch (name any smell associated with the disaster, such as gas, mold, burn smell) during or after the disaster?	___	___
	5. If in the disaster, were you able to help yourself or someone get to a safer place during (the disaster)?	___	___
	6. Did you go to a shelter before, during, or after (the disaster)?	___	___
	7. Have you had a chance to help others in any way since (the disaster)?	___	___
	8. Do you have an adult that you can talk with about your thoughts and feelings about your losses?		

Note. It may be best to stop the questions temporarily and redirect the assessment to focus on the death and life of the person who died and the relationship to the child. See the case example in the chapter illustrating this.

FIGURE 12.1. *(cont.)*

child regulate his or her distress level during the assessment, to help the child feel more in control, and to prevent the child from becoming overwhelmed during the assessment phase. During the assessment, the child needs to know that he or she may simply point to "yes" or "no," and that he or she has the right to pass when answering the questions and may signal this to the clinician by simply raising his or her hand. These questions may also be asked of the parent or caregiver about the child's experience and about the parent's own experiences (consult Figure 12.1).

When the child has experienced the death of someone close in the context of a natural disaster, there may be numerous disaster recovery adjustment issues, sadness, or depression related to the losses and the death, and, in some cases, traumatic elements may cause and maintain posttraumatic stress symptoms or other anxiety disorders. It is important to ascertain in the assessment the areas for targeted clinical intervention. After asking children about their disaster-specific experiences, it may be helpful to ask three questions (Salloum, 2006) to identify the initial clinical focus. Of all of the things that you indicated have happened:

1. Which one bothers you the most?
2. Which one makes you feel the saddest?
3. Which one is the hardest to talk about?

It is necessary to understand the importance of the deceased person to the child and briefly assess what he or she knows about the death. If the child was close to the person who died, assessing the meaning of the loss and the child's knowledge and perception about the manner of the death may need to take temporary precedence over assessing other disaster-specific factors (e.g., the questions in Figure 12.1). Also, standardized instruments measuring anxiety, including posttraumatic stress, depression and grief, can help to provide a more targeted intervention. Information about different types of disaster-specific screening tools and psychological assessment instruments may be found at the National Center for Childhood Traumatic Stress (*www.nccts.org*).

Brief Assessment Example

An illustration of the assessment process is provided in the following dialogue between a clinician and a 10-year-old African American boy who survived Hurricane Katrina.*

---

* This example is disguised with a pseudonym and changes in details to protect confidentiality.

Content/Transcript

Rationale/Analysis

CLINICIAN: Did someone you know die during or after the Hurricane Katrina?

Ask directly about death. State "someone you know" rather than asking only about family members or friends. When the death is due to a disaster that the child experienced, the death may become more salient for the child, perhaps leading to survivor's guilt, fear, threat, and/or realization of the destruction of the disaster.

CHILD: Yes, the water got my neighbor. She didn't want to leave and would not come with us. When we came back, my mom found her in the mud. It smelled real bad.

The child has an understanding of the manner of the death and relates potentially distressing details.
The child may be referring to the person as the "neighbor" because the clinician does not know the person or the child was not close to the person, or the child is avoiding talking directly about the person. Assess the relationship of the child to the deceased. Later, assess avoidance, intrusive images, and feelings of guilt.

CLINICIAN: I want to hear more about what you saw when you came back and when your mom found your neighbor, but first, I would like to know, what was your neighbor's name?

Let the child know that you want to hear more about the death and that it is OK to talk about it. Before asking more about the manner of death, see whether the child can talk more about the person, his or her life, and their relationship to begin to understand the meaning of the loss.

CHILD: Ms. Patrice. She always lived next to us ever since I was born. I went to her house after school until my mom got home from work. After she helps me with my homework, we make snow cones and sell them to the other kids in the

The child begins to explain who he deceased person was to him, the roles she played in his life, and a positive memory. The clinician needs to monitor for the child's level of distress as he reminisces about the deceased.

neighborhood. She was a lot of fun.

CLINICIAN: It sounds like you and Ms. Patrice were close and you spent a lot of time with her. Can you tell me more about when the two of you would make snow cones and sell them?

Acknowledge the importance of the relationship. Assess whether the child is able to engage in recalling a positive memory, without automatically going to the manner of death. Monitor the child's affect: Is he able to retell the positive memory with detail and positive emotion, or is he recounting it as if he is thinking about other thoughts with constricted affect?

CHILD: *Looking down (no eye contact) with a sad facial expression* and *mumbling.* We just used to make them.

Reality of the loss. The child's affect is congruent with the content and he is not able to continue. Body language changes to express feelings of sadness and the reality of the loss. The clinician still needs to assess intrusive thoughts and images, avoidance, arousal, and guilt.

CLINICIAN: You know, you are very brave to have shared a little with me about what you have seen and your relationship with Ms. Patrice. When someone close dies, it is normal to have a lot of different feelings about the loss of the person and also how the person died. I would like to take a moment and ask you some questions about your experiences, thoughts, and feelings. These questions are based on what other children have told us they have experienced after someone close dies. Not everyone has all of these reactions, so I want to see how you are doing.

Highlight the child's strength in being able to talk with the counselor about the loss. Acknowledge and normalize the range of thoughts and emotions due to the loss and trauma. Continue assessing disaster-specific experiences. Assess for anxiety and depression using standardized instruments. Determining the child's posttraumatic stress related to the death includes assessing level of guilt, intrusive imagery, other reexperiencing symptoms, avoidance, and trauma triggers.

GTI for Children

Rather than provide a session-by-session outline, the next three sections provide an overview of general topics within GTI that are common to many grief- and trauma-focused therapies. These topics are organized within three main overlapping components: (1) resilience, (2) restorative retelling, and (3) reconnecting. For specific details of each session, see Salloum (2006).

Due to the postdisaster demands of recovery on parents, consistently transporting children to weekly therapy sessions is often difficult. Therefore, GTI for children (with about six children per group) may occur in schools or agency-based settings, with one or two individual parent meetings. Additional family-based treatment may follow for those who continue to suffer severe clinical levels of distress and impairment in functioning.

Resilience

The beginning of treatment focuses on promoting coping skills and helping bereaved children learn ways to regulate their emotions. Topics to address include (1) anger management; (2) relaxation including deep-breathing exercises, muscle relaxation, and guided imagery; (3) supportive people; (4) education about grief and traumatic reactions, including the connections between thoughts, feelings, body reactions, and behaviors; (5) recognition of family support and changes; (6) culturally relevant rituals for anniversary dates, holidays, and significant days (e.g., the birthday) of the deceased; (7) the role of spirituality; (8) disaster-specific education, including preparedness; (9) upsetting and comforting dreams and strategies for sleeping well; and (10) ways to increase a sense of safety. These topics can be divided up among the six sessions based on children's needs and preferences. Clinicians are to build upon the strengths and resources identified in the assessment to moderate distress and to build the children's coping capacities.

Restorative Retelling

Retelling is more than just having the child, as a distant observer with constricted affect, tell the story about how the person died. "Restorative retelling" helps the child create a more coherent narrative of the life of the person who died, of the relationship between the child and deceased, and of the manner of the death. Children are provided an avenue to tell their story of life before, during, and after the disaster and/or death. This retelling helps the child to organize what is often a fragmented story. Engaging the child in retelling his or her story is often an empowering experience for the child. Retelling may begin during the resilience-building component, but the child is provided three sessions in which retelling is the main focus. During the retelling, it is important to amplify alternative stories (non-trauma-focused stories) that highlight the child's bravery, strengths, and hope. The systematic process of drawing, discussing, writing, and having others serve as supportive observers or witnesses helps the child to express intrusive death and/or trauma images that may be occurring and to connect his or her thoughts and feelings to a more coherent story. This process is individualized, allowing the child to choose where he or she wants to begin the story. To help the child construct his or her story, worksheets labeled *before, during,* and *after* are provided to the child as part of the *My Story* book.

A child may choose to begin with telling about the life of the person who died and who this person was to the child, or the story may begin right before the disaster, with the details leading up to the death. In individual meetings with a mental health clinician, the child is provided the opportunity to draw, discuss, and write about the worst moment. This often entails the death imagery, regardless of whether the child witnessed the death or not. The individual meetings are also designed to address the unique clinical needs of the child, such as tailoring stress management strategies, assessing level of guilt, developing coping strategies for traumatic reminders, and addressing cognitive distortions. A brief example from a boy whose grandmother died during Hurricane Katrina is included below to illustrate the process of having the child draw, discuss, write and share his story about his experience before, during, at the worst moment, and after the event. Due to limited space only an overview of the child's story is presented.

Before the Storm

James, a 9-year-old African American male, drew a picture of the outside of his grandmother's house, with windows, a door, grass, and trees. The clinician responded, "Tell me about your drawing." The boy explained that everyone in his family used to go to his grandma's house and have "Sunday lunches at her house with all of my cousins." The clinician continued asking questions about James's relationship to his grandmother, such as "Can you share something special that she taught you?" He replied, "She taught me how to pray and always told me I was going to go college." After the discussion, the clinician transcribed James's story about his grandmother and the fun he used to have at her house with all of his cousins. He shared with the other group members the story about his relationship with his grandmother and read his story proudly.

When the Storm Happened

For the drawing of "when it happened" James drew a picture of his grandmother and uncle in water with their hands in the air and their mouths open, yelling for help. Again, the clinician asked, "Will you tell me about your drawing?" James explained that his grandmother and uncle had to leave due to the rising water, but that his grandma got too hot and could not make it. He stated, "They got to the highway away from the water, but she passed out and died." He explained that he was at his house during the storm and that his house was not flooded, but the wind had torn off part of the roof. The clinician asked additional questions, such as where James was in his house when part of the roof blew off, what he and his mother did to try to protect themselves, what other sounds he heard, what he remembers thinking when he heard them, how he was feeling when he heard these sounds, and whether at any time he noticed his body feeling different. During this discussion, the boy's bravery was highlighted by the clinician, who amplified James's ability to remain calm during the storm and to help his mother also stay calm when they heard the roof tear off. He remembered telling her, "We just got to stay here in the bathroom and keep praying, and we will be all right." After the discussion, James wrote a story to accompany his drawing and shared it with the other group members. He wrote, "When everything happened I was scared that we wouldn't make it, but we did. My mom kept telling me we were going to be OK, and I told her we were going to be OK, and we kept praying. I knew my grandma would be OK, because she was with my uncle. Our house did not flood, but part of the roof flew off. We sat in the bathroom during the storm but my uncle and my grandma had to swim through the water. I was glad my uncle was with my grandma, because he is strong. They needed help, because they had to go through the water. He carried her out of the water, but it got too hot for her."

Worst Moment

In an individual session James was asked to draw the worst moment (or the part he identified in the assessment that was hardest to talk about). He drew a picture of his grandma, dead on the street, and his uncle holding her body, yelling for someone to help. The clinician, looking at the drawing, said, "Tell me about your drawing." James stated, "When she got too hot and didn't have any water, she died in the street." He explained that he was proud of his uncle for walking miles in the water and carrying his grandmother, but he was angry that nobody came to help them. The clinician acknowledged and validated James's angry feelings. James reported that he often imagined her lying in the street and people just walking around trying to survive and nobody helping. He stated that he was sorry that his uncle had to see her die, but he was glad that his uncle was with her. When asked what he imagined happened when she died, James stated that he was not sure, but he thought his "uncle prayed over her body as she died." The images of his uncle praying seemed somewhat to counterbalance the horrific images of his grandmother lying dead in the street. James stated that it made him "feel good" to know his uncle was there and praying. The clinician suggested that when the image of his grandma lying in the street entered James's mind, he should remember that his uncle was with her and prayed over her.

The clinician explored questions feelings of guilt by asking questions:

> "Do you think you did something that in any way caused your grandmother to die?"
> "Do you think anyone is mad at you because of what happened?"
> "Are you mad at anyone because of what happened?"

Because of these direct questions, James was able to share that he was angry with his mother for not having his grandmother stay with them during the storm. He was able to discuss this and realize that while he thought this and felt angry with his mother, the reality was that they had taken precautions by having his uncle stay with his grandmother, and that there was no way for his mother to know that the water was going to rise at his grandmother's house and not theirs.

After the Storm

In his drawing entitled *After the Storm,* James drew a picture of a house and a school, with a sun both smiling and frowning. The clinician said, "Tell me about your drawing." James stated that his uncle was now living with them in their new house, but his uncle did not like it when James talked about his grandmother. He talked about all of the changes since the storm, such as attending a new school. He explained that the sun is shining and there is no more water, and he is "a little happy now" because he is back in school, the roof on his house is fixed, and his mother takes him out to dinner sometimes. However, James stated he is still sad because his grandmother is not with them anymore, his uncle seems different, and some of his cousins have not come back to the city.

Further discussion included questions:

"Tell me more about the house you drew and what happens inside."
"Tell me about the sun's smile and frown."
"What changes do you like, and what changes are still hard?"
"What would your grandmother tell you now?"
"What would you want to tell her?"

After this discussion, James wrote a story about telling his grandmother about his life now, after the storm, and he was able to share this with the other group members.

In the next component of reconnecting, James was able to share more about his memories of this grandmother and talk about the role she played, and will continue to play, in his life, such as his use of prayer and his goal of going to college. He was able to share all of his drawings and writings with his mother and eventually to share these with his uncle also.

Reconnection

Reengaging in activities that interest the child begins in the initial sessions and continues throughout the intervention. After a disaster, safe recreational opportunities that existed before the disaster may be limited. Therefore, it is important to begin to identify the child's prior and current interests and to find ways to connect him or her to activities. Also, bereaved families confronted with disaster recovery tasks may need to be encouraged to find time for the family to take breaks and engage in pleasurable activities.

A priority is connecting the child to supportive people, since research suggests that this is one of the essentials for coping well. Similar to getting connected with community activities, such as relief agency recreational programs, sports, afterschool programs, clubs, church groups, and so on, the child must feel connected with supportive people. If GTI is being provided in a group format, other children in the group may serve as supports. Children are asked in the assessment who can they can talk with about their thoughts and feelings about their loss and everything that has happened in the disaster. If the child is not able to identify someone, the main focus of the intervention becomes trying to cultivate supportive adults, preferably a parent or family members.

Reconnecting also involves connecting with the positive memories of the deceased. Using the same processing format of drawing, discussing, writing and having others serve as witnesses to children's stories, children are encouraged to explore topics, such as favorite memories, things they miss most, and/or happy times together. The internalized relationship with the deceased may serve as a support for the child.

During this time of reconnecting, positive aspects about the child's current situation are acknowledged, and threads of hope and optimism about the future are elicited by having the child draw, discuss, and write about current things he or she likes about life and hopes for in the future. At the end of the intervention, children are encouraged to share all of their drawings and writings with their parent (or caregiver), allowing the parent to serve as a witness and to encourage parental emotional support and open communication.

CONCLUDING COMMENTS

Challenges and Guidelines

Children experiencing CTG have unique symptoms and responses that are rooted within their cultural context. For example, the grief responses of many African Americans may be more demonstrative than those of Chinese Americans (Nader, Dubrow, & Stamm, 1999). In addition, the meaning of "traumatic death" varies greatly among cultures. Some Vietnamese may view it as a curse that requires exorcism of spirits, while some European Americans may view it as "God's appointed time to go." Therefore, when implementing GTI, mental health clinicians must develop multicultural competencies, including self-awareness, knowledge of cultures, and skills that are sensitive to specific cultures (Sue, Arredondo, & McDavis, 1992; Webb, 2001).

Some children need developmental adaptations to GTI based on their age. For example, younger children benefit from infusion of play therapy procedures of providing therapeutic toys and puppets, and facilitating restorative retelling through play (Baggerly, 2007; Baggerly & Exum, 2008). Older adolescents may prefer to use creative writing or drama therapy during their restorative retelling.

If children's symptoms persist after GTI is implemented, clinicians may need to provide or make referrals for ongoing individual psychotherapy. Family counseling may also be needed to adapt interactional patterns and strengthen the family system. Clinicians may need to provide social justice advocacy to obtain equity in resources and children's rights within social systems (schools, government agencies, insurance, etc.) (Constantine, Hage, Kindaichi, & Bryant, 2007).

Repeatedly hearing graphic stories of death and trauma can cause mental health clinicians to develop "compassion fatigue." This phenomenon is defined by Gentry (2002) as the synergistic effect of primary traumatic stress from the clinician's own prior trauma, secondary traumatic stress from hearing the client's story, and burnout. To prevent compassion fatigue, mental health clinicians should develop a compassion fatigue resilience plan. Helpful components of such a plan are developing a personal/professional mission statement, maintaining a nonanxious presence, self-soothing, exercise, healthy eating, spiritual rituals, self-validation, connecting with supportive peers, counseling for self, and supervision (Gentry, 2002; Maschi & Brown, Chapter 17, this volume).

Hope and Resilience

Thousands of children worldwide experience devastating traumatic grief due to the death of loved ones in natural disasters every year. However, there is hope for children and families, because the human spirit is strong and resilient. Healing can be facilitated by caring, trained, skilled professionals who understand (1) the prevalence and increasing rate of natural disasters; (2) children's common and atypical symptoms; (3) risk and resilience factors; (4) a range of immediate, short-term, and long-term psychological interventions; (5) GTI procedures; and (6) guidelines for challenges. Clinicians should commit to being a part of the healing by implementing these strategies to create a caring community for children and families who experienced a loved one's death due to a natural disaster.

DISCUSSION QUESTIONS AND ROLE-PLAY EXERCISES

Discussion Questions

1. Contrast the potential symptoms of the following children who had a family member killed during an earthquake: (a) a 5-year-old European American boy living with his single mother, who has a disability, and two siblings in public housing; (b) a 10-year-old African American girl who lives with her mother and father in an upper-middle-class home; (c) a 13-year-old Mexican American girl who lives with her parents and grandparents in a lower-middle-class home; and (d) a 17-year-old boy who is a refugee from Darfur and lives with his mother in public housing. Which child is most at risk? Explain.

2. Which immediate, short-term, and long-term interventions would you recommend for these children? What cultural adaptations would you recommend?

3. Discuss a research study design for GTI. Specify participants, instruments, control or comparison group, methods, duration, and data analysis.

4. Based on this chapter, what systems changes and interventions would

you recommend to the Federal Emergency Management Agency (FEMA) and the Department of Health and Human Services (DHHS)? What systems changes and interventions would you recommend to your local government and community agencies, as well as school districts?

5. Develop and describe your compassion fatigue resilience plan. How would you guard against countertransference of deaths that you have experienced? What will be the most difficult part for you in working with children who experienced traumatic grief? What will you do to prepare?

Role-Play Exercises

1. Role-play a clinician implementing the GTI assessment process with a 5-year-old European American boy who lives with his single mother, who has a disability, and two siblings in public housing.

2. Role-play a clinician implementing the GTI resilience phase with a 10-year-old African American girl who lives with her mother and father in an upper-middle-class home.

3. Role-play a clinician implementing the GTI restorative retelling phase with a 13-year-old Mexican American girl who lives with her parents and grandparents in a lower-middle-class home.

4. Role-play a clinician implementing the GTI reconnection phase with a 17-year-old boy who is a refugee from Darfur and lives with his mother in public housing.

REFERENCES

Abramson, D., Redlener, I., Stehling-Ariza, T., & Fuller, E. (2007). *The legacy of Katrina's children: Estimating the numbers of at-risk children in the Gulf Coast states of Louisiana and Mississippi* (National Center for Disaster Preparedness Columbia University Mailman School of Public Health Research Brief 2007:12). Retrieved August 19, 2008, from *www. ncdp.mailman.columbia.edu/files/legacy_katrina_children.pdf.*

Abramson, D., Stehling-Ariza, T., Garfield, R., & Redlener, I. (2008). Prevalence and predictors of mental health distress post-Katrina: Findings from the Gulf Coast child and family health study. *Disaster Medicine and Public Health Preparedness, 2,* 77–86.

American Academy of Pediatrics. (n.d.). *Psychosocial issues for children and families in disasters: A guide for the primary care physician.* Elk Grove Village, IL: Author.

Baggerly, J. (2007). International interventions and challenges following the crisis of natural disasters. In N. Webb (Ed.), *Play therapy with children in crisis* (3rd ed., pp. 345–367). New York: Guilford Press.

Baggerly, J. N., & Exum, H. (2008). Counseling children after natural disasters: Guidance for family therapists. *American Journal of Family Therapy, 36*(1), 79–93.

Cohen, J. A., Mannarino, A. P., & Deblinger, E. (2006). *Treating trauma and traumatic grief in children and adolescents.* New York: Guilford Press.

Constantine, M. G., Hage, S. M., Kindaichi, M. M., & Bryant, R. M. (2007). Social justice and multicultural issues: Implications for the practice and training of counselors and counseling psychologists. *Journal of Counseling and Development, 85,* 24–29.

Federal Emergency Management Agency. (2008). *Disaster information.* Retrieved August 19, 2008, from *www.fema.gov/news/disasters.fema.*

Gentry, J. E. (2002). Compassion fatigue: A crucible of transformation. S. Gold & J. Faust (Eds.), *Trauma practice in the wake of September 11, 2001* (pp. 37–61). New York: Haworth Press.

Herman, J. L. (1997). *Trauma and recovery.* New York: Basic Books.

Jones, R. T., Frary, R., Cunningham, P., Weddle, D. J., & Kaiser, L. (2001). The psychological effects of Hurricane Andrew on ethnic minority and Caucasian children and adolescents: A case study. *Cultural Diversity and Ethnic Minority Psychology, 7*(1), 103–108.

Knabb, R. D., Rhome, J. R., & Brown, D. P. (2005). *Tropical Cyclone Report Hurricane Katrina 23–30 August 2005* [National Hurricane Center]. Retrieved August 15, 2006, from *www.nhc.noaa.gov/pdf/TCR-AL122005_Katrina.pdf.*

La Greca, A. M. (2008). Interventions for posttraumatic stress in children and adolescents following natural disasters and acts of terrorism. In R. G. Steele, T. D. Elkin, & M. C. Roberts (Eds.), *Handbook of evidence-based therapies for children and adolescents: Bridging science and practice* (pp. 121–141). New York: Springer Science.

La Greca, A. M., Silverman, W. K., & Wasserstein, S. B. (1998). Children's predisaster functioning as a predictor of posttraumatic stress following Hurricane Andrew. *Journal of Consulting and Clinical Psychology, 66,* 883–892.

Nader, K., Dubrow, N., & Stamm, B. H. (1999). *Honoring differences: Cultural issues in the treatment of trauma and loss.* Philadelphia: Brunner/Mazel.

Perry, B., Pollard, R, Blakely, T., Baker, W., & Vigilante, D. (1995). Childhood trauma, the neurobiological adaptation and "use-dependent" development of the brain: How "states become traits." *Infant Mental Health Journal, 16*(4), 271–291.

Pynoos, R. S., & Eth, S. (1984). The child as witness to homicide. *Journal of Social Issues, 40*(2), 87–108.

Rosenfeld, L. B., Caye, J. S., Ayalon, O., & Lahad, M. (2005). *When their world falls apart: Helping families and children manage the effects of disasters.* Washington, DC: National Association of Social Workers Press.

Rynearson, R. (2001). *Retelling violent death.* Philadelphia: Brunner/Routledge.

Salloum, A. (2004). *Group work with adolescents after violent death: A manual for practitioners.* Philadelphia: Brunner/Routledge.

Salloum, A. (2006). *Project LAST (Loss and Survival Team) elementary age grief and trauma intervention manual.* Unpublished treatment manual.

Salloum, A. (2008). Group therapy for children experiencing grief and trauma due to homicide and violence: A pilot study. *Research on Social Work Practice, 18,* 198–211.

Salloum, A., & Overstreet, S. (2008). Evaluation of individual and group grief and trauma interventions for children post-disaster. *Journal of Clinical Child and Adolescent Psychology, 37*(3), 495–507.

Scheuren, J. M., le Polain, O., Below, R., Guha-Sapir, D., & Ponserre, S. (2008). *Annual Disaster Statistical Review: The numbers and trends 2007.* Brussels: Centre for Research of the Epidemiology of Disasters.

Silverman, W. K., & La Greca, A. M. (2002). Children experiencing disasters: Definitions, reactions, and predictors of outcomes. In A. M. LaGreca, W. K. Silverman, E. M. Vernberg, & M. C. Roberts (Eds.), *Helping children cope with disasters and terrorism* (pp. 11–34). Washington, DC: American Psychological Association.

Speier, A. H. (2000). *Psychosocial issues for children and adolescents in disasters* (2nd ed.). Washington, DC: U.S. Department of Health and Human Services.

Spence, P. R., Lachlan, K. A., & Burke, J. M. (2007). Adjusting to uncertainty: Coping strategies among the displaced after Hurricane Katrina. *Sociological Spectrum, 6,* 653–678.

Stacey, K., & Loptson, C. (1995). Children should be seen and not heard?: Questioning the unquestioned. *Journal of Systemic Therapies, 14*(4), 16–31.

Sue, D. W., Arredondo, P., & McDavis, R. J. (1992). Multicultural counseling competencies and standards: A call to the profession. *Journal of Multicultural Counseling and Development, 20,* 64–88.

U.S. Fire Administration. (2007). *Residential structure fires statistics.* Retrieved November 12, 2007, from *www.usfa.dhs.gov/statistics/national/residential.shtm.*

Vernberg, E. M., La Greca, A. M., Silverman, W. K., & Prinstein, M. J. (1996). Prediction of posttraumatic stress symptoms in children after Hurricane Andrew. *Journal of Abnormal Psychology, 105*(2), 237–248.

Webb, N. B. (2001). (Ed.). *Culturally diverse parent, child, and family relationships: A guide for social workers and other practitioners.* New York: Columbia University Press.

Webb, N. B. (2004). (Ed.). *Mass trauma and violence: Helping families and children cope.* New York: Guilford Press.

Weems, C. F., Pina, A. A., & Costa, N. M. (2007). Predisaster trait anxiety and negative affect predict posttraumatic stress in youths after Hurricane Katrina. *Journal of Consulting and Clinical Psychology, 75,* 154–159.

White, M., & Epston, D. (1990). *Narrative means to therapeutic ends.* New York: Norton.

PART IV

INTERVENTIONS WITH BEREAVED CHILDREN

CHAPTER 13

Cognitive-Behavioral Therapy and Play Therapy for Childhood Trauma and Loss

JANINE SHELBY

Despite strong empirical support for the use of cognitive-behavioral therapy (CBT) to treat anxiety and depression in both youngsters and adults, recent discussion in the child CBT literature has identified problems in the developmental fit between CBT and young children. For example, some cognitive skills (e.g., the ability to shift one's cognitions, engage in causal reasoning, or perceive self in relation to others) are inherent in both cognitive-behavioral theory and treatment, but the extent to which young children can engage in such cognitive tasks has been questioned (Grave & Blissett, 2004; Ollendick, Grills, & King, 2001; Southam-Gerow & Kendall, 2000; Stallard, 2002). Other issues related to childhood development have also been raised, including the concern that CBT's reliance on verbal and didactic—as opposed to experiential and active learning—methods may not be developmentally sensitive for many children (Shelby & Berk, 2009). In contrast to CBT, there is little question in the literature as to play therapy's developmental sensitivity, though there is also far less research to support its efficacy for distressed children. Recently, an increased interest in blending CBT with play therapy (PT) has emerged (Drewes, 2009; Knell, 2009; Shelby & Berk, 2009). Though this discussion is not new, having appeared sporadically in the literature for more than 15 years (Gil & Johnson, 1993; Grave & Blissett, 2004; Knell, 1993; Schaefer, 1999; Shelby, 2000; Shelby & Felix, 2005; Webb, 2007), there is now heightened interest in fostering greater integration among pedagogy, child development, PT, and evidence-based treatments. In both CBT and PT literature, there is widespread agreement that treatments for young children should be developed, modified, or blended, such that the therapies are developmentally sensitive and research-based or evidence-informed.

A blend of CBT's key treatment ingredients with PT's developmentally sensitive orientation would seem to be a complementary and innovative union, but to what extent are these treatments already merged? It is commonplace in the PT literature to find descriptions of young children whose play sessions emphasize, or at least involve, alterations in cognitions and behaviors, though these phenomena may not be described using CBT theory and terminology.

In this chapter I speculate that PT has strong cognitive elements, and that the cognitive aspects of CBT for young children may be enhanced by the use of PT. To create a context for the discussion, I describe a poignant case of a young trauma survivor with a terminal illness. After a few sessions, the boy's initial course of CBT was shifted to a type of PT that fit within the broad class of child-led PT approaches. I responded to the child's play with fundamental PT techniques, such as description, reflection, and interpretation of his play narratives and play themes. I offered empathy; reflected the characters' feelings, dilemmas, and actions; and "mourned" with my young patient when his characters did not "survive" their quests. Occasionally, I asked questions with content designed to suggest the potential for a sense of mastery, adaptive coping, or other adaptive responses. My remarks about the child's play remained within his play metaphor. For the most part, the boy led his own play narratives, with minimal direction from me. He spontaneously found solutions to the problems he faced in his play scenarios, and solace and gratification in his play, even when the themes he played were exquisitely sad.

A fundamental premise of this chapter is that similar alterations of cognitive processes are likely to occur among young children during the course of several distinct forms of PT (e.g., psychodynamic, humanistic, and prescriptive). The child's cognitive experience, as demonstrated in his play narrative, is compared to the cognitive processes hypothesized to occur in CBTs. Though conceptual rather than empirical in nature, this chapter is intended to explore specific ways in which PT might achieve primary CBT goals, such as the alteration of cognitions and cognitive processes.

THE CASE OF NATHAN

Nathan was a 7-year-old boy with a keen sense of humor and a great yearning for adventure, despite his frequent hospitalizations. Nathan's life-threatening illness was advanced, and his prognosis tended to be whispered rather than spoken by the adults in his world. Nathan's mother and older sisters were usually at his bedside and did their best to instill hope, provide comfort, and lend psychological support. Yet there were topics that were difficult for him to discuss with them. A certain pessimism descended when Nathan's condition was assessed, and there were clear boundaries between what Nathan experienced and what he and his family could bear to express with words. Some among the medical staff referred to him as avoidant, and were concerned about his difficulty discussing his illness. Therein was the sanctity of his play sessions, which I describe in more detail in the following pages. Therapeutic play gave Nathan power, irrespective of his prognosis, his family's pain, and his own grief over the loss of his future life. This power, comingled with the comfort he found in his family's support, was sufficient to help Nathan endure what he faced as he lived and as he died.

One of my first impressions of Nathan was that he loved to play. Nathan's hospital room was littered with toys. We initially discussed pain management techniques, coping strategies, and various problem-solving methods. I explored behavioral activation strategies (e.g., assisting him to engage in as many pleasurable activities as possible) and assessed for misattributions regarding his illness. I further provided psychoeducation, psychological support, and family-based interventions. In short, I covered the standard curricula designed to assist hospitalized youngsters like Nathan. He was usually patient and cooperative and seemed to benefit from some of the strategies and interventions he was provided. Yet Nathan preferred to play rather than to verbalize the salient themes in his experience. Regularly, he implored, "Now can we play?" I began to ponder how to make his treatment more engaging, and how to weigh a child's preference against the more empirically sound but less developmentally engaging treatments available to assist youngsters like him. So, I reconsidered my standard treatment protocol. He had asked me to play with him, so I did.

During the first weeks of our therapy, Nathan's custom during our sessions was to build an impressive array of castles. He explained that the inhabitants lived safely behind sturdy walls in castle cities that stretched into the clouds. Without directly ascribing his play themes to his illness, Nathan's play depicted the course of his illness with remarkable clarity and intent. One play narrative recurred frequently during the first weeks I knew Nathan. With figurines surrounding him in his bed, Nathan pretended that all the young men of the city were called to serve in the military under the High General's command, so they could protect their castles. In special training activities, these brave young men learned to ride gallant white stallions, on which they performed amazing equestrian feats. The General, who rode with the most skill on the best white stallion, taught the younger men valuable lessons of both riding and valor.

The General, the men, and their horses made powerful armies. Attacks by invading gray knights were frequent but unsuccessful. During these play sessions, the young heroes on their white stallions proclaimed victory over the invaders again and again. During the many raging battles in his play, cowards always lost conflicts to brave men, and hopelessness transformed itself to triumph. In Nathan's world of fantasy, miracles were yet possible, awkward young men grew to become thriving soldiers, and fear receded into the mist outside his fortressed walls. As his body deployed its own defense, Nathan's pretend defenders boldly protected the castles nestled in the mountains near the clouds. This was the world he understood, and the one in which I believe he found considerable hope and comfort.

His family members relished Nathan's descriptions of the battles, which he enjoyed embellishing in the stories he told them after our meetings. After I suggested that she do so, Nathan's mother became adept at reiterating the themes of persistence, bravery, and survival that dominated his play themes. During this phase, Nathan's play, and the corresponding tales he told about it, created a safe medium of communication for Nathan and his family. Nathan's play also served another important purpose. As he suffered and sought hope to withstand his ordeal, Nathan's play proved to him that his survival was, at least, a *possible* outcome of a heinous and devastating war.

During the next phase of his illness, Nathan's play began to change in its tone. The dreaded gray knights began overtaking the fortress walls. The gray knights began to capture the kingdom, piece by piece. On their white horses, the defenders battled fiercely to protect their castles and their cities. The wars often raged across many sessions. During these days of our play, the defenders tried one strategy after another to save their kingdom. They showed bravery and quickness of wit, and endured much suffering. Despite their best effort, the battles were lost in one disappointing fight after another. In one poignant battle, the General, who was high atop the mountain in the clouds, received word that the kingdom was falling. Upon hearing this dreaded news, the General rushed to his stable to release his beloved white horse so that, at least, the horse could escape. With the command "Away my good horse!", the horse jumped without its master over the city's walls, where it escaped into the remoteness of distant mountains.

As the world of castles and soldiers continued to crumble at the hands of the invaders, the medical professionals responsible for Nathan's care believed that he was near the end of his life. As he struggled to survive, even the once-compelling world of play no longer held as much intrigue for him. Castles now rested in the corner of his hospital room. Soldiers lay relieved of their duties on the window sill. Cities in the clouds no longer spread across his bed. Nathan was too fatigued to play when I visited him, but he sometimes reminisced with me about his castles and his stronger days of battle. When his medical situation became particularly bleak, I told Nathan that the decision about how to face the next battle was solely his. I described how history was full of exceptional generals, some of whom had won after long, bitter battles and others of whom had not emerged victorious but were long remembered for their heroism. "Really?" Nathan asked. He looked relieved, so I continued to speak to him using terms appropriate for his metaphor. I said that surrendering and defending were two different ways to be brave, and that each way was as brave as the other. In a family meeting the next day, Nathan and I described to his family how the "General" was trying his best to figure out what to do in the midst of so many recent defeats. No one used the word "death," but everyone understood what Nathan intended to convey, and Nathan remained fully communicative and descriptive regarding the topic of his "battle." The meetings with Nathan and his family were filled with grief, but I was grateful that he had found a metaphor that allowed us to speak about the challenges that he faced.

As the destiny of the falling kingdom emerged for Nathan, he began to ask for a castle, the General, and horses to be placed on his bed, though he rarely found the energy to play. "Hey," he said, stopping me as I left his room one afternoon near the end of his life. "You can tell other kids about the white horse." He continued slowly, deliberately, and pensively, "You know, at least, the white horse gets away." Then, he recited his own play narrative, in which—in the midst of a losing battle—the General made his way to the stable high atop a mountain. Nathan described how it took the General a long time to reach the mountaintop, as if it were more arduous to find his last white horse in this iteration of the play narrative. At last, the General found his horse, and he reminded the stallion that it had to go on without him. Then, speaking as the General, Nathan said, "Away my good horse!" He repeated his command a couple of times before I joined him. "Away my good horse," we pronounced together softly and sadly. At this conjoint decree, Nathan issued a subtle but peaceful smile.

In my next meeting with him, I struggled with my own opposition to his illness. I wondered aloud whether, upon reaching his horse, the General needed to do anything else. I silently hoped that the General could ride the last white horse to a safe vantage point, where he could build an even stronger castle to withstand the battles that besieged him. I commented on the fact that there had been many battles before, and that by now the General was very good at figuring out the best thing to do. After a period of silence, I finally wondered aloud whether anything at all could make him more comfortable that day. Nathan responded by asking for a castle and some of his toy walls. When I handed them to him, he said plainly, "I don't *want* these anymore [as if to say, 'I don't need these now; they can't help me']. Just the horses from now on, OK?" I realized what he was telling me. There would be no more battles; the General would not survive. My task was to bear witness to the heroic General and the escaping horse. Weeks before, Nathan had figured out how the play narrative ended. In his play, he came to terms with his mortality, and now, in the terms of his metaphor, Nathan was slowly making his way to the stable to release his stallion. He looked fatigued, so I concluded our session. "Just the horses," I echoed. "You need the horses from now on. At least, you can send a horse to a safe place. Maybe, that is how there is escape from the invaders, even when it seems that there is no escape." He nodded with tranquil satisfaction when I asked whether I understood him correctly, and he held my gaze for a few seconds longer than usual. Then, he handed me the castle to put away, and closed his eyes.

When I left Nathan's room, I felt the profound sadness of his impending death. I longed to spare Nathan, and the impossibility of doing so roused my own sense of inadequacy and despair. As I recognized and accepted my reactions, my despair gave way to a renewed willingness to tolerate the sadness and grief that pervaded my work with Nathan. I realized my powerlessness over the course of Nathan's illness, but instead of dwelling on what I could not control, I focused myself on knowing him in the full depth of his experience, and on the privilege of doing whatever I could to make his pain easier to bear. In this way, my empathy evolved into the courage to accompany him through whatever he needed.

While he slept in his hospital bed that evening, I returned to Nathan's room. His sleeping body seemed implausibly small for someone who had played with such mightiness. I took a single white horse out of the box that contained his toy horses and left it for him at his bedside table. I wanted him to have a tangible reminder that his special white horse could be freed to roam whatever mountains exist in the clouds beyond this life.

Apart from a couple of brief visits while he was heavily sedated, I never saw Nathan awake again. His family was instructed to make a white horse available to him, when he desired one. I visited Nathan several times while he slept. Once, a white horse lay near Nathan's hand, as if the horse had been in Nathan's grasp before sleep had released both of them. I paused at the sight of Nathan in his hospital bed. I thought of him as the General, now preparing his own white horse for escape. That evening, I lingered in his quiet, dimly lit room, remembering the hours in which he had been a boy at play with castle cities and valiant warriors. Through his play, Nathan had prepared himself and his family for the battle, as well as for the outcome. In his play and verbalizations about his play narratives, Nathan had rehearsed this moment many times. As I watched him sleep, I realized what Nathan would have wanted me to do. I summoned all my courage but produced little more than the whisper, "Away my good horse." Then, more powerfully came "Away my good horse!", which I declared for Nathan as a final command on his behalf.

Nathan's mother was with him when he died a few days later. After Nathan's death, I sent his family the most regally decorated toy white horse I could find. They told me that they hung it in a memory box in their hallway. As for me, it has been more than 15 years, and I continue to keep a small plastic likeness of the horse with which Nathan and I played. It reminds me of him. It reminds me to be brave. It reminds me that a long time ago, a courageous boy knew that playing would help him find closure and peace as he found ways to link his illness to his life, his life to his death, and his death to his memory. Finally, it reminds me that—although knowledge about PT's effectiveness is incomplete—PT holds enormous value for at least some young children.

HOW SIMILAR ARE COGNITIVE THERAPY AND PLAY THERAPY?

In Nathan's case, a PT approach was used with a youngster who preferred to play rather than speak directly about his illness, anxiety, problems, and emotional conflicts. Apart from the use of toys and the emphasis on play, there was considerable overlap between the objectives of traditional CBT and the PT with Nathan. In Nathan's PT sessions, four of the six most common cognitive components in child CBTs (as noted by Spence, 1994) were present, including the following: (1) problem-solving; (2) self-statement modification; (3) stress inoculation training; and (4) cognitive restructuring. (The remaining two components, self-control and social skills training, were less salient to Nathan's presenting concerns.) In his play narrative, Nathan identified and processed his emotions and reactions to his illness, he generated and tested hypothetical solutions to his problems, and he experimented with various methods of managing or coping with distress. In the play narratives he created for his pretend soldiers, Nathan demonstrated (i.e., through his characters' actions and statements) various coping methods to deal with adversity and tolerate discomfort. As his illness worsened, he reassessed his situation and shifted both his play and cognitions away from battle and toward closure.

In addition to the cognitive aspects of his play, there were behavior-ally mediated benefits as well. The act of playing itself was often help-ful to Nathan, in that it provided a means of behavioral activation, a behavioral coping strategy (i.e., distraction), as well as a tangible way in which he could experiment with altering his cognitions (e.g., charac-ters engaged in cognitive reframing). Also, the play metaphor provided an important medium in which Nathan could communicate the experi-ence of his illness to his family. Notably, Nathan usually played first and then verbalized some of the issues, solutions, or coping efforts he had discovered or developed during his play. So several elements of CBT were present during Nathan's play-based treatment, but in addition to these components, Nathan's play offered benefits that go beyond CBT-targeted goals. Nathan was comforted and gratified by his creativity. He derived pleasure from his play, and he experienced a sense of empower-ment from developing ingenious solutions to the problems he posed dur-ing his play narratives.

How much overlap exists between PT and CBT? It is reasonable to assume that when there are positive changes in a child's affect during PT sessions, these changes are usually related to changes in the child's cog-nition or behavior. Thus, CBT's fundamental premise about the interre-latedness of thoughts, behavior, and affect holds true for play therapists. It is not clear whether the specific process (e.g., cognitive shifting) by which these cognitive alterations occur is also shared by both PT and CBT therapists, but if so, the treatments may differ more in terms of their packaging and delivery than their content. To examine this issue, it would be helpful to "dismantle" CBT and PT to separate the core treatment components from the methods through which the treatment curricula is delivered. Is it possible that PT is a more developmentally sensitive but less defined and researched relative of CBT?

DISMANTLING THE KEY INGREDIENTS OF COGNITIVE-BEHAVIORAL THERAPY AND PLAY THERAPY

To address the question as to how closely related CBT and PT are, a review of the specific elements, or key ingredients, of each treatment is included in the following pages. A number of authors have discussed and explored the key ingredients of CBT's therapeutic success, but PT's change agents are not well understood. CBTs, at least those written for adults, have defined therapeutic gain in terms of altering two primary ingredients: cognition and behavior. Several authors in the PT field have proposed a diverse array of key ingredients, usually referred to as "curative factors," but little consensus emerges across the diverse theoretical orientations of play therapists. The discussion that follows focuses on specific key ingredients that are directly related to the components of individual sessions with young children. An exhaustive review of all the factors related to positive psychotherapy outcomes for children (e.g., the involvement of adult caregivers in the child's treatment) is beyond the scope of this chapter.

Cognitive-Behavioral Therapy

The question as to *whether* CBTs are effective for anxious or depressed adults and older children has been affirmatively answered in a compelling body of research. Thus far, research regarding CBTs for children younger than 8 years old has been limited. The therapeutic gains for adults and older youth are thought to be related to both key ingredients of the approach (i.e., behavioral and cognitive alterations). In the cognitive portion of CBTs, clients learn to alter their thoughts, and the ways in which they think about their thoughts (i.e., metacognition) by engaging in mental techniques such as reinterpreting or reframing the cognitions. At least with older youth and adults, CBTs have emphasized specific aspects of cognition (e.g., "mediated thoughts" and "cognitive shifting"). The *behavioral* components of the treatment do not pose developmental challenges to the underlying theory given that behavior appears from birth, and there is a logical link between behavior and corresponding changes in emotion or mood. However, the *cognitive* components of the treatment are more problematic. In their review, Grave and Blissett (2004) identify several issues regarding the fit between CBT interventions for young children and childhood development, including the following: (1) whether young children have the cognitive developmental capacity to use CBT; (2) the role of cognitive development in the therapeutic process (e.g., the CBT rationalist paradigm base requires a range of cognitive skills that young children may not fully possess, such as self-reflection, information processing, language, reasoning, and memory); and (3) the models underpinning the therapeutic approaches do not fully account for normative cognitive development (e.g., cognitive errors are normative for young children, but cognitive errors are targeted for intervention in most CBTs). As a result of these issues, the assumption that cognitive shifts produce a corresponding change in emotion or mood is much less theoretically "tidy" when applied to young children. In fact, some have questioned whether cognitive shifting plays a key role in therapeutic gain from CBTs for young children (Grave & Blissett, 2004). Others have emphasized behavioral over cognitive factors as accounting for therapeutic benefit to children (Mahoney & Nezworksi, 1985).

So, the question of how central the alteration of thoughts is to therapeutic gain for young children has yet to be answered. Perhaps, cognitive shifting may not be as fundamental to childhood CBT gains as it is
to gains made by adults. Another possibility is that cognitive shifting
is important to the success of CBT in young children, but CBT's typical methods of teaching and learning may make it difficult for young
children to engage in and achieve cognitive shifts. Thus, it may be the
method (i.e., verbally based, didactically oriented) rather than the skill
itself that is cognitively taxing for young children.

Play Therapy

Research on PT's efficacy for distressed children is limited. Historically,
play therapists have not emphasized research, and specific, manualized
forms of PT have rarely been compared to CBT. Therefore, the use of PT
has not been *disproven*, it simply has not been adequately researched.
Whereas CBT is a specific, defined therapy with similar treatment for-
mats, components, and procedures, PT is a broad term that loosely
encompasses many forms of PT, including CBT (see Knell, 1993; 2009)
and several other treatments. To further complicate the issue, there is
also overlap between CBTs and some PTs given that some CBTs use play-
based interventions as a vehicle to achieve CBT goals (Asarnow, Scott,
& Mintz, 2002; Knell, 1993; Podell, Martin, & Kendall, 2009; Shelby
& Berk, 2009; Webb, 2007).

PT is only beginning to establish its research base, and empirical
examination of PT's key ingredients is extremely limited. The 2008 Association for Play Therapy (p. 2) definition describes PT as "the systematic
use of a theoretical model to establish an interpersonal process wherein
trained play therapists use the therapeutic powers of play to help clients"
but no specific elements of PT's "therapeutic power" are named. Several authors have hypothesized which qualities might be related to PT's
therapeutic value. Schaefer and Drewes (2009) discuss a comprehensive
list of therapeutic powers based on Schaefer's (1999) work, including
the following: self-expression; access to the unconscious; direct and
indirect teaching; abreaction; stress inoculation; counterconditioning of
negative affect; catharsis; positive affect; sublimation; attachment and
relationship enhancement; moral judgment; empathy; power/control;
competence and self-control; sense of self; accelerated development; creative problem solving; fantasy compensation; reality testing; behavioral
rehearsal; and rapport building. Landreth's (1991) definition of PT suggests that the key ingredients might be as follows: (1) the use of play
materials; (2) the therapeutic relationship; and (3) the expression, identification, and discovery of various aspects of affect, cognition, history,
and behavior. Drewes (2009, p. 4) described PT as providing "power

and control that comes from solving problems and mastering new experiences, ideas, and concerns." Although the specific definitions of PT's key ingredients vary, their authors share the assumption that cognitive processes help to foster therapeutic change.

TOWARD SYNTHESIS OF COGNITIVE-BEHAVIORAL THERAPY AND PLAY THERAPY

There has been general agreement in the CBT literature that treatments for children should be more developmentally sensitive, but few specific recommendations emerge as to how to modify treatments for younger children. Attempts to integrate cognitive developmental level into CBT generally involve the following suggestions: (1) Rely less on complex techniques or techniques that require advanced cognitive skills; (2) rely less on verbal methods; and (3) add more pictures, story-based representations, or metaphors depicting therapeutic tasks. Some authors suggest an emphasis on behaviorally active learning techniques (Grave & Blissett, 2004; Shelby & Berk, 2009). In their critical review, Grave and Blissett (2004) sound as though they are justifying the use of PT—though they are merely arguing for increased use of metaphor, analogies, and stories in child CBT protocols—when they cite Friedberg (1994):

> Abstract concepts (e.g., causal mediators), can be given concrete form, and introspection can take place externally. Reasoning can be demonstrated using creative and engaging analogy and metaphor. Egocentrism becomes a therapeutic advantage, with the child's story representing a projection of his own thoughts, beliefs, and self-representation. . . . The limitations of domain-specific knowledge, memory, and motivation are easily overcome with an interesting and exciting story using the child's protagonists, settings, and storylines. (p. 416)

Grave and Blissett (p. 417) go on to emphasize that therapists should find appropriate metaphors around which children can build therapeutic narratives, which again seemingly endorses PT's traditional use of play narratives. In any event, there is an interesting parallel between century-old PT practices and endorsements arising from the CBT literature to use less verbal and more concrete, metaphoric, and child-created narratives.

A Note Regarding Metaphors

The recommendation to use therapeutic metaphors and analogies is widespread, but a small caveat is in order. Several authors, including myself, have made attempts to include metaphors in child treatments to enhance developmental sensitivity. As a result, a diverse group of metaphors exists in CBTs (e.g., "Running Thoughts Off My Land"; "Bad Thought Monsters"; "Zen Warriors," who help to fight maladaptive thoughts; "Touching Monster"; "Coping Menus"; or "Coaches," who provide alternative self-statements). Though designed to be developmentally sensitive, treatment developers face challenges when they propose metaphors that will be used by a diverse array of children from different geographic regions, cultures, religions, and socioeconomic groups. As a result, some metaphors selected for inclusion into manualized treatments may be unfamiliar, frightening, or even objectionable to youth and their caregivers. This is not to discourage the use of metaphors and analogies, but to make a stronger case for considering the use of a child's *self-generated* metaphor, when possible, to reduce the possibility of a metaphor–child "misfit." There may be times when children may be more skilled at generating appropriate metaphors for themselves than therapists or manual authors would be, and a child's self-initiated metaphors may be qualitatively superior to the "one-size-fits-all" metaphors predetermined by professionals.

Caveat Regarding the Generalizability of Nathan's Case

Nathan was, admittedly, adept at resolving his own psychological issues, and the PT portion of his treatment progressed with a minimal level of clinical intervention. Not all children achieve this kind of benefit from their play. For example, children who engage in repetitive, posttraumatic play lacking spontaneous resolutions and adaptive problem-solving skills may require a more directive, skills-focused approach. Even so, many of these children might benefit from play-based efforts to integrate psychoeducation, cognitive aspects of treatment, and skills training into the children's own play narratives and play-based metaphors, to the fullest extent possible.

Substance or Packaging?

It would be interesting to explore whether the typical devices used to deliver CBTs (e.g., the use of workbook assignments, written exercises, and verbal discussions—or even verbally described metaphors) add to or detract from the treatment's success with young children. Similarly, research is needed to discern whether PT's delivery techniques (e.g., child's self-generated metaphor; use of play materials; and instructional methods involving experiential, active learning methods) show advantages or disadvantages compared to traditional CBT delivery methods. Until this research is conducted, clinicians are left to draw their own conclusions, to consider making developmentally sensitive modifications to CBTs when necessary, and to attempt to find a balance between treatments that are developmentally sensitive and those that are evidence based but, perhaps, less developmentally sensitive.

CONCLUDING COMMENTS

Questions remain about the relative impact of the cognitive elements of CBT interventions with young children, and the extent to which therapeutic change is cognitively or behaviorally mediated. In this chapter, I speculated that some forms of PT share several core components with CBT, and that the phenomenon of cognitive shifting among young children may occur more readily in PT than in verbally mediated treatments. Perhaps, there is less difference between the key ingredients of both the treatments, when they are successful delivered, than some have recognized. Given the advice in the CBT literature to achieve greater developmental sensitivity in CBTs, as well as the emerging discussion of CBT's misalignment with development, it is surprising that PTs have not been integrated into CBTs to a greater extent. However, the PT field has yet to establish a strong research base to define and support its various forms of treatment. Whereas play therapists are called upon to empirically examine the efficacy of PT, explore the key ingredients of PT, and integrate evidence-based treatments into their practice, cognitive-behavioral therapists would benefit from considering PT's century-long tradition of developmental sensitivity, and most young children's preference to engage in play- rather than verbally based interventions.

As a final note, I hope that Nathan's case stimulates further discussion of a greater CBT–PT blend. Based on the number of times he asked me whether we could play yet, I think he would be pleased with that legacy.

DISCUSSION QUESTIONS AND ROLE-PLAY EXERCISES

1. In what ways were Nathan's "cognitive shifts" depicted in his play?
2. What are some possible reasons that Nathan preferred to engage in play-based treatment over more verbal modes of treatment?
3. What would the therapist have needed to do to assist Nathan if PT had not been effective in bringing about cognitive shifts (e.g., if Nathan had merely played defeat in battle repetitively, persistently, and without resolution, gratification, or more positive affect over a sustained period of time).

4. What are some ways in which therapists can deal with their own sense of sadness during treatment of a child like Nathan? If you had been Nathan's therapists, how would you have transformed your grief into something positive?

5. Role play: Imagine a scenario in which you are the therapist engaged in PT with a 6-year-old girl who has a terminal illness. After many weeks of engaging in play narratives, in which the child masters her fears by searching for cures from a magical tree, she begins to engage in less optimistic play narratives. In one session, she plays a scenario in which her character realizes that she will never find the tree she has been searching for to make the play character well. In a role-play activity, respond as if you were the therapist. After completion of this portion of the activity, discuss the extent to which the therapist's responses both conveyed empathy and encouraged the child to find some sense of resolution or comfort.

REFERENCES

Asarnow, J. R., Scott, C. V., & Mintz, J. (2002). A combined cognitive-behavioral family education intervention for depression in children: A treatment development study. *Cognitive Therapy and Research, 26*, 221–229.

Association for Play Therapy. (2008). About APT. Retrieved March 16, 2008, from *www.a4pt.org/ps.aboutapt.cfm?ID=1212*.

Drewes. A. (2009). *Blending play therapy with cognitive behavioral therapy: Evidence-based and other effective techniques.* Hoboken, NJ: Wiley.

Gil, E., & Johnson, T. C. (1993). *Sexualized children: Assessment and treatment of sexualized children and children who molest.* Rockville, MD: Launch Press.

Grave, J., & Blissett, J. (2004). Is cognitive behavior therapy developmentally appropriate for young children?: A critical review of the evidence. *Clinical Psychology Review, 24*, 399–420.

Knell, S. J. (1993). *Cognitive-behavioral play therapy.* Northvale, NJ: Aronson.

Knell, S. J. (2009). Cognitive-behavioral play therapy: Theory and applications. In A. Drewes (Ed.), *Blending play therapy with cognitive behavioral therapy: Evidence-based and other effective techniques* (pp. 117–133). Hoboken, NJ: Wiley.

Landreth, G. (1991). *Play therapy: The art of the relationship.* Muncie, IN: Accelerated Development.

Mahoney, M. J., & Nezworksi, M. T. (1985). Cognitive-behavioral approaches to children's problems. *Journal of Abnormal Child Psychology, 13*, 467–476.

Ollendick, T. H., Grills, A. E., & King, N. J. (2001). Applying developmental theory to the assessment and treatment of childhood disorders: Does it make a difference? *Clinical Psychology and Psychotherapy, 8*, 304–314.

Podell, J. L., Martin, E. D., & Kendall, P. C. (2009). Incorporating play within a manual-based treatment for children and adolescents with anxiety disorders. In A. Drewes (Ed.), *Blending play therapy with cognitive behavioral therapy: Evidence-based and other effective techniques* (pp. 165–178). Hoboken, NJ: Wiley.

Schaefer, C. S. (1999). Curative factors in play therapy. *Journal for the Professional Counselor, 14*(1), 7–16.

Schaefer, C. S., & Drewes, A. (2009). The therapeutic powers of play and play therapy. In A. Drewes (Ed.), *Blending play therapy with cognitive behavioral therapy: Evidence-based and other effective techniques* (pp. 3–15). Hoboken, NJ: Wiley.

Shelby, J. S. (2000). Brief therapy with traumatized children: A developmental perspective. In H. G. Kaduson & C. E. Schaefer (Eds.), *Short-term play therapy for children*. New York: Guilford Press.

Shelby, J. S., & Berk, M. J. (2009). Play therapy, pedagogy, and CBT: An argument for interdisciplinary synthesis. In A. Drewes (Ed.), *Blending play therapy with cognitive behavioral therapy: Evidence-based and other effective techniques* (pp. 17–40). Hoboken, NJ: Wiley.

Shelby, J. S., & Felix, E. (2005). Posttraumatic play therapy: The need for an integrated model of directive and nondirective approaches. In L. A. Reddy, T. M. Files-Hall, & C. Schaefer (Eds.), *Empirically based play interventions for children* (pp. 79–104). Washington, DC: American Psychological Association.

Southam-Gerow, M. A., & Kendall, P. C. (2000). Cognitive-behavior therapy with youth: Advances, challenges and future directions. *Clinical Psychology and Psychotherapy, 7*, 343–366.

Spence, S. H. (1994). Practitioner review: Cognitive therapy with children and adolescents: From theory to practice. *Journal of Child Psychology and Psychiatry, 35*, 1191–1228.

Stallard, P. (2002). Cognitive behavior therapy with children and young people: A selective review of key issues. *Behavioral and Cognitive Psychotherapy, 30*, 297–309.

Webb, N. B. (Ed.). (2007). *Play therapy with children in crisis: Individual, family and group treatment* (3rd ed.). New York: Guilford Press.

CHAPTER 14

Conjoint Caregiver–
Child Treatment Following
a Parent's Death

PATRICIA VAN HORN

This chapter presents developmental frameworks for understanding the phenomenology of young children's grief and for helping children cope with the death of a parent. Grieving children must learn to accept the physical reality of the parent's permanent absence, to cope with trauma and loss reminders, and to regain a positive developmental trajectory by forming new attachments that substitute for the lost parent, without replacing the memory of that unique, loving relationships. Two controversies attend work with children bereaved in early childhood. The first deals with the question of whether young children, in fact, have the capacity to grieve; the second, with the proper sequencing of clinical work when the parent dies suddenly and violently. In this chapter I discuss these issues and, using clinical examples, offer concrete strategies for helping young children who lose a parent to death.

GRIEF IN EARLY CHILDHOOD

Too often adults believe that toddlers who have little language do not understand what is happening and will forget about their lost parent if not reminded. Theoreticians differ in their beliefs about young children's capacity for mourning, with some holding the view that children under 5 years of age lack both the cognitive ability to understand that death

278

is final and the emotional maturity required to tolerate the process of relinquishing a beloved parent before establishing an affective bond with a new attachment figure (Freud, 1960; Spitz, 1960), and others arguing that grief and mourning can occur even in the absence of these skills (Bowlby, 1960, 1980; Furman, 1974; Hofer, 2003). In addition, parents and clinicians refer to children's resilience, suggesting that children have an innate quality that helps them recover quickly and completely from stressful events. The more realistic views of resilience in childhood, however, suggest that it is an interactive process (Cicchetti & Rogosh, 1997), with children able to mobilize their internal resources for coping with stress through the support of trusted adults (Lieberman, Compton, Van Horn, & Ghosh-Ippen, 2003).

In fact, young children's grieving for a lost parent affects every aspect of their functioning and development, with the negative effects mitigated only when surviving adults close to them provide sufficient support.

Case Example

When Carla was 15 months old, her father stabbed her mother to death. Carla was placed in foster care because no family member was able to take her in. At the family's request a social worker brought Carla to the funeral, where she confronted several large photographs of her mother that were on display in the church. One family member who attended the funeral reported that Carla walked up to the photographs, stroked them with her hands, kissed them, and began to cry. A family member carried Carla away from the pictures and back to a social worker, who took her out of the room. No one, however, offered Carla any explanation of what had happened to her mother.

Several weeks later, when Carla was 17 months old, her social worker arranged for a clinician to assess her emotional well-being. The social worker told the clinician that she expected that Carla would be doing well, because she seemed to be developing typically at the time of her removal from home. The clinician met with Carla and her foster mother, Mrs. James, in their home. On her first visit, the clinician asked whether Carla asked for her mother. Her foster parent responded that she did not believe Carla remembered her mother. She said, "She doesn't ask for anyone—not her mother or father or sister. And we haven't said anything about them. I don't know what to say." Mrs. James said, however, that she had no objection to the clinician's speaking with Carla about her family.

When she returned the next week, the clinician showed Carla the picture of her mother, and Carla glanced at it only briefly, showing no sign of recognition, before she put it aside. The clinician said, "That is a picture of your mommy. A sad thing happened to her. She got so hurt that the doctors couldn't help her get better. They tried very hard, but she was too hurt and she died." The clinician told Carla that her mommy could not come to see her anymore, could not walk or talk or play, because she died. She said that Carla's mommy had loved her very much and that she did not want to die, but she got too hurt. Carla listened silently and without any expression on her face. She continued to sit quietly and the clinician handed her a baby doll. She held it briefly, then tossed it aside and looked in the clinician's bag of toys for something else. She found a toy baby bottle and put it in her mouth and sucked on it. The clinician said, "You are still a little baby, too, and you need someone to hold you and feed you. Your mommy used to hold you and feed you. It is so sad that she can't do it any more." At that, Carla crawled into the clinician's lap.

Mrs. James, Carla's foster mother, repeated that Carla did not seem to think about her mother. She did not search for her or respond to her name. She said that, to her, Carla seemed much younger than her 17 months. She had no language. She did not babble. She did not point to things that she wanted, but simply accepted what was given to her. She was willing to be picked up and held once she was familiar with a new person, but she did not actively seek to be hugged or cuddled. Mrs. James said that Carla had warmed up to the clinician faster than she warmed up to most people, and together they speculated that this might be because the clinician talked about her mother and Carla's wish to be a baby again and to be cared for. The foster mother continued, "The thing I worry about is, she doesn't seem to have a little personality. It's like she never learned to be a baby. She doesn't know who she is."

In fact, it seemed that Carla's development across multiple domains had halted with her mother's death. Her separation from her mother was sudden and complete, and it left her withdrawn, and without language or desire. The fact, however, that she responded when the clinician spoke of her mother, and of Carla's wish to be cared for gave promise that with intervention and support, Carla's developmental momentum might be restored.

CHOOSING PATHS FOR INTERVENTION:
TRAUMA AND LOSS

Children, whatever their age, who lose a parent to death are faced with a dual task. They must recall and hold in their minds the love of the deceased parent with whom they will always identify. Simultaneously, they must form allegiances to someone new who will love and care for them, and offer a secure base from which they can explore and grow. Unless children succeed in these tasks, their development will be compromised; psychological intervention with bereaved children focuses on helping them say goodbye to their lost parent without relinquishing their love for that parent, and on forming new attachments.

The challenge that bereaved children face is compounded, however, when the parent's death is sudden and violent. The process of grieving always involves summoning up comforting and sustaining memories of the lost person. After a traumatic death, the bereaved child must incorporate within his or her memory of the lost parent the terrifying sights and sounds that surrounded the death. This begs the question: How is the child to remember her parent without being terrified by the shocking and violent memories that accompanied the death? The wish to avoid the feelings of shock and horror that these memories bring interferes with children's ability to think about their lost parents and interferes with the retrieval of warm, loving memories that will comfort them over time. Because shock and trauma interfere with the grieving process, therapists working with traumatically bereaved children are generally advised to conduct their treatments sequentially: to address first and help the child deal with issues of trauma, then to approach the feelings connected with loss (Cohen, Mannarino, & Deblinger, 2006; Webb, 2007).

For very young children, however, the demands of intervention may be different. Young children form their sense of self around the patterns of care they receive. The way they are handled, rocked, and spoken to is integrated into their core beliefs about who they are. These patterns of caregiving are specific to the caregiver; if the caregiver disappears from the child's life, a young child loses some of his or her basic sense of identity. Further, young children are completely dependent upon their parents or other caregivers for protection from stress and danger. They lack independent coping mechanisms that allow them to maintain neuroposychological regulation, and to sustain an organized and coherent sense of self while undergoing the stress of the grieving process (Hofer, 1996, 2003; Lieberman et al., 2003). For these reasons, the death of a parent, when it occurs in the first 5 years of life, before the child has established an autonomous sense of self, independent of the parent's protection and care, constitutes in itself what Bowlby (1980) called the "trauma of loss." The revised edition of the *Diagnostic Classification of Mental Health and Developmental Disorders of Infancy and Early Childhood* (Zero to Three, 2005) recognized the vulnerability of young children's psychological integrity when it determined that, for these children, a trauma occurs not only when the physical integrity of the child or another is threatened, as mandated by the *Diagnostic and Statistical Manual of*

Mental Disorders (American Psychiatric Association, 2000), but also when the threat is to the psychological integrity of the child or another (Zero to Three, 2005). Bereaved infants, toddlers, and preschoolers face multiple challenges, regardless of whether their parents die in shocking acts of violence, witnessed by the child, or peacefully, after an illness. Clinically, young bereaved children are shocked and overwhelmed, and behave in ways that are mysterious and troubling to their new caregivers, whether these are family members grieving their own loss, or foster parents called in to provide shelter and love to newly homeless children who are strangers to them. Sometimes the children appear desperately upset, crying and searching for their lost parent. At other times, they play as if nothing had happened. Some of these children have the task of processing memories that are traumatic in the classic sense: memories of scenes of shocking and overwhelming violence in which their parents died. But even the children who do not have such memories, children who do not witness their parent's death or those whose parents die of illnesses that take them slowly and gradually, have suffered such an assault to their own psychological integrity that they carry with them the shocked and shattered air of survivors of violent trauma.

USING CHILD–PARENT PSYCHOTHERAPY
TO TREAT EARLY CHILDHOOD BEREAVEMENT

The dual goals of treatment with bereaved children, helping children grieve their lost parents and integrate memories of the lost parent into their ongoing sense of self, and helping them find and begin to feel secure in new attachments that will sustain their continued development, are relationship-based goals. Although there are a variety of modalities in which intervention can be offered, including consultation with the child's surviving family members and/or child care providers, for children who need clinical intervention after a parent's death, the most parsimonious way to attain these goals is to treat the child conjointly with the caregiver who is undertaking the child's care after the death of the parent. A clinical focus on strengthening that relationship serves the child in two ways. First, it helps to build a strong coregulating relationship upon which the child can rely to help him or her endure, without psychological disintegration, the strong feelings that attend the grieving process. Second, it helps to solidify the attachment that will guide the child's future development. Child–parent psychotherapy is described more fully elsewhere, both as it is used to treat bereaved children (Lieberman et al., 2003) and to treat other traumas (Lieberman & Van Horn, 2005, 2008), as is the empirical support for its effectiveness (Cicchetti, Rogosh, & Toth,

2000; Cicchetti, Toth, & Rogosh, 1999; Lieberman, Ghosh Ippen, & Van Horn, 2006; Lieberman, Van Horn, & Ghosh Ippen, 2005; Lieberman, Weston, & Pawl, 1991; Toth, Maughan, Manly, Spagnola, & Cicchetti, 2002; Toth, Rogosch, Manly, & Cicchetti, 2006). This chapter briefly outlines the assessment philosophy and treatment domains of child–parent psychotherapy.

Assessment

Best practice suggests that a thorough assessment may require several hours of interview and observation (Zero to Three, 2005). Information may be gathered from interviews with family members, the current primary caregiver, and collateral sources, such as day care providers. It should include direct observation of the child's interactions with the current primary caregiver, and an interactive session between the assessor and the child, in which the child may offered the opportunity to play out associations to the parent's death. The assessment should focus on factors that affect the child's bereavement process, and should elicit information about the following nine domains:

1. *The child's emotional, social, and cognitive functioning before and after the death.* This domain includes temperamental propensities, the child's ability both to relate to others and to function autonomously within cultural norms and with a manageable amount of anxiety, and delays in cognitive development that may impede the grieving process.

2. *What the child knows about the death and details about how it happened.* It is important to know what and how the child was told about the parent's death and to know what additional or different facts the child may have overheard from adult conversations. Adults may have been unaware of the child's presence during these conversations or may have underestimated the child's capacity to understand, so it is important for the assessor to ask how the death has been discussed among adults.

3. *Traumatic reminders.* Understanding whether traumatic reminders are playing a disruptive role in the child's development (Pynoos, Steinberg, & Piacentini, 1999) requires careful observation of the child's behavior and careful inquiry into what adults involved with the child have observed. Young children may not be able to explain what has caused their distress; when they respond with excessive distress to seemingly benign stimuli, the assessor should investigate to determine whether there exists a detail that may remind the child of the trauma. Distress from reminders can disrupt children's neuophysiological functioning, making it more challenging for them to manage their feelings.

4. *The nature of the child's relationship to the deceased parent.* It is important to understand the place of the dead parent in the child's life. Did the child rely on the parent for basic routines of caregiving? Was the parent the child's preferred source of comfort in times of illness or stress? Did the parent have a special role as a treasured playmate? The child can be expected to grieve over specific activities associated with the lost parent and to experience these activities as reminders of the lost parent. The child may also reject the new caregiver's efforts at performing these routines and activities.

5. *The child's current relationships.* At least one supportive adult needs to be available to support the child, and to provide safety and security during the mourning process. One important function of the assessment is to understand who is performing that function and how well the surrogate caregiver, or caregivers, and others in the child's life are able to preserve routines that the child associated with the lost parent, and to use those routines not as occasions for conflict when the child is rejecting, but as opportunities to talk with the child about the dead parent, and how that parent would still wish to be with the child.

6. *Continuity versus disruption of daily routines.* Continuity and predictability facilitate the child's mourning process. Mourning, on the other hand, is made more difficult by sudden changes in the family's circumstances. Adaptation to new circumstances is difficult for bereaved children, because they have lost the security of their relationship with the lost parent, and because surviving adults, also striving to cope with loss and change, are less available to help the child.

7. *Cultural and family traditions and beliefs about death and dying.* The assessor needs to understand the family's beliefs, how these beliefs are being transmitted to the child, and what part the child is playing in the rituals surrounding the death. When a clinician becomes involved with the family immediately after the death, the first issue of concern is often whether the child should attend the funeral. Helping the family find an answer to this question demands sensitive balancing of a number of factors. Will an infant or toddler too young to process what is happening be overwhelmed by the emotions of grieving adults? Will the sight of the parent's unresponsive body in an open casket be beyond the child's comprehension? How much value does the family place on participation in the funeral and other rituals as an essential part of saying goodbye to the lost parent? When family members decide that they want to include a very young child in these rituals, the best solution is often to have available an adult who is familiar to the child and responsive to the child's needs: to answer questions and possibly take the child out for a break if the ritual becomes too much to handle (Webb, 2002).

8. *The family's child-rearing values and plans to care for the child.* The assessor will need to understand whether there is unanimity or conflict among extended family members about how to care for the child. Conflicts can be especially bitter and intractable when there are questions involving who is to blame for the parent's death. If outside agencies, such as child protection agencies, become involved, the question of who will ultimately care for the child may remain unanswered for many months as court proceedings prolong the uncertainty. To be helpful in these circumstances, clinicians must understand the following: (a) whether an adult is available who can become a new primary attachment figure for the child; (b) whether that adult is motivated to and has the support resources necessary to carry out the role of primary caregiver; (c) the nature of the previous relationship between this adult and the child; and (d) the adult's ability to empathize with the child's shifting feelings.

9. *The surviving caregiver's response to the death.* It is to be expected that the new caregiver will be grieving the loss of the child's parent and, in his or her grief, may be less emotionally available to the child. This difficulty is compounded when the new caregiver witnessed the sudden or violent death of the child's parent and was traumatized by those circumstances. Under these conditions, speaking about the death during the assessment or treatment, taking part in treatment, managing the daily routines of the child's care, and even the child's presence may become traumatic reminders for the new caregiver. The assessor needs to inquire into these circumstances with tact and sensitivity, and, as the assessment period evolves into treatment, be prepared to support the new caregiver in coping with his or her own trauma response and help the caregiver be maximally responsive and available to the child.

Although a good assessment is a critical basis for good treatment, the intent to conduct a thorough assessment should not stand in the way of needed intervention. Bereaved family members may need to process their *own* feelings about the loss before they can focus on the child's needs. They may have practical questions to which they want immediate answers that get in the way of a smooth assessment. Clinicians should view the assessment period as a time of relationship building and early intervention, as well as a time of information gathering.

Using the Assessment Information

At the end of the assessment period, the clinician should meet with the concerned adults in the family to offer feedback that focuses on strengths, as well as vulnerabilities. This feedback session will be more effective if the assessor has shared this information with the family as it emerged during the assessment. Under these circumstances, the feedback session presents an opportunity to revisit and weigh alternatives that have already been raised and discussed, and the family is not overwhelmed with new information or taken by surprise by the clinician's recommendations.

Recommendations for treatment meet with less resistance if they are framed in terms of the family's needs and of wishes or goals that family members have expressed for the child. Any recommendation should include a frank discussion of what the clinician reasonably believes can be accomplished, a plan for periodic reassessment, and a proposed duration of treatment.

INTERVENTION WITH BEREAVED CHILDREN: THE DOMAINS OF CHILD–PARENT PSYCHOTHERAPY

Child–parent psychotherapy revolves around joint sessions between a child, or children, and a caregiver, in which the focus is on translating the child's and the caregiver's emotional experiences, so that they become understandable for one another. This requires of the clinician the capacity to attend simultaneously to the caregiver's and the child's subjective experiences and to the emotional tone of their interactions with one another and with the clinician. At times, the caregiver's needs may become so urgent that the clinician feels unable to pay adequate attention to the child, or vice versa. These occasions will not detract from the overall goals of treatment, however, if the clinician bears in mind that the work is ultimately intended to help the child by enhancing the caregiver–child relationship. Although the caregiver is an indispensable partner in the treatment, the treatment is for the child.

Play and Giving Words to Feelings

The message that the treatment is for the child is conveyed primarily by the central place of play in the clinical sessions. Play becomes the vehicle for understanding the child's internal world, including his or her beliefs and anxieties about safety, relationships, and loss. It is important for the clinician to choose toys that the child can use to express a variety of needs. Children who have witnessed the violent death of their parents may need toys that they can use to process those memories; all bereaved children need toys that they can use to work through themes of separation and loss, going away and coming back, and damage and repair. Dolls and human and animal family figures are often central to this play, as are art materials, emergency vehicles, and medical kits. Withdrawn children need toys, such as soft balls or clay, that can encourage them to begin again to take part in physical activities. Children also need a way to calm themselves after play that is about worrying and upsetting material. Blowing bubbles, listening to music, or taking time out to snuggle in a caregiver's lap are all essential parts of child–parent sessions.

Books and games are also useful components in child–parent psychotherapy. Bibliotherapy can be an important part of children's recovery. Many books can serve as a starting point for conversations between caregiver and child about the feelings connected with death. Peekaboo and hide-and-seek are classic games through which infants and young children can explore and gain some control over their feelings about going away and coming back.

Case Example

Marie was 17 months old when her mother died of a drug overdose. Because there were no other family members available to take her in, Marie was placed in foster care and came to child–parent psychotherapy with her foster mother. For many sessions, one of her favorite toys was a board book with tabs that she could slide in and out to make characters in the story disappear and reappear. As Marie sat on her foster mother's lap, they looked at the book together, paying little attention to the story but allowing Marie ample time to make each character come and go as many times as she wanted. Her foster mother said, "See, they go away, but they come back—just like I do when I go to work. I always come back to you." The clinician added, "It's so sad that your mommy can't come back. But people almost always come back when they go away."

Developmental Guidance

Often the most effective intervention is the simplest: offering information that helps the caregiver understand the child's needs. This can be an intervention in its own right, and involves the clinician meeting with adults in the family, without the child, to help them support the child during the mourning process. Developmental guidance, offered as an intrinsic part of child–parent sessions, can help the caregiver understand the child's behavior in a developmental context.

Case Example

Juliet lived with her mother and grandmother, Mrs. Arnold. Juliet's mother had serious bipolar disorder and had been hospitalized several times for suicidal ideation. Shortly after Juliet's third birthday, her mother committed suicide by hanging herself. Although Juliet did not see her mother's body, she heard her grandmother and other relatives speak about the way her mother died. She heard them say that her mother had killed herself, or hanged herself. Mrs. Arnold, however, who was unable to find a way to speak that truth directly to Juliet, told Juliet that her mother died because she was sick. After her mother's death, Juliet continued to live with Mrs. Arnold. During the assessment, Mrs. Arnold expressed her distress about Juliet's behavior, which shifted between searching tearfully for her mother and playing as if nothing had happened, in a way that her grandmother could not explain. Juliet also spoke of her mother's death in ways that her grandmother could not understand, sometimes saying tearfully, "I didn't do it . . . I didn't do it."

Developmental guidance was a helpful intervention in this case. Addressing Juliet's play, which to Mrs. Arnold demonstrated that Juliet neither cared about nor missed her mother, the clinician explained that very young children have so much growing to do that they sometimes seem to have a short attention span for grieving. She empathized with Mrs. Arnold's distress at seeing Juliet laugh and play when Mrs. Arnold herself was so immersed in grief at her daughter's death. She reminded Mrs. Arnold of times when Juliet, too, was sad: "For adults that sorrow just doesn't seem to go away. For some little children, it's like the sadness comes suddenly sometimes and overwhelms them and at other times all their energy goes into growing and learning."

The clinician also used developmental guidance to help Mrs. Arnold understand Juliet's tearful cries of "I didn't do it." She suggested to Mrs. Arnold that two different things might be behind what Juliet was saying. First, young children assume that everything important that happens to them is somehow connected to them. Mrs. Arnold responded that her daughter's death had been connected to Juliet in a strange way: Juliet's mother had used Juliet's toy jump rope to hang herself. Mrs. Arnold quickly told the clinician, who was hearing this remarkable fact for the first time, that Juliet couldn't know this. She said, "Juliet didn't see her mother hanging. She was at day care. All that was gone by the time she got home." The clinician wondered aloud whether it was possible that Juliet had heard adults in the family talking about how her mother had died. Mrs. Arnold said that this was possible. The clinician responded that if Juliet had overheard such a conversation, it might be very confusing for her, in view of the fact that she had been told that her mother died because she was sick, and that in her confusion she might have assumed responsibility for the use of her toy. This intervention set the stage for

Mrs. Arnold's decision that it might be better to tell Juliet what had really happened. She worked with the clinician to find simple language that Juliet could understand. When Juliet next said, "I didn't do it," the clinician helped Mrs. Arnold tell her, "Of course, you didn't do it. Your mommy was sick, and her sickness made her forget that people can solve her problems. She was so sad, and she didn't think she could feel better, so she killed herself. But it wasn't because of you. It wasn't your fault. It was because your mommy was sick."

Placing Juliet's behaviors in a developmental context helped both Mrs. Arnold and Juliet better understand Juliet's emotional predicament. As the explanation began to sink in, Juliet asked her grandmother, "You're sad. Are you going to die, too?" Mrs. Arnold said, "No. I'm sad about your mommy just like you are. But I know that in time I'll feel better. I won't forget that. I'll still miss her, but I'll feel better."

Concrete Assistance with Problems of Daily Living

This domain of intervention is particularly important when family members are suffering the stress of bereavement and their emotional resources are stretched thin. If the surviving caregiver is not the child's other biological parent, the caregiver may need help to be appointed the child's guardian or to find convenient child care or other supportive resources that allow him or her to care for the child. If the child is placed in foster care, the foster parent may need support in advocating for the child to have pictures of family members, keepsakes of the lost parent, and even toys and clothing from home.

Case Example

Two-year-old Sammy's mother was stabbed to death, and his father was arrested for the crime. The family home was a crime scene; Sammy was taken to foster care with nothing but the clothes he was wearing. The clinician assigned to the case worked with the child welfare worker and the police to arrange for photograph albums, possessions belonging to Sammy and each of his parents, and the stuffed animals and blankets from his bed to be taken from the house and given to Sammy in a way that did not interfere with the criminal investigation. The clinician also laminated pictures of Sammy's mother and father, so that he could have them to keep without worrying that they would be torn and destroyed, and helped the foster mother find a special box to store and easily transport many of the items to Sammy's new caregiver when a permanent home was found for him.

Intervention with Preverbal Children

Even very young children can use symbolic play to cope with their loss. A clinician who understands young children's emotional needs, working with a caregiver, can use the communication in the play of even children with little or no language, to help them hold on to treasured memories of their lost parents and confront the permanence of their loss.

Case Example

As Carla, introduced earlier, became more comfortable in her foster home, and turned more to her foster mother, Mrs. James, for comfort, her play became more focused. When the clinician came into her home, Carla immediately pulled the baby doll from the bag of toys and began to rock and coo to it, to feed it with the bottle, and to wrap it tenderly in a blanket. The clinician said, "Your mommy took such good care of you. When you take care of the baby, you remember your mommy and all the things she did for you. It's so sad that she can't be here to take care of you now." Mrs. James also became more comfortable speaking with Carla about her loss. She told Carla that her mommy was in heaven watching over her. She said, "Your mommy misses you. She wishes she could be here, but she got too hurt and the doctors couldn't help her." By the end of every session, Carla would be cuddled on Mrs. James's lap, playing with a board book with tabs that allowed characters in the story to be pulled out, then tucked away again. As Carla turned the pages and made the characters appear and disappear, her foster mother helped her say "hi" and "bye-bye" to them. The clinician said, "You can make them go away and come back. You wish you could make your mommy come back."

One day, after several weeks of treatment, Carla watched as the clinician drew a picture. The clinician said, "Here you are, and here is your mommy." Before she could continue, Carla took the picture and deliberately tore the paper through the picture of her mother. Then she looked at her foster mother and said, "Band-Aid." The clinician said, "Your mommy's is hurt and you want to make her better." Mrs. James brought a box of bandages and handed one to Carla, who put it carefully across the picture of her mommy and then said, "More." One at a time, Mrs. James handed the Band-Aids to Carla, who carefully placed them on the picture, until the picture of her mother was covered with bandages. The clinician said, "It's so sad that your mommy can't get better and come back. You miss her and you want to help her, but she was too hurt." Carla crawled into Mrs. James's lap.

Carla had very little language to express her feelings, but her play made her needs clear: She needed to hold the memory of her mother's care, to process her anxiety about loss, and to express her wish that her mother could be made better and come back to her. As she felt safer in Mrs. James's home and more confident that she could be comforted there, all of these needs emerged in her play.

Goodbyes: Breaks in Treatment and Termination

Endings have a place of central importance in the treatment of bereaved children. Every "goodbye" with a child who has lost a parent to death needs to be handled with special care. The ends of sessions, breaks in treatment caused by illness or vacations, and the end of treatment itself all have the potential to recapitulate the child's original loss. They also carry the potential for repair, if they are managed well.

Rituals that give children a way to anticipate and to become active participants in the separation rather than passive victims of it are especially important for ending sessions. The rituals and reminders can be as varied as the child's needs and the clinician's imagination. The most compelling ritual for some children consists simply of putting the toys away together and saying "goodbye" to each toy. This ritual worked well for Carla, who, at the beginning of treatment, was not saying words. Still, she waved at each toy as she dropped it into the clinician's bag, and later was able to say "bye-bye" to each one. By the time the bag was filled and the clinician had repeated her reassurance that she would be back the next week, Carla was ready to go to her foster mother for a hug and walk to the door with the clinician without crying. Some children have a more difficult time with separation and need a concrete reminder to help them grasp the fact that the separation from the clinician will not be permanent, and that he or she will return. One little boy traded cars with his therapist at the end of each session, giving her one of his small cars to keep in her bag, and taking one of her cars to keep on the table next to his bed. Every week, when the therapist came, he would proudly return the car and tell her that he had taken good care of it. Every week, when she left, he would choose another car to be his companion for the week, and make sure that the therapist had a car, so that she could remember him. Other children may be satisfied with a tangible reminder of the session rather than an actual toy. One little girl always took three sheets of colored paper from the playroom when she left. Her grandmother said that she drew on the paper when she got home, then taped the pictures to her bedroom wall. Another boy was comforted by a photograph of his favorite toy.

Longer separations require more elaborate rituals. Calendars, for example, can help children visualize how long a clinician's vacation will last. Clinician, caregiver, and child can work together to create the calendar during a session, marking with stickers the date of the last session before the vacation, the date of the clinician's return, and important dates in between. With the caregiver's permission, the child can take the calendar home and, every night at bedtime, cross off the day that is ending. If the clinician will be away for several weeks, it may be useful, again, with the caregiver's permission, to send the child a card during the absence as a reminder that the clinician is still alive, and still thinking of him or her.

This ongoing sense of permanence becomes even more critical as treatment ends. Again, the need is for the child to understand that though the clinician will not be coming to play every week, he or she is still alive and still thinking of the child and the caregiver. As bereavement cases terminate, the last several sessions can be used to build a memory book that contains pictures of the child, the caregiver, the clinician, and favorite toys. It is also useful to write one or more cards or letters together during the closing sessions that the clinician can mail to the child at predetermined times in the weeks and months after treatment has ended. Finally, clinicians can encourage the caregiver to bring the child back for a visit a month or two after treatment ends. All of these strategies help bereaved children grasp the difference between the permanent loss of their parent and other goodbyes.

INTERVENTION WITH BEREAVED CHILDREN: THE THERAPIST'S EXPERIENCE

Clinical work with bereaved children is difficult and emotionally draining. The clinician must be open to the depth and breadth of children's suffering. If he or she defends herself against children's feelings, she will communicate to children that their losses are too great to be borne and their feelings of grief and rage are too much, too dangerous, to be tolerated. On the other hand, the clinician needs to maintain some sense of clinical distance from the children's grief and not take it on as his or her own personal suffering. This is true, of course, for all psychotherapists, offering any type of therapy. Often, however, the emotional intensity of doing bereavement work with very young children takes clinicians by surprise. Because of their developmental stage, young children's emotions are not well modulated under the best of circumstances. When they are suffering from the loss of caregivers who were once the center of their world, children's feelings become more intense and difficult to manage. It is the clinician's job to understand the source of those feelings, to validate the child's experience, and to help the child understand and cope with these powerful feelings—tasks that can be very taxing and evoke feelings of helplessness and despair as the clinician faces the inevitable truth that he or she cannot possibly grant the child's most deeply felt wish—that the lost parent will return. The child's despair may awaken the clinician's own sorrow over past losses and anxiety over traumatic experiences. Clinicians may also find themselves feeling angry at the child's current caregivers for their perceived failure to provide adequate care and support the child, or having vivid fantasies of adopting and raising the child him- or herself. All of these feelings may interfere with the clinician's ability to remain grounded and secure in his or her capacity to work with the child and caregivers, or may be enacted in unconscious ways. Chapter 17 in this volume deals with this topic in detail.

Working with bereaved children demands more than specific knowledge about the emotional needs of young children, and the impact of trauma and loss on their development. It also requires substantial maturity on the part of the clinician, supportive consultation and supervision, so that the clinician is not working in isolation, and sustaining relationships and routines for self-care away from work.

CONCLUDING COMMENTS

There is by now substantial observational and clinical evidence that the death of a parent is a shattering loss for a young child. With ongoing support from caring adults, children can recover from this loss in the sense that they can form new attachments to support their unfolding developmental needs.

DISCUSSION QUESTIONS AND ROLE-PLAY EXERCISES

1. The most difficult part of helping a young child and his or her surviving caregivers deal with a parent's death can be finding the language to speak about such a difficult topic. This chapter contains some examples, but there are many other ways to talk about death.

   In group discussion or role play, develop examples of simple, truthful, and concrete language that does not inundate the child with too many details that he or she is too young to process.

2. Supervision and consultation are essential supports for therapists working with bereaved young children and their families. Discuss potential challenges that may emerge in supervision and ways for the supervisor to guide the clinician.

REFERENCES

American Psychiatric Association. (2000). *Diagnostic and statistical manual of mental disorders* (4th ed., text rev.). Washington, DC: Author.

Bowlby, J. (1960). Grief and mourning in infancy and early childhood. *Psychoanalytic Study of the Child, 15,* 9–52.

Bowlby, J. (1980). *Loss: Sadness and depression.* New York: Basic Books.

Cicchetti, D., & Rogosch, F. A. (1997). The role of self-organization in the promotion of resilience in maltreated children. *Development and Psychopathology, 9,* 797–815.

Cicchetti, D., Rogosch, F. A., & Toth, S. L. (2000). The efficacy of toddler–parent psychotherapy for fostering cognitive development in offspring of depressed mothers. *Journal of Abnormal Child Psychology, 28,* 135–148.

Cicchetti, D., Toth, S. L., & Rogosch, F. A. (1999). The efficacy of toddler–parent psychotherapy to increase attachment security in offspring of depressed mothers. *Attachment and Human Development, 1,* 34–66.

Cohen, J. A., Mannarino, A. P., & Deblinger, E. (2006). *Treating trauma and traumatic grief in children and adolescents.* New York: Guilford Press.

Freud, A. (1960). A discussion of Dr. John Bowlby's paper "Grief and mourning in infancy and early childhood." *Psychoanalytic Study of the Child, 15,* 53–62.

Furman, E. (1974). *A child's parent dies: Studies in childhood bereavement.* New Haven, CT: Yale University Press.

Hofer, M. A. (1996). On the nature and consequences of early loss. *Psychosomatic Medicine, 58,* 570–581.

Hofer, M. A. (2003). The emerging neurobiology of attachment and separation: How parents shape their infants' brain and behavior. In S. Coates, J. L. Rosenthal, & D. S. Schechter (Eds.), *September 11: Trauma and human bonds* (pp. 191–211). Hillsdale, NJ: Analytic Press.

Lieberman, A. F., Compton, N. C., Van Horn, P., & Ghosh-Ippen, C. (2003). *Losing a parent to death in the early years: Guildelines for the treatment of traumatic bereavement in infancy and early childhood.* Washington, DC: Zero to Three Press.

Lieberman, A. F., Ghosh Ippen, C., & Van Horn, P. (2006). Child–parent psychotherapy: Six month follow-up of a randomized control trial. *Journal of the American Academy of Child and Adolescent Psychiatry, 45,* 913–918.

Lieberman, A. F., & Van Horn, P. (2005). *Don't hit my mommy!: A manual for child–parent psychotherapy with young witnesses of family violence.* Washington, DC: Zero to Three Press.

Lieberman, A. F., & Van Horn, P. (2008). *Psychotherapy with infants and young children: Repairing the effects of stress and trauma on early attachments.* New York: Guilford Press.

Lieberman, A. F., Van Horn, P., & Ghosh Ippen, C. (2005). Towards evidence-based treatment: Child–parent psychotherapy with preschoolers exposed to marital violence. *Journal of the American Academy of Child and Adolescent Psychiatry, 44,* 1241–1248.

Lieberman, A. F., Weston, D., & Pawl, J. H. (1991). Preventive intervention and outcome with anxiously attached dyads. *Child Development, 62,* 199–209.

Pynoos, R. S., Steinberg, A. M., & Piacentini, J. C. (1999). A developmental psychopathology model of childhood traumatic stress and intersection with anxiety disorders. *Biological Psychiatry, 46,* 1542–1554.

Spitz, R. (1960). A discussion of Dr. John Bowlby's paper "Grief and mourning in infancy and early childhood." *Psychoanalytic Study of the Child, 15,* 53–62.

Toth, S. L., Maughan, A., Manly, J. T., Spagnola, M., & Cicchetti, D. (2002). The relative efficacy of two interventions in altering maltreated preschool children's representational models: Implications for attachment. *Development and Psychopathology, 14,* 877–908.

Toth, S. L., Rogosch, F. A., Manly, J. T., & Cicchetti, D. (2006). The efficacy of toddler–parent psychotherapy to reorganize attachment in the young offspring of mothers with major depressive disorder: A randomized preventive trial. *Journal of Consulting and Clinical Psychology, 74,* 1006–1016.

Webb, N. B. (Ed.). (2002). *Helping bereaved children* (2nd ed.). New York: Guilford Press.

Webb, N. B. (Ed.). (2007). *Play therapy with children in crisis* (3rd ed.). New York: Guilford Press.

Zero to Three: National Center for Infants, Toddlers, and Families. (2005). *Diagnostic classification of mental health and developmental disorders of infancy and early childhood (DC:0–3R)* (rev. ed.). Washington, DC: Author.

CHAPTER 15

Bereavement Groups and Camps for Children

An Interdisciplinary Approach

PRISCILLA A. RUFFIN
SARAH A. ZIMMERMAN

One of the most painful experiences in life is the death of someone dear. For adults with sufficient coping skills and well-developed cognitive and language abilities, the aftermath of the death of a family member or friend presents a serious challenge. The death of a loved one poses even greater challenges for children who have yet to develop the cognitive understanding of what it means to die or the language ability to express the powerful emotions of grief.

Grieving children are in crisis. Life has been disrupted by a painful and traumatic event that has thrown the family into a turmoil (Kirwin & Hamrin, 2005; Turner, 1999). Chaos comes not only from the pain and confusion caused by someone loved and cared about having disappeared, but the loss also often marks the end of the belief that the world is safe and predictable (Turner, 1999; Zambelli & DeRosa, 1992). After a death, children yearn for the family to return to being just like everyone else's as they struggle to cope with an everyday existence that has irrevocably changed (Granot, 2005). Grieving children need to work through essentially the same issues as those of grieving adults: accepting the reality of the death, facing the pain of the loss, and making the emotional adjustments necessary to continue on with life and make new and meaningful attachments (Fox, 1988; Lohnes & Kalter, 1994; Worden, 1996).

While a child's capacity to comprehend the reality of death will be influenced by his or her stage of development, a grieving child has additional developmental tasks of mastering the complex challenges brought on by grief and transforming the lost relationship from face-to-face interaction to reexperiencing the person in memory (Cohen & Mannarino, 2004; Leighton, 2008; Oltjenbruns, 2001). Children's and adolescents' reactions to the emotions accompanying grief, when left unrecognized and unattended, may become lasting and impact negatively on their well-being and the successful development of future relationships (Cohen & Mannarino, 2004; Farber & Sabatino, 2007; Kirwin & Hamrin, 2005; Worden & Silverman, 1996).

Professionals who understand the unique ways children experience grief are able to develop programs to help youngsters acquire the coping mechanisms needed to manage the pain of grief and to teach children how to articulate their feelings to caregivers (DiSunno, Zimmerman, & Ruffin, 2004; Ruffin & Zimmerman, 2007). These vital skills help the child and the family cope over time with the painful feelings associated with loss and grief (Turner, 1999).

A combination of theoretical frameworks, including developmental, behavioral, cognitive, and psychodynamic theories, can be applied to establish an interdisciplinary bereavement therapy program that will successfully meet the emotional and psychoeducational needs of grieving children (Leighton, 2008). This chapter presents the Ruffin–Zimmerman model, a therapeutic program for the treatment of children's grief based on a blend of theoretical frameworks selected for relevance to the treatment of children's grief to provide therapists from a variety of disciplines an understanding of the concepts behind the operation of a children's bereavement therapy program and a bereavement camp (Ruffin & Zimmerman, 2007). The Ruffin–Zimmerman model described here incorporates the traditional tasks of grief work from William Worden (1996); Sandra Fox's (1988) tasks for grieving children; D. W. Winnicott's (1965) facilitating environment; Mary Turner's (1999) ideas about primitive fear and magical thinking in children under stress; Irvin Yalom's theory on the interpersonal interaction with the here and now and curative factors inherent in the process of group therapy (Yalom & Leszcz, 2005); Erik Erikson's (1963) eight ages of man; Jean Piaget's theory of cognitive development (Piaget & Inhelder, 1969); Edith Kramer's (1993) art therapy; and the play therapy of Virginia Axline (1969) and Nancy Boyd Webb (2007).

GROUP THERAPY

Group therapy is one of the preferred interventions for aiding grieving children (Mitchell et al., 2007; Webb, 2002). Universality and peer support are two of the essential curative factors at work in a children's bereavement group (Bacon, 1996; MacLennan, 1998; Mitchell et al., 2007; Tonkins & Lambert, 1996; Yalom & Leszcz, 2005). Children do not like feeling different from peers and respond positively to being in the company of others who are experiencing similar situations (Bacon, 1996; Glazer & Clark, 1999; Webb, 2002). Being one among many whose lives have been disrupted by the death of a loved one helps the child begin the process of normalizing grief and integrating the loss into everyday life. Being an empathic witness to the emotional pain of peers boosts a child's self-esteem and aids participation in the group activities (Lohnes & Kalter, 1994).

The Ruffin–Zimmerman model of children's bereavement therapy has the following seven objectives: (1) to help children to "normalize" grief (DiSunno et al., 2004; Glazer & Clark, 1999; Lohnes & Kalter, 1994; Schuurman, 2008); (2) to aid the development of coping mechanisms and to model self-soothing techniques (Ruffin & Zimmerman, 2007; Turner, 1999); (3) to aid children in acquiring the language necessary to express the emotions of grief (DiSunno et al., 2004; Farber & Sabatino, 2007; Turner, 1999); (4) to aid the process of individuation as children acquire the skills to manage new and complex emotions independent of a parent or guardian (Erikson, 1963); (5) to acquire an appreciation of remembering and honoring the past (Silverman, Nickman, & Worden, 1992); (6) to begin the lengthy process of reintegration of the memory of the lost person into children's everyday experience (Cohen & Mannarino, 2004; Lohnes & Kalter, 1994); and (7) to educate adults about the importance of helping children with grief work (DiSunno et al., 2004; Ruffin & Zimmerman, 2007).

A central objective of the Ruffin–Zimmerman model is to help children acquire the language necessary to express the new and confusing emotions that follow a tragic event and the accompanying turmoil of loss and grief (DiSunno et al., 2004). One of the curative factors inherent in telling and retelling one's story of grief and loss is to provide structure and meaning to the experience (Gilbert, 2002; Yalom & Leszcz, 2005). Without language to express feelings and fears, children are unable to tell the adults in their lives what they are thinking and feeling, which often leads parents, teachers, and caretakers to misjudge the depth of children's emotional pain and need for nurturance and support (Gilbert, 2002; Kirwin & Hamrin, 2005; Oltjenbruns, 2001; Ruffin & Zimmerman, 2007; Turner, 1999). During the group sessions, the therapist plays a vital role in helping children acquire the language necessary to name and articulate feelings. During play and guided activities, the therapist assigns words to the feelings being expressed or acted out, which also serves to validate the sense of loss.

A child's acquisition of the language to express the emotions of grief has a double benefit. Not only are the children able to participate in group activities at a higher level while gaining age-appropriate knowledge about death, loss, and grief, but they also then bring their new found language skills home or to school where meaningful dialogues can begin (Glazer & Clark, 1999; Ruffin & Zimmerman, 2007). The children are able to express feelings with words, allowing adults to grasp children's level of comprehension about the death and understand the impact of the death in changing their everyday lives. Adults are then able to respond to the children with needed empathy and support.

Case Example

Six-year-old Andy came to a bereavement group a few months after his father had been killed in a collision while driving home from work. Andy did well in the group, eagerly participated in the activities, and was often observed offering support to the other children. His mom called the therapist to say how thankful she was to have Andy in the bereavement group. Before coming to group, he had not talked much about his father's death. Now that they were talking, Andy's mom was finding out what Andy was really thinking. She did not realize her son did not know his father was dead. She had told him that his Dad was in heaven and thought he understood. One day, Andy asked if she knew you had to be dead to be in heaven. Was his mom ever surprised! In the group, Andy was learning the language of grief and beginning to understand death as irreversible. Bringing his new knowledge and verbal skills home and talking with his mother, Andy and his mom were now partners, sharing their grief together and processing what happened to change so drastically their lives (Glazer & Clark, 1999; Turner, 1999).

At a time when a child's need for parental attention has never been greater, a parent who is lost in grief has little energy to recognize and attend to the emotional needs of a grieving child (Corr & Corr, 1996; Glazer & Clark, 1999; Kirwin & Hamrin, 2005; Pynoos, 1992; Ruffin & Zimmerman, 2007). A benefit for the families of children who attend a bereavement group is that the leader and group members act as a surrogate support system, providing emotional holding while attending to children's grief and confusion at a time when families are under tremendous stress and parents or guardians are unable to respond to children's need for reassurance and comfort (Glazer & Clark, 1999; Zambelli & DeRosa, 1992).

Children are keenly aware of signs of distress in a parent or caregiver. When the family is in a state of acute grief, the child may act as if all is well out of fear of bringing on tears and adding to a parent's burden of sadness. An impartial adult, the group leader, does not respond emotionally to a child's expressions of pain, freeing the child to disclose feelings without fear of causing distress.

ART THERAPY

In the Ruffin–Zimmerman model of bereavement therapy, art therapy techniques are an integral part of the treatment plan and are used to help children express the emotions of grief. Art embodies symbolic expression, and creating a piece of art allows grieving children to express painful thoughts and feelings without the use of words. Guided by the therapist, children quite naturally and enthusiastically enter into the creative process and produce drawings, paintings, and sculptures revealing the emotions, frustrations, and fears that accompany grief (DiSunno et al., 2004; Lohnes & Kalter, 1994). Engaging in a creative process is soothing and helps the children begin to make sense out of what seems disorderly, forming a basis for discussion of their interpretation of a new reality (Kramer, 1993).

PLAY THERAPY

Play is a child's natural medium of expression (Axline, 1969; Glazer & Clark, 1999; Webb, 2007). In a bereavement care setting, with a few simple tools and lots of imagination children reconstruct traumatic or distressing events in a safe and controlled environment. By play acting the event and perhaps fantasizing a different outcome, children begin to process and relieve the emotional distress of grief (Glazer & Clark, 1999; Pynoos, 1992; Turner, 1999; Webb, 2007). Through repetitive play acting, children redeem what may be felt as a failure and regain hope for the future (Erikson, 1963). For example, a child may be distressed by thinking not saying goodbye as Dad went off to work caused something bad to happen, or, influenced by magical thinking, a child may believe that something he or she did or did not do caused the death. Replaying the event helps the child reconstruct and transform the experience and correct misperceptions, and it aids in the development of problem-solving skills (Axline, 1969; Kramer, 1993; Webb, 2007).

In bereavement play therapy, children often fantasize a reunion, recreate the intact family, or express confusing feelings. Using play with puppets or stuffed animals as distancing objects and games as displacement activities helps grieving children manage traumatic reminders and often relive the important last memory of the person who died (Lohnes

& Kalter,1994; Pynoos, 1992). Under the watchful eyes of the therapists, the children are carefully guided in the process and are helped to put words to feelings. Symbolic play allows us to view what the child is thinking and understand what he or she knows about the events surrounding the death, giving us the opportunity to clarify confusion and intervene appropriately (Webb, 2007). When a child witnesses a violent death, that child during play may repeatedly and unconsciously reenact a part of the experience in an effort to self-soothe, lessen the feelings of helplessness, and ease the extreme emotional trauma (Pynoos, 1992).

Case Example

Four-year-old Maggie came to a bereavement camp 2 years after her mother was murdered. She was there when her mom was shot in the head by a boyfriend, who then turned the gun on himself. Maggie was found by a police officer, who had been called by neighbors to investigate the sounds of gunfire.

Maggie lived with her maternal grandparents, who, while overwhelmed with sorrow and grief, were struggling to help Maggie, whose behavior was becoming more troubling. She was acting out, unable to focus on completing even the simplest task and was combative with the other children in her preschool.

To the camp therapists, Maggie's behavior revealed the extent of her psychological trauma. She was exhibiting signs of repetition compulsion manifested in a "game" she repeatedly played. With smiles and laughter, but also with aggression, Maggie smeared food, soapsuds, paint, clay, milk, or water on her head, in her hair, and over her face, and she tried to do the same to others.

Skilled observation by practitioners experienced in the treatment of children's grief linked Maggie's behavioral symptoms to the trauma she had witnessed 2 years earlier. A bereavement camp was not the therapeutic setting to effect lasting change for this child. However, her grandparents now understood the family's need for long-term treatment for traumatic grief. Attending the bereavement camp was the entry point to therapy for this family.

Through art and in their play, young children tell us the story of the loss and their grief (Gilbert, 2002). Activities to aid children in play therapy are unlimited and use a variety of simple tools and props, such as puppets, dolls, games, and paints and paper. It is important to have materials on hand for children who have been impacted by disasters such as a plane crash, flood, tornado, hurricane, or war to help them reenact events as they understand them (Lohnes & Kalter, 1994). After the September 11, 2001 terrorist attacks, we prepared for bereavement groups and Camp Good Grief by having a supply of large and small building blocks that the children could use to reenact the planes hitting the World Trade Center and the Pentagon. For the older children, journaling or letter writing can be cathartic, and it gives us a glimpse into what they are thinking and just how much pain they are experiencing.

Case Example

In a bereavement group for 8- to 10-year-olds in their neighborhood school, the children wrote letters to the person who died. A 10-year-old child's note to his dad read, "I love you. Little Joey's getting big and starting to talk a lot. You know, I really don't know what you died from. I wasn't listening when the nurse told me you were dead."

A girl's note to her brother read, in part, "Ever since you're gone, life is like HELL for me. First you then Grandma. I don't know if I can take anymore. Please remember I love you, goodbye and don't worry."

A child who missed her mother wrote, "I love you, I wish you were here. I can't stand it when I don't hear your voice any more. I feel lonely. I hate it that I couldn't say goodbye. I cry every night because you died, I miss your cooking and your face. R.I.P."

And another child's letter shows need for forgiveness as she wrote, "I miss you and Grandpa and I want to know if you are mad at me for saying goodbye and if you are I am very sorry."

SCHOOL-BASED BEREAVEMENT GROUPS

Schools are an ideal venue for a children's bereavement group. Parents have trust in their children's school, which is a familiar and comfortable environment for the children. Begin by introducing to school administrators, guidance counselors, and social workers the concepts of holding a bereavement group. Provide literature to validate and support the concept. Offer to hold an in-service workshop on children's grief to teachers and to provide training for guidance staff who may be interested in coleading the groups. Once approval has been obtained, involve the guidance counselors in the selection process; they will recruit and screen the group members. Provide teachers with information to introduce the group to the children. Send a letter to parents explaining the purpose of the program, and obtain written parental permission for the children to attend the group. Excerpts from a letter to parents drafted by the administrative office of one school read, in part:

"We are aware of many youngsters in our school who have recently experienced a loss. We have invited a social worker from East End

Hospice to provide interested students with help in this regard. This is a wonderful opportunity for students to have a supportive environment, with counselors who specialize in loss and grief. Those who have participated in the past have found it to be a great help. Please discuss this program with your child to see whether he or she would want to participate."

The therapists and coleaders facilitate the groups, provide materials and refreshments, and follow up with the guidance counselors and parents, if and when an issue arises.

FORMAT FOR CHILDREN'S BEREAVEMENT THERAPY GROUPS

It is preferable to place preschool, latency-age children and adolescents in separate groups (MacLennan, 1998; Tonkins & Lambert, 1996). When that is not possible, the addition of a coleader is recommended to work with the different age groups so that participation in developmentally appropriate activities occurs smoothly within the session. When working with children in groups, the use of a coleader facilitates the process and helps to make efficient use of the limited time the children spend in a group (Bacon, 1996). The coleader helps with practical matters, such as distributing materials or leading an activity, freeing the therapist to observe or to spend one-on-one time with a disruptive child or one who is having difficulties. Under usual circumstances, a trained volunteer with appropriate experience is an ideal coleader for children's bereavement groups. However, certain conditions preclude the use of volunteers and require a second therapist to colead the group safely and efficiently. In school populations in which the children's home environments are known to be chaotic, a second therapist helps to address the impact of complex issues on children's ability to process the information presented in the group.

The children's groups meet for a total of eight weekly sessions, each lasting 45 minutes to 1 hour, at a time most convenient for the school. The group size is best limited to eight participants, 10 as a maximum. Providing the children's bereavement groups as a service to the community will promote attendance.

Use of the Ruffin–Zimmerman model's goals for a children's bereavement therapy program structures the format of the groups; the first session sets the tone. The group's purpose is explained and ground rules are agreed upon (Samide & Stackon, 2002). Using the go-around method, group members introduce themselves, and the therapist may encourage them to say a word or two about the person who died. Because children do most of their grief work not by talking but through activities, the majority of group time is taken up with guided exercises, which are always followed by discussion. Group exercises help to break down resistance and give the children an opportunity to distance emotionally from feelings, making it safer to express powerful emotions. By the end of the session, the children have worked hard and, as a reward, the group ends with a snack of cookies and juice.

The format for the remainder of the sessions is similar. The therapist introduces a topic and conducts exercises that cover issues such as managing the feelings that accompany grief, changes since the death, funerals and memorials, problem solving, honoring memories, and exploring what the future may hold. Exercises are always followed by discussion and perhaps brainstorming as the children learn to help and to comfort each other while managing their own grief. The final group meeting has more of a celebratory tone. After a review of the sessions, the children relate what they have discovered over the weeks and now know what they would say to others who are grieving. The session ends with a pizza party, and the children receive a certificate of achievement for attending group.

There is no sameness in group therapy. Although the process and outcomes are similar, every group develops its own working style. The content and flow of a children's bereavement group is influenced by many variables, including the environment where the group is held, the culture and norms of participants, and concurrent stressors in the children's lives at home and in school. The challenge for the therapist is to remain flexible and maintain fluidity to facilitate the process and work toward achieving the group's goals.

The aim is for the group to be viewed as a place where disclosure is safe, where children know they will be listened to and have their experiences validated (Lohnes & Kalter, 1994; MacLennan, 1998; Yalom & Leszcz, 2005). No matter how chaotic or disruptive the children's lifestyles may be, the therapist models consistency by being present at a time when children's needs for understanding and compassion are the greatest. As one middle-school-age child, who had a reputation for being angry and disruptive in and out of the classroom, remarked after he attended every group session following the death of his mother, "This is the only place where I'm not in trouble."

CHILDREN'S BEREAVEMENT CAMP

The basic tenet of a children's bereavement camp is to bring youngsters together for a brief time in a therapeutic environment to facilitate acquisition of the coping skills and language necessary to express the feelings associated with grief and bereavement, and to begin an ongoing process of integrating the loss into their everyday lives (Farber & Sabatino, 2007; Ruffin & Zimmerman, 2007; Webb, 2002). One of the most important variables when developing a children's bereavement program is the environment where care will be rendered (Winnicott, 1965).

While it is generally known that attending camp promotes children's self-esteem and builds confidence (Farber & Sabatino, 2007), the camp setting also lends itself nicely to the special needs of bereaved children. The universal themes of grief and bereavement bring children together with the purpose of engaging in developmentally appropriate activities designed to promote an understanding of the feelings associated with grief and to help children gain the skills and confidence needed to cope with the aftermath of the death of a friend or loved one (Farber & Sabatino, 2007; Turner, 1999; Yalom & Leszcz, 2005).

Children have little tolerance for the painful and confusing emotions associated with grief. To control exposure to these strong and unfamiliar feelings, children's outward expressions of grief generally come in short spurts. To ease discomfort, they distract themselves with friends or play (Lohnes & Kalter, 1994; Oltjenbruns, 2001; Webb, 2002). A camp setting allows grief work to be balanced with fun, thereby meeting the children's need for a kinetic reprieve from painful emotions, while providing information about the feelings associated with grief as children acquire the language skills necessary to gain the attention of caregivers (Ruffin & Zimmerman, 2007; Schuurman, 2008). Equally important, a bereavement camp provides campers with valuable exposure to models of self-soothing techniques that, once learned, will benefit them throughout their lifetime.

With camp as the therapeutic setting, a grieving child is joined by peers in a variety of activities geared to the camper's developmental age and cognitive ability. Group and art therapy sessions are carefully paced to promote expression of thoughts, exploration of feelings, discussion of circumstances surrounding the death and fears for the future, and to help children develop strategies to cope with changes in their lives since the death. During a day at camp, group and art therapy sessions are combined with a wide variety of recreational activities. Sports, games, and arts and crafts provide for children the needed relief from exposure to painful thoughts and feelings (Samide & Stockton, 2002). Time spent in recreational activities promotes group cohesiveness, helps to rebuild a child's self-esteem, and reduces feelings of isolation, which is often an overlooked accompaniment of grief in children.

Camp Good Grief was purposefully designed as a day program. As a result of 12 years of experience, we recognize a double benefit to utilizing the day camp model to help children and families cope with the enormity of grief. First, returning home to family and familiar surroundings each night after a day of exploring powerful emotions comforts the children. Second, using newly acquired language skills, campers share the events of the day with parents and caregivers, which promotes a much needed dialogue among family members. Caregivers often report being surprised by the ease with which their campers talked about feelings and the impact the death has had on their lives. In their everyday lives, the message children often receive is not to talk about the death or their grief (Glazer & Clark, 1999). At camp, we see and feel the children's relief on the very first day as they realize that here they are not different, that everyone at camp has had someone they care about die, and it is OK to talk about it. A bereavement camp should be a memorable experience, one upon which children reflect back to remember days full of fun and laughter, while they engaged in a variety of stimulating activities, surrounded by new friends and caring adults.

Therapists

Careful selection of therapists is critical to the success of any therapeutic children's bereavement program; however, it is even more so when compiling the team of therapists for a bereavement camp. At Camp Good Grief, to conform with the Ruffin–Zimmerman model of an approach to the care of grieving children, the interdisciplinary treatment team includes therapists from a variety of practice bases and disciplines, including a selection of advanced practice social workers with experience in hospice or end-of-life care; psychiatric nurse practitioners experienced in pediatric care; school social workers; art therapists; and child psychologists and psychiatrists with experience in a community, school, or child treatment center. All have worked with children in a fluid environment and are better able to recognize and take advantage of the fleeting therapeutic moments when a child reveals a thought or a feeling, or seeks a private answer to a lingering question.

With grieving children as the focus of care, therapists are required to have a working knowledge of child development and be proficient in the treatment of children's grief, bereavement, emotional trauma, and facilitation of the group process. In addition, therapists must present a positive attitude and have desirable personal characteristics, such as a high level of energy, the ability to facilitate emotional expression gently and foster hope for the future in the children and families (Mitchell et al., 2007; Webb, 2002).

The death of a loved one presents children with a crisis, and children's ability to master developmental tasks in times of crisis is challenged and may be delayed or even stop (Fox, 1998; Oltjenbruns, 2001; Webb, 2002). Applying Winnicott's theory of creating an ideal holding environment, therapists at a bereavement camp have a vital role in nurturing and providing children with good-enough mothering in the psychotherapeutic context (Winnicott, 1965).

Use of Volunteers at Camp

A team of volunteers and professionals is needed to staff a children's bereavement camp adequately. There are a great many tasks to be done and any number of children to supervise. Careful selection, training, and supervision of volunteers to staff a bereavement camp, while challenging and labor intensive, is critical to the success of the program. A pool of volunteers from a wide variety of age groups, genders, and professional backgrounds adds a vast richness to the camp experience. Interacting with volunteers of all ages and genders increases the opportunity for the children to reexperience a meaningful moment with a lost parent, grandparent, or sibling.

Case Example

Five-year-old Teddy's dad was killed in the 9/11 terrorist attack on the Twin Towers. At camp one day, just as the lunch bell rang, Teddy asked volunteer Mike to give him a ride on his shoulders to the lunchroom. As Mike lifted Teddy onto his shoulders, the boy smiled and told Mike that his dad always gave him rides on his shoulders. With tears in his eyes, Mike proceeded to bounce Teddy on his shoulders as they made their way to the lunchroom.

In the Ruffin–Zimmerman interdisciplinary model of a children's bereavement program, camp therapists, staff, and volunteers are required to complete an approved course in grief and bereavement, which ensures that all those who come in contact with children and families are thoroughly versed in issues of the treatment of children's grief.

Under the supervision of the coordinators and camp directors, volunteers are charged with a variety of responsibilities. Some colead a small group in conjunction with the therapist; others are in charge of the free-time activities. Volunteers provide supervision, help with lunch, and sometimes offer a special something to a struggling camper.

Case Example

Volunteer Lucille was coleading group therapy sessions for the 6- to 8-year-olds. During one session when campers were engaged in a discussion, suddenly one of the boys, Allen, jumped up and ran from the group. Lucille followed him as he ran, until he scrambled into the crawl space under a dormitory. Lucille caught up to Allen where he was hiding and began gently to coax him out, telling him that they could talk about whatever he was thinking or feeling. No amount of coaxing worked; he would not budge. Lucille got down on all fours and crawled under the building to join Allen. Together they lay in the dirt with all sorts of bugs crawling under, over, and above them. Allen turned to Lucille and said, "I knew you would find me. No one looks for me anymore." With that they both came out from under the building. Allen was comforted, knowing that someone would go to great lengths to find him, and Lucille was glad she overcame her aversion to creepy crawlers to reach out in a meaningful way to help this child reexperience genuine caring from another adult (Schuurman, 2008).

Teenage volunteers bring a special vitality to a camp. Teens age 14 and up are solicited from area schools to volunteer at camp. Volunteering at a children's bereavement camp is a serious undertaking, and a rigorous application process helps to define a young applicant's commitment. Teen volunteers are assigned meaningful activities, such as helping the therapists in the small groups or being with the children during free time to assist with sports, games, and other activities. In return, they earn a letter from the organization, documenting their community service and recognizing them for joining the larger community of people who care. For some teen volunteers, time spent at a children's bereavement camp defines a career path and brings greater insight into a personal experience.

Case Example

They sat at a table in art therapy, one 6 years older than the other. James, a camper, was building a boat out of clay, and David, a volunteer, was helping to mold a piece of clay for the boat James was sculpting. They continued to work after the others left, quietly sharing each other's company. Six months earlier, James had last seen his father leaving on a fishing boat; now he was reconstructing his memory. David knew the power of memories; his dad had died 2 years earlier. On this day, in complete understanding that comes from having an experience in common, they shared their grief. After camp, remembering the quiet challenge of helping a grieving child, David said, "Sometimes you just want someone to sit by you, not try to make it right, but to just sit and let you feel your feelings."

Adequate supervision is important for those engaged in the emotionally demanding atmosphere of grief work at a children's bereavement camp. Therapists and coleaders benefit from having an opportunity each day to debrief, problem-solve, and receive the support and guidance necessary to ward off compassion fatigue and leave camp each day with a feeling of accomplishment. Volunteers are closely supervised and supported by the therapists, camp directors, and volunteer coordinators.

Structure and Organization

Campers are grouped by age, with an ideal number of 8–11 campers to a group. Each group is assigned a therapist as the leader, a volunteer coleader, and two to three adult or youth volunteers. Careful consideration was given to forming segregated groups for children at high risk for traumatic grief, such as those who lost a loved one in the 2001 terrorist attacks or witnessed a death. Given our knowledge of the group process, and knowing that children react negatively to feeling different than their peers, in addition to observing the empathetic nature of grieving children's attitudes toward one another, we concluded that the children at risk for traumatic grief would benefit greatly from support received from peers who are also grieving. After 12 years of experience treating grieving children, this has proven to be a valid conclusion (Ruffin & Zimmerman, 2007).

Among the more practical lessons learned was to assign a color to each group. T-shirts, hats, name tags, wristbands, and group mascots are all color coordinated. From primary colors for the youngest to more trendy tie-dye or camouflage for the 12- to 16-year-old campers, color coordinating the groups promotes cohesiveness and certainly aids in gathering the children for activities, lunch, and therapy sessions.

Camp Good Grief is in session for five consecutive days, Monday through Friday. Each day a theme or a task is assigned and carried out through the day's activities in both group and art therapy, and modified appropriately to suit the developmental ages of the various groups. In a camp environment, the art therapists work in conjunction with the group therapists to design activities to reflect the theme of the day.

In the Ruffin–Zimmerman model, the activities and exercises for children's bereavement groups are flexible and may be modified to suit the developmental ages of participants. Each session is assigned a theme to correspond with an adaptation of a combination of Fox's (1988) tasks for grieving children (understanding, grieving, commemorating, and going on) and Worden's (1996) tasks of mourning for children (to accept the reality of the loss, to experience the pain of the loss, to adjust to an environment where the deceased is missing, and to relocate the dead person within one's life and find ways to memorialize the person).

For example, the first day of camp is structured around Fox's task of understanding and Worden's task to accept the reality of the loss. General introductory themes for the first day include becoming acquainted, engagement, and identifying the common purpose. During group therapy on the first day, the children create a list of group rules. Younger groups of campers are given a bear, which is used as a distancing object to comfort and soothe a camper while talking in a group session. The children take ownership of their group mascot by naming and decorating their bear with a camp hat or necklace made in arts and crafts. It is not unusual to see the toughest acting boy hold the bear close to his chest while talking in the group.

The older campers make good use of a Native American talking stick. During tribal councils, the talking stick is a symbol of the speaker's importance, and it commands the respect and the attention of listeners. The campers handle the talking stick with reverence. Holding the talking stick gives one the permission to speak and the honor of being listened to and also serves to prompt a camper who may be reluctant to participate (Locust, 2008).

Art therapy continues the dialogue started in group therapy, dispelling the taboo of talking about the death. Using modeling clay, children are asked to make a model of a memory. The children make beautiful and moving clay models of their memories: A mom with the wings of an angel holding a child on her lap; a father's baseball mitt, and a brother's fishing pole are just a few of the clay memories the children have made over the years.

The feeling tone at the start of day 1 at camp is that of uncertainty and fear of the unknown. As the day progresses, the mood is transformed and the campers' relief is almost palpable as they come together, understanding that everyone at camp is just like them. Something terrible happened and all their lives have changed. By the end of the day, campers are feeling connected and eager to return in the morning.

Day 2 of camp is all about feelings. This day, the children start to acquire the language to express feelings and begin the process of normalizing their grief. Day 3 epitomizes the working phase of therapy (Yalom & Leszcz, 2005). The children are confronting feelings and voicing fears. Painful emotions that emerge may be observed in the children's irritability or acting-out behaviors.

Art therapy on this day connects feelings to the loss. Each child makes a mask that shows the feeling face he or she presents to the world on the outside versus feelings that are private and hidden from view painted on the inside. The masks vividly contrast the turmoil and internal emotions some of these children are feeling with the cool colors of calm in the painted face they present to the world.

The challenge for therapists is to help the children with containment, to gain control over feelings by use of language and self-soothing techniques (Turner, 1999). Sometimes children use this time to reveal something they needed to keep secret.

Case Example

Sam's dad was killed in the 9/11 terrorist attack on the World Trade Center. During the first session, Sam did not share in the group, but he appeared to want to be part of the group process. He would glance at the therapist whenever he thought he was "caught" joining the fun. It was as though his story was not to be told. During group one day, Sam suddenly blurted out that his dad had been killed in the terrorist attack. Unable to control his words, his anxiety went up, his eyes got wide and he looked as if he wanted to gulp back the words. He glanced at the other kids; the group simply continued on. Sam's face was filled with relief. He had taken a chance in telling the secret and nothing had changed. The group responded with calm acceptance. There could not have been a better time for Sam to unburden himself by sharing his secret.

The feeling tone on day 3 is one of irritability. The children seek relief from the stress of painful feelings by increasing their activities, testing limits, and occasionally some good old-fashioned mischief making. Art therapy presents ideas about using art materials to contain feelings by creating a safe place, decorating a box to depict a special place where the children go in their hearts and minds when they need solace.

On day 4, the themes are gaining mastery over new challenges, developing internal connections to the lost person, and beginning the termination process in earnest. Each child brings a memento, a special something that reminds him or her of the person who died to share with the groups. The children reverently tell the story behind their mementos. Dad's fireman's helmet, Mom's wedding ring, Grandma's button box, or the Christmas present crafted in woodworking shop that Dad never got to see, are just a few of the treasured objects children have brought to share with the group. These transitional objects are an important connection to the persons they have lost (Corr & Corr 1996; Silverman et al., 1992; Yalom & Leszcz, 2005).

A group exercise can be a very powerful and cathartic experience. In one exercise designed to help the children feel connected to the person who died, the kids are given a large shell, such as a clamshell, and a marker, with instructions to write a message to the person who died on the shell. At Camp Good Grief, situated on a body of water, the children go to the shore and, if they so choose, throw their shell far into the water.

One little boy, with a bit of magical thinking, was comforted by believing his very special message to his mother was received.

Case Example

Jake was 4 years old when his mother was murdered. There were troubling domestic issues within the family, and he had been living with his father for about a year at the time his mother was killed. His mom often missed visitation dates, without calling to tell him she was unable to visit.

The summer following his mother's death, Jake came to camp. On this day, the children were asked to write a message to the person who died on the inside of a seashell. The children took their shells to the beach and tossed them as far as they could into the water to send a message to their special person. Before Jake threw his shell into the water, he explained why he'd written his phone number on his shell. "Now," said Jake, "Mom will know where to find me."

The feeling tone for day 4 is generally quiet and introspective as the children share their precious mementos. They are beginning to accept and to cope with the strong feelings and emotions associated with their grief. They have bonded with their peers and anticipate the separation, knowing that tomorrow is the last day of camp.

The format changes for day 5. It is family day, the day the kids take charge. The campers arrive with their parents or guardians in tow and eagerly show them around. In spite of having been prepared by the coordinators and reading the book *Jeremy Goes to Camp Good Grief* (DiSunno et al., 2004), which describes the camp process and activities, after observing the transformation in their children the families are distant at first not wanting to disturb whatever magic that has made such a difference for their children. To break the ice, the day starts with a bang. A DJ plays the latest disco and party music, and a conga line is soon organized. With straw hats, bandanas and, colorful paper leis, families are pulled into the game and are soon laughing having fun doing the Chicken Dance at warp speed.

Later the parents gather with the therapists for a private talk. The children have learned new language and have gained confidence to express feelings. Families are encouraged to keep the dialogue going, to talk to their children about grief and loss. Some families are referred for further counseling, and some children will attend a bereavement group later in the year at school. Given that children grieve anew at each developmental stage, some of them will be returning to camp next summer (Kirwin & Hamrin, 2005; Worden & Silverman, 1996). Everyone is encouraged to stay in touch.

Group therapy on the last camp day is all about modeling termination. The children gather in their groups one more time; e-mail addresses and phone numbers are exchanged. Each child is given a small teddy bear as a reminder of the time at camp, and with hugs all around, group comes to an end.

In art therapy, the children share with their parents the projects they have made during the week. The project for this day is to create a tangible memorial to the person who died. It may be a stepping-stone made of cement for the garden, with imprints of hands and Mom's name spelled out in pretty rocks. Or a flag for the porch, decorated with feathers and sequins in memory of Grandma, or with cork and fishing line just like Dad's.

After a picnic lunch, the children, who have been practicing throughout the week, put on a talent show. Hula Hoops, a bit of ballet, some jokes, a magic act, lip-synching to the latest tune, and card tricks are met with whistles and wild applause. After the show, everyone gathers for the last singing of the camp song; goodie bags are handed out and goodbyes are said, a happy and sad time for everyone. Shortly after camp ends, families are sent evaluation forms, which provide a picture of what the children and their parents benefited from most, and changes for future sessions are suggested. The children usually mention adding a food item to the already kid-friendly menu, but their answers to questions of what they liked most or least about camp are revealing. For most, being able to talk about the person who died and learning about feelings are what they liked best. One child remarked, "I learned that being sad is OK." There are lots of positive comments on the activities, and one child even suggested we schedule in time for a nap.

The parent evaluations express gratitude for the camp, the therapists, and how the process benefited their children. So many are surprised that their children came home each afternoon, as one mother put it, "so happy!" There are frequent comments about the value of the children getting together with others who have had similar experiences. One parent said her son understood that some people felt worse than he did; another said her daughter felt that she belonged and was recognized. One mother wrote, offering thanks for "an amazing week at camp. It was the happiest I have seen him in a long time. As we move through our sadness, camp will be one of the most healing stops along the way."

An unrecognized benefit of organizing a bereavement camp is an upsurge in community awareness and interest in helping grieving children. Camp Good Grief started the first year with 29 children, four therapists, and eight volunteers and 12 years later hosted 120 children, with help from 75 volunteers and 12 therapists. In a short time, the bereavement camp captured the attention of the community and became a local tradition, relied upon to help grieving families. Counselors, clergy, physicians, teachers, friends, and neighbors refer families to camp to help the children after a loved one dies. From modest to the most generous donations, support for the camp comes from all sectors of the community. Organizing a bereavement camp brings a community together to raise awareness of the importance of attending to children's grief and helping grieving families reorganize and continue on with life after a tragedy.

CONCLUDING COMMENTS

Attending a bereavement group or camp often begins the process of discovery for a grieving child. After the death of a loved one, a bereavement program provides children with support and information needed to adapt to a new and changed world and to master the powerful feelings associated with loss and grief. Coming together in a structured environment that offers a variety of activities balancing work with fun, and with the oversight of qualified professionals, brings about a dual effect that facilitates both the child's and the family's bereavement process. An interdisciplinary bereavement therapy program for children, such as the Ruffin–Zimmerman model described herein, applies carefully selected conceptual frameworks from a combination of disciplines chosen for demonstrated ability to aid children in acquiring the language and skills needed to begin to gain mastery over the feelings associated with grief, and start the ongoing process of integrating the loss into their everyday lives. The goal of this children's bereavement program is to minimize what too often are the overwhelmingly negative consequences of loss for children, by providing the tools of language and knowledge, and the courage to visualize a future with renewed strength and confidence, bolstered by lasting positive memories of the past.

DISCUSSION QUESTIONS AND ROLE-PLAY EXERCISES

1. When leading a children's bereavement group, it is important for the therapist to be prepared to answer children's questions. If a child were to ask you to explain what happens when someone dies, how would you answer, and what criteria would you use to frame your response? Would you answer differently if asked by a 5-year-old, a 9-year-old, or a 13-year-old? If so, explain how and why.

2. A primary goal of a children's bereavement program is to help children acquire the language to express the emotions of grief so that caregivers

can respond to their need for comfort and understanding. What are some of the methods the therapist can use to teach children the language of grief?

3. Children often have a kinetic response when confronted with powerful feelings, and this is nowhere more apparent than in a bereavement camp setting. Explain the characteristics that are necessary for a therapist to practice effectively in what often is the organized chaos of a bereavement camp. How does camp as the therapeutic setting differ from bereavement therapy provided in an office or a school, and what adjustments would you need to make in your practice to be effective as a therapist at a bereavement camp?

4. Simulate a group therapy exercise that is designed to help participants get in touch with a memory. Have the group sit in a circle. After guiding participants through a simple relaxation exercise using a modeling clay product, ask group members to model an object that reminds them of someone they love who has died. Ask for volunteers who are willing to show what they have created and to describe the memory it holds for them, being sure to help participants process this information as you move through the group.

5. Role play: Six-year-old Andy was astonished to learn that a person had to be dead to be in heaven. Fearful of saying the wrong thing, parents often ask the therapist for help to find the right words to answer a child's questions about death. Using role-play, practice what advice you would give Andy's Mom, and how you would respond to Andy and his discovery.

REFERENCES

Axline, V. (1969). *Play therapy* (rev. ed.). Boston: Houghton Mifflin.

Bacon, J. (1996). Support groups for bereaved children. In C. A. Corr & D. M. Corr (Eds.), *Handbook of childhood death and bereavement* (pp. 285–303). New York: Springer.

Cohen, J. A., & Mannarino, A. P. (2004). Treatment of childhood traumatic grief. *Journal of Clinical Child and Adolescent Psychology, 33*(4), 819–831.

Corr, C. A., & Corr, D. M. (Eds.). (1996). *Handbook of childhood death and bereavement*. New York: Springer.

DiSunno, R., Zimmerman, S., & Ruffin, P. (2004). *Jeremy goes to Camp Good Grief*. Westhampton Beach, NY: East End Hospice.

Erikson, E. (1963). *Childhood and society* (2nd ed.). New York: Norton.

Farber, M. L. Z., & Sabatino, C. A. (2007). A therapeutic summer weekend camp for grieving children: Supporting clinical practice through empirical evaluation. *Child and Adolescent Social Work Journal, 24,* 385–402.

Fox, S. S. (1988). *Good grief: Helping groups of children when a friend dies*. Boston: New England Association for the Education of Young Children.

Gilbert, K. R. (2002). Taking a narrative approach to grief research: Finding meaning in stories. *Death Studies, 26,* 223–239.

Glazer, H. R., & Clark, M. D. (1999). A family-centered intervention for grieving preschool children. *Journal of Child and Adolescent Group Therapy,* 9(4), 161–168.

Granot, T. (2005). *Without you: Children and young people growing up with loss and its effects.* London: Jessica Kingsley.

Kirwin, K. M., & Hamrin, V. (2005). Decreasing the risk of complicated bereavement and future psychiatric disorders in children. *Journal of Child and Adolescent Psychiatric Nursing, 18*(2), 62–78.

Kramer, E. (1993). *Art as therapy with children* (2nd ed.). Chicago: Magnolia Street.

Leighton, S. (2008). Bereavement therapy with adolescents: Facilitating a process of spiritual growth. *Journal of Child and Adolescent Psychiatric Nursing, 21*(1), 24–34.

Locust, C. (2008). The talking stick. Retrieved September 26, 2008, from *www.aciacart.com/stories/archive6.html.*

Lohnes, K. L., & Kalter, N. (1994). Preventive intervention groups for parentally bereaved children. *American Journal of Orthopsychiatry, 64*(4), 594–603.

MacLennan, B. W. (1998). Mourning groups for children suffering from expected or sudden death of family or friends. *Journal of Child and Adolescent Group Therapy, 8*(1), 13–22.

Mitchell, A. M., Wesner, S., Garand, L., Gale, D. D., Havill, A., & Brownson, L. (2007). A support group intervention for children bereaved by parental suicide. *Journal of Child and Adolescent Psychiatric Nursing, 20*(1), 3–13.

Oltjenbruns, K. A. (2001). Developmental context of childhood: Grief and regrief phenomena. In M. Stroebe, R. O. Hansson, W. Stroebe, & H. Schut (Eds.), *Handbook of bereavement research: Consequences, coping, and caring* (pp. 169–198). Washington, DC: American Psychological Association.

Piaget, J., & Inhelder, B. (1969). *Early growth of logic in the child.* New York: Norton.

Pynoos, R. S. (1992). Grief and trauma in children and adolescents. *Bereavement Care, 11*(1), 2–10.

Ruffin, P., & Zimmerman, S. (2007). *A parent's guide to children's grief.* Unpublished manuscript. Westhampton Beach, New York, East End Hospice.

Samide, L. L., & Stockton, R. (2002). Letting go of grief: Bereavement groups for children in the school setting. *Journal for Specialists in Group Work, 27*(2), 192–204.

Schuurman, D. (2008). Grief groups for grieving children and adolescents. In K. J. Doka & A. S. Tucci (Eds.), *Living with grief: Children and adolescents* (pp. 255–268). Washington, DC: Hospice Foundation of America.

Silverman, P. R., Nickman, S., & Worden, J. W. (1992). Detachment revisited: The child's reconstruction of a dead parent. *American Journal of Orthopsychiatry, 62*(4), 494–503.

Tonkins, S. A. M., & Lambert, M. J. (1996). A treatment outcome study of bereavement groups for children. *Child and Adolescent Social Work Journal, 13*(1), 3–21.

Turner, M. (1999). Tackling children's primitive fears during the grieving process. *Bereavement Care, 20*(2), 22–25.

Webb, N. B. (Ed.). (2002). *Helping bereaved children: A handbook for practitioners* (2nd ed.). New York: Guilford Press.

Webb, N. B. (Ed.). (2007). *Play therapy with children in crisis* (3rd ed.). New York: Guilford Press.

Winnicott, D. W. (1965). *The maturational process and the facilitating environment: Studies in the theory of emotional development.* Madison, CT: International Universities Press.

Worden, J. W. (1996). *Children and grief: When a parent dies.* New York: Guilford Press.

Worden, J. W., & Silverman, P. R. (1996). Parental death and the adjustment of school-age children. *Omega: Journal of Death and Dying, 33*(2), 91–102.

Yalom, I. D., & Leszcz, M. (2005). *The theory and practice of group psychotherapy* (5th ed.). New York: Basic Books.

Zambelli, G. C., & DeRosa, A. P. (1992). Bereavement support groups for school-age children: Theory, intervention, and case example. *American Journal of Orthopsychiatry, 62*(4), 484–493.

CHAPTER 16

Storytelling
with Bereaved Children

DONNA O'TOOLE

Stories are not merely a nice or fun decoration added to the real
stuff of mental development. They are, in many respects, the real
stuff of mental development. . . . Through stories children construct
a self and communicate that self to others.
                                          —ENGEL (1995, p. 206)

A Poem for the Way of Words

There were days when people gathered stories
As they gathered coal and wood—
To make safe and warm the hearth and home.
Their stories were told so they might live and learn.
The words spoken and heard
Were medicine—transforming fear into hope,
Bringing order from chaos—
Rearranging danger into courage, desire, determination.
And still today the stories live amongst us,
Changing lead into gold,
They call us back to the fires' edge.
For even when we think ourselves to be alone,
When darkness threatens loss of sense and sight,
The stories wait—long lines of children wise beyond their years,
Waiting to be called upon, to be heard, to heal, to cradle fear.
These stories come back to us in many ways,
As images unbridled and unbidden by need,
For they are a part of us that does not die.
Memories eternal. Remember, their embers are glowing in the night.
                                          —DONNA O'TOOLE (copyright 2008)

FINDING OUR WAY THROUGH STORIES:
A TRANSGENERATIONAL JOURNEY

Storytelling is as ancient as human civilization. Although the use of story for healing, awareness, instruction, and hope was once obscured by the persuasions and popularity of analytical psychology, cultures across the globe once again recognize the richness and value of story. Today professionals of various disciplines, including those of us working on behalf of bereaved and seriously ill children, once again rely upon ancient and contemporary stories as a way to move forward, to offer connections and courage, and to share information and insight.

Neuroscientists and professional storytellers tell us why story works. They propose that we have returned to stories because deep in our cerebral cortex we know that stories matter (Haven, 2007). Stories realize and validate the power and ability to find meaning even in the face of grief and adversity. Modern culture and modern life offer countless stories of superheroes and everyday children who have faced unthinkable losses as children, and who found themselves to be empowered to go forward with hope, compassion, and power through facing their grief and extracting meaning from the loss of their loved ones. The Harry Potter books by J. K. Rowling (1998, 1999, 2000a, 2000b, 2004, 2006, 2007) provide a popular and beloved series of such stories, in which Harry Potter, a bereaved orphan, searches to rediscover his lost parents. As in other stories of children who have suffered grievous loss, Harry's determination to face challenge and his capacity to seek meaning and hope with imaginative courage pay off (Haven, 2008). Children enjoy these fairytales and superheroes, and they also use stories they make up or extract from other family members in their search for safety, validation, and meaning in their own lives.

Stories in which characters face loss and adversity until they gain competence and transformation also resonate with adults. In 1995 Barack Obama, whose father was absent from his daily life as a child, wrote the story of his grief, hopes, fears, and uncertainties as he struggled to understand, recover, and restory his life. The real-life stories he told in *Dreams from My Father* (Obama, 1995) and in *The Audacity of Hope* (Obama, 2006) fostered the belief that a bewildered, bereaved boy of color could and did grow strong and smart enough to become President of the United States of America.

Through research, practice, and science, we have come to understand the power of story to create and shape reality. Our stories, even when they contain trauma, need not be feared (Johnson, 2004). Story is how we organize, remember, and make meaning. In story we navigate our way through the world, learning how to ameliorate the loss and grief of challenges and change.

Parents and caregiving adults can introduce therapeutic stories and books to children as they live with their grievous losses from toddlerhood to adolescence and beyond. New developmental stages and significant life events may call into being a search for new, age-appropriate meaning. Stories allow us to weave continuity and uncertainty into new awareness and images, granting self-empowerment. Likewise, professionals in various disciplines have discovered storytelling and story sharing as a motivational and informational tool.

In my 40 years of work, study, and practice in the field of loss and grief, death and dying, story and storytelling have allowed me to value the extension of the boundaries of psychological theory by embracing story as a valuable and practical life art form, a form inherently known and available to all people. Story can surely be named as folk art, but it is so much more. Story, as I am speaking of it here, is also more than what has become known in counseling circles as a theory of narrative practice. Story is in a class of its own and is more than narrative. As I have said, story is the way our brains are wired. Whereas a narrative can be a chapter from a story, an experience, a portion of a whole, story is an evolving process with specific content elements. Story has inquiries, quests, dangers, and conclusions. Stories have form (Haven, 2007), and through story we come to know and make sense of the world. Through story we face or shrink from the challenges and joys of life. Human beings who are inherently meaning makers resonate to stories as a natural way to navigate the challenges brought about by loss throughout the lifespan. Stories can imprint solutions, guide our quests, and emerge as beacons of light in times of darkness and despair.

My Personal Experience:
On How Story Changed My Life

The story *Aarvy Aardvark Finds Hope* (O'Toole, 1988) came to me 6 months after the death of my 21-year-old son Matthew. I still feel in my bones the contrast of the light streaming through my kitchen windows on a November afternoon when the aardvark appeared into the great void of the sadness I was feeling. During the previous several weeks I had been experiencing the pain of intense longing for my son. Now, while I was at work writing a graduate thesis on the value of using creative expression in times of grief, the story of a bereaved animal, an aardvark who named himself Aarvy Aardvark, came to me. I did not consciously think this story into being. Rather, the story came to me, unbidden, persistent, and image filled. It was more the experience of movement and knowing through my body than through my head.

So intense was the story that I could not block it from awareness. Thus, Aarvy's story simply unfolded before and strangely beyond my eyes. Finally I picked up a pad of paper and a pen as the words of the story, without effort or thought, flowed onto the pages. How long did it take? I do not know. Time changed and time stood still, until I realized I was sitting in the dark with only a small light shining from another room. I had in my hands a treasure. A story. I checked each word as if I were a new mother checking my baby's fingers and toes. The story told everything, even more than I knew. It was a life-changing story without footnotes. From where had it come? How did it happen? This new kind of knowing was for me an experience of words, yet an experience that our language is inept to describe. The story, which at first I kept hidden from others, was eventually shared and much later published as *Aarvy Aardvark Finds Hope*.

Gradually, as I read, reread, and shared the Aarvy story with others, I discovered the deeper meanings embedded in the story. I found many intergenerational factors of my own life history in Aarvy's story. Here were situations that spoke not only to the loss and death of my infant daughter and 21-year-old son but also to layers of loss I had experienced as a child when my father abandoned our family. As I turned *Aarvy Aardvark Finds Hope* around in my mind, shadows of my own child-hood losses emerged into light. Miraculously, it seemed, I was restorying myself with poignant memories and newly discovered meanings, insight, and hope.

Over time, and through the feedback of many others who came to know and appreciate *Aarvy Aardvark Finds Hope*, I have come to value Aarvy's story as timeless and universal. Aarvy's story demonstrates the possibility that grief that is realized, expressed, validated, attended to, and witnessed can be a natural healing, even transformational, process. New experiences with children and adults led me to courses and confer-ences with skilled, veteran storytellers. Eventually I incorporated story-telling into my own international teaching related to loss, pain, healing, and transformation.

Mama Mockingbird's Story

Mama Mockingbird (Wood, 1998) is another modern folk story that demonstrates how stories can emerge from sorrow, transforming sad-ness and quickening hope. Shattered by the sudden death of her grown son Scot Kenneth Wood in 1982, and at times doubting whether her

322 INTERVENTIONS WITH BEREAVED CHILDREN

"pieces" would ever get back together again, Saunie Wood was walking the hills near her home when the story of *Mama Mockingbird* came to her, as she says, "through the wind." Like Mama Mockingbird in her story, Saunie was in search of the lost vitality and joy of the life she had known when her son was living. In the story, Mama Mockingbird's son suddenly dies. Mama Mockingbird and her family cry and cry. They cry so long and so hard that they forget how to sing. Later, as Mama Mockingbird sets out on a journey to find her song, she says to her family, "I have lost my son, but I do not think I was meant to lose my song."

Like me, Saunie was at first startled by the power of the story that came to her. For a long time she hid her story and told it to no one, as had I. One day a counseling friend gave Saunie a copy of *Aarvy Aardvark Finds Hope*. She so resonated to Aarvy's story that, as a gift, Saunie sent me a taped version of her story *Mama Mockingbird*, and gave me permission to share and tell the story as I saw fit. Although Saunie is a gifted storyteller herself, *Mamma Mockingbird* was then too painful and personal a story for her to tell.

Gradually Saunie's pain was lifting. The story that was given to her, as she said, "through the wind" was heard by others through my telling and recognized for its depth and beauty. The *Mama Mockingbird* story (Wood, 1998) uses the natural world as a metaphor for the nature and naturalness of the healing process of grief. Once again, a healing story offered comfort and meaning long before the author had a cognitive understanding of its meaning.*

Adults are not the only ones who have used stories to quicken hope and to guide them toward understanding and a reduction from suffering. My son Matthew Schmidt, as a 19-year-old, and 5-year-old Joeri Breebaart further demonstrate how even the very young can find their way through loss with story making and storytelling.

Matthew's Story

Although he was pale, thin, and often seriously ill, Matthew wrote about himself in a different and powerful way—as "Super Cystic" (Schmidt, 1981). Matt was born with cystic fibrosis, a hereditary disease that adversely affects the internal secreting functions of the body. To help himself and others dealing with the boredom, homesickness, and fear

---

* Saunie's story *Mamma Mockingbird*, told in her own voice, is available on a CD of healing stories for children entitled *Stories of Lead, Stories of Gold* (O'Toole with Wood, 2002).

that young children feel when they enter a hospital for treatment, he developed a coloring book of characters who faced up to and outwitted the challenges of their disease.

Super Cystic had many powerful friends and cohorts (see Figure 16.1). There was an inventive nurse named Fabulous Fran Fibrosis, as well as IV Man, Bob the Breather, Carol Capsule, Polly Pounder, Ralph Respiratory, and Erving Enzyme. Together Super Cystic and his mighty and wise companions battled the powerful bad guys—the bugs—Boris Bacteria and Nasty Pneumonia.

Although often hospitalized and ill, Matt lived with integrity, imagination, and humor to age 21. His brief life challenged and inspired me and many others to live life creatively and fully. A year after his death, Matt's coloring book was posthumously published by a pharmaceutical company (Schmidt, 1981), which made it available, so that other youngsters with cystic fibrosis might have a greater understanding of the nature of their illness, thereby fostering in these young patients hope and personal empowerment.

Joeri's Story

But, we might ask, can even very young children make use of story as a part of their healing process? The true story of Joeri Breebaart and his father Piet Breebaart gives insight. The following paragraphs are excerpts from the foreword of their book, *When I Die, Will I Get Better?* (Breebaart & Breebaart, 1993).† Here Piet tells in his own words what happened after his son Remi died suddenly of meningitis when he was 2 years, 8 months old; at the time Joeri, who shared a bedroom and had been very close to his brother, was 5:

> In the weeks after the funeral, Joeri was not only sad, but also very withdrawn and often angry. He was confused and disturbed by the loss of Remi and the concept of death and dying. He couldn't really talk about Remi's illness and death, and we had a hard time trying to reach Joeri and understand his feelings. We looked for children's books on death but there wasn't much that appealed to us.
>
> About six weeks after Remi's death, Joeri and I came to talk about Joe Rabbit. Joe was an invented character about whom we used to tell stories to Remi at bedtime. For Joeri, Joe Rabbit stood for Remi. Joeri himself was Fred Rabbit, Joe's brother. Joeri said it was impossible to make up stories about Joe Rabbit now, since Remi was dead. I then suggested making up a story in which Joe would die. That was fine with Joeri.

---

† Reprinted with permission from the McGraw-Hill Companies.

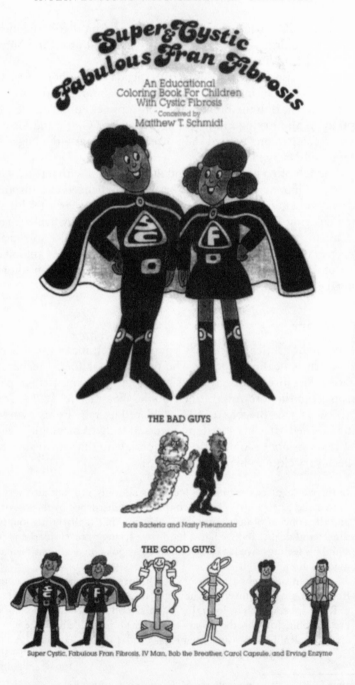

FIGURE 16.1. Illustrations of Super Cystic and cohorts. From Schmidt (1981). Reprinted by permission of Organon Inc.

Joeri created the story himself and told me what he wanted to be drawn for each illustration. I wrote down the story and made the drawing, sometimes the same day, sometimes a few days later.

It was important to Joeri that I followed his indications. When, for example, I had made a fox for a doctor, Joeri protested, for the fox would eat the rabbits. No, Joeri said, the doctor ought to be an owl. There were also days, when Joeri didn't want to talk about it.

The story describes Joeri's own experience. We entitled the story, *When I Die, Will I Get Better?* It tells how Remi got ill, how he died, the funeral, the loss, the coming to terms with the sadness. For us it meant a possibility to talk about it all with Joeri. It wasn't threatening this way. Joeri talked about the rabbits, and about us.

This healing process took about four weeks, and Joeri was very proud of the result. He told his teacher he had made a book about rabbits. Later he could tell her it was about his brother. He took the book to school and his teacher read it out loud in class. This meant a great deal to Joeri. (Breebaart & Breebaart, 1993, p. 2)

It meant a great deal to Piet, Joeri's father, as well. Healing stories reach across the generations. Just as I found comfort in witnessing my son's creative capacity for restorying hope by helping himself and others imagine strength and wholeness in the midst of illness and disease, so too was Joeri's father Piet comforted. As he watched and listened, and as he illustrated the words that Joeri told him to depict the death of his brother, he was bonded in a process that moved from the pain of unbearable silence to that of a new type of presence, one of remembering. Story making and storytelling allow the essence of a life to be savored, honored, known, and remembered.

Stories that carry themes of resilience and wholeness can assist healing during times of loss and grief (Taylor, 1996; Dwivedi, 1997). Stories weave or reweave lives together. A healing story can clarify and validate, as well as provide new information and insight. A story theme can resonate across races, ages, and circumstances, illuminating connections and lessening isolation and uncertainty (Taylor, 1996).

Those of us wishing to help bereaved children grieve and grow can enhance our abilities to coach and validate these children by expanding our storytelling, story-making, and story-sharing abilities. We can use stories to address unique circumstances and needs, and to encourage insight, imagination, and understanding. Through such stories we can break down isolation, quicken hope, and normalize the many intense ups and downs of the grief process. Although stories do not keep children from hurting, they may keep them from hurting for the wrong reasons, and from feeling strange and alone. We can help children restore (restory) hope for a more meaningful, happier tomorrow.

THE ROLE OF RESILIENCY AND HARDINESS
IN RESTORYING

Resilience and hardiness research provides a scaffold through which we can elicit and stimulate healing stories. The research on hardiness and resilience (O'Connell Higgins, 1994; Flach, 1988; Walsh, 2006; Kobasa, 1985) can strengthen our confidence in helping children through story forms. This research documents how children and adults positively transform loss and adversity into life-enhancing ways of being. Resilient persons are those who have weathered great gales and storms in life, emerging from these trials as hope-based rather than fear-based individuals (Schneider, 2000). Rather than being diminished by their losses, they are made stronger. They feel somehow enhanced by the rough circumstances they have integrated into the tapestry of their lives.

As the Skin Horse in the story *The Velveteen Rabbit* tells us, this restorying—this integration of the chapters of a life—does not happen as an event but as a process:

> It doesn't happen all at once. You become. It takes a long time. That's why it doesn't happen to people who break easily, or have sharp edges, or who have to be carefully kept. . . . [But] once you are *Real* you can't be ugly, except to people who don't understand. (Williams, 1922/1995; emphasis added)

Helpers, or "interaction agents" (a term I prefer), who desire to assist bereaved children need to know what can go right (resilience, positive reformulation, and transformation), as well as what may go wrong (complicated grief and pathology). We are called to differentiate grief experiences that may naturally reoccur across the lifespan from complicated grief that is often overdiagnosed as depression (Schneider, 2000). For all professionals working with bereaved children, I recommend a thorough review of the work of Therese Rando (1993) and John Schneider (2000), as well as perusal of current developmental literature. I hope this book will also serve as a resource for many.

In choosing potentially healing stories to tell and share with children and their families, I look for tales that exhibit the following elements I have extracted from the literature as key traits of those who possess hope-based, resilient personalities:

- Examples of hopefulness in characters that find or maintain an enduring belief in the possibility of fervent wishes. In challenges of doubt and fear, these characters face (rather than avoid) the unknown. They proceed through grief not without fear and uncertainty but with the help of some small, inner, hopeful voice. They are moved by determination rather than held back by mistrust or resignation.

- Characters and story elements that display personal, nonjudgmental awareness and acceptance of needs, emotions, values, and mental and physical states.
- Characters with intact personal boundaries.
- Characters who express their needs and feelings assertively as a hallmark of personal choice rather than coercion, manipulation, or judgment.
- Characters who display congeniality—the ability to engage and be engaged.
- Stories that demonstrate remembrance and commemoration in ordinary life or through recognized rituals. These stories tangibly or symbolically recognize and make real the loss, its value, and meaning.
- Some story elements that honor or demonstrate affinity, a connection or kinship to something greater and/or beyond the self.
- Elements that demonstrate and encourage active imagination— the willingness and capacity to dream and to conceive of ideas and possibilities and mystery, all of which offer the possibility of an unfolding, ongoing, and changing story rather than a certain, absolute end or solution.
- Stories that favor forgiveness and awareness over blame and shame. Forgiveness here implies the ability to accommodate to the imperfection of oneself and of others.

Annotated lists of storybooks for children and adolescents facing loss and bereavement can be found in the Compassion Books catalog (O'Toole, 2009) and in Corr (2000), Corr, Nabe, and Corr (2000), and O'Toole (1995).

GRIEVING AS A LIFE SKILL

From the cradle to the grave, loss and grief are part of life. Young people need to understand various responses to loss across the lifespan. By understanding how grief manifests itself through thought, emotion, behavior, and spiritual questioning and meaning making, children can learn to build awareness, acceptance, and competence.

Grieving can be thought of as a life skill that can be shared and learned (O'Toole, 1989). Adults can use teachable moments of grief in many ways: to normalize the experience of grief (e.g., for the death of a pet); to witness, to validate, and to label a child's feelings of loss (e.g., a move to a new home), without judging those feelings; and to model and guide ways of externalizing (and ultimately integrating) feelings that avoid harm to the child or to others.

Adults who have themselves navigated loss have an important and crucial role in modeling and holding hope for bereaved children (Jevne & Miller, 1999). It is possible for children to overcome great adversity and grievous losses, and thrive. Maintaining hope and being able to imagine a meaningful future lie at the foundation of positive outcomes from a grievous loss (Schneider, 2006).

STORY AS A MEANING-MAKING PROCESS

A storied or narrative view of life recognizes that grief can be a lifetime process—a spiral of feedback loops rather than a single event that follow a prescribed path. A metaphor, a theory, or a stage model of grief, extrapolated from the experiences of many, may present a valuable road map of grief but is unlikely to show the exact terrain any individual child or adult will travel as each experiences his or her own grief process.

Story, as a topic of inquiry, presents an enormous playing field. For both the storyteller and the story listener, narrative approaches involve all aspects of self (mind and body, spiritual and social), often simultaneously. Therefore, story approaches are inherently holistic in nature and difficult to analyze by separating elements. They emerge at the intersection of experience, emotion, and language as a meaning-making process.

From a *spiritual* perspective, one in which meaning making and personal spiritual development are included and valued, both story and grief provide a cornucopia of lifelong opportunity. As we process our losses across the lifespan through experience and selective attention, and as we alter and elaborate on stories that unfold, we are creating the "true" story—the meaning of our life. Moreover, the key to transforming losses into something positive lies in embracing our memories. In this way we remember ourselves (Harvey, 1996)—or, in story terms, we restory (and restore) ourselves.

Narrative approaches are child- or individual-centered. From a narrative point of view, a person whose intention is to be part of a healing process for a grieving child (or family) plays the role of interaction agent rather than expert. Using their current awareness and intuitive insights, the children and adults play with story possibilities to explore and cocreate connections, change, and healing.

Additionally, using storytelling as a way of processing a loss experience calls for a leveled playing field. Storytelling is an interaction process between the teller and the listener. This process evolves over time with flow and mystery rather than through fixed, stable expectations that are certain and provable. Story approaches imply a collaborative rather than a hierarchical process. Both the listener and the teller are affected by the telling. Both are changed by the process. Since possibilities are offered but not prescribed, choice abounds. The locus of control is shared and internal. In this approach, authority is often based on intuition and personal experience rather than on objective formulas or power.

Naming an event, designating it as a specific vignette, a story, or a chapter of life, gives it importance. By naming, writing, and telling our stories, we lay claim to their rightful place in our memory. Matt's and Joeri's stories as told, written, and titled remind us that those we care about give life quality and meaning long after they are gone from our sight.

Stories can also cause us to explore our personal histories. From the story of Aarvy Aardvark, who loses his entire family at a very young age, I can explore memories of abandonment I felt as a young child when my father left our family. By working with Aarvy's story I have been able to realize ways that my entire family and I were forever changed by this loss.

My mother is no longer living, but from the vantage point of Aarvy, a profoundly bereaved creature, I can explore my relationship with my mother. Why did she grow to mistrust imagination and guide me to value facts rather than also to entertain fiction? As I remember my mother, I also remember my sister Sharon, 5 years my elder, who was tireless in enthusiastically reading fairytales or making up stories to delight and entertain. Now, as a storyteller myself, I feel deeply connected to my sister Sharon. Through sharing family stories with Sharon I have come to understand that, in her mind, I am her child, not my mother's. She cared for me, watched over me. Sharon has five other children, but now, in her 70s, she thinks of me as her first child. As we come to accept how we each created meaning and story, we can wonder about the different themes we created as children in a family experiencing many profound losses of the Great Depression and World War II. Whether recognized or not, storytelling and story sharing are intergenerational processes of continuity with a cast of thousands—those known, and those yet to be discovered.

THE ROLE OF STORY ALTERATION
AND STORY CHOICE

The selection of a story for telling or reading to bereaved children can be both science and art. Selecting a story takes awareness, knowledge, and a sensitivity to the individual needs and developmental aptitudes of your audience. However, once you are familiar with various materials and stories, it is likely to take only a short time to determine whether a particular book is appropriate and satisfactory. You may even experience yourself as capable of making up stories on the spot to match particular situations. Doris Brett's book *Annie Stories* (1988) is an excellent resource that shows how brief but poignant made-up stories can help children cope with a variety of real or anticipated loss situations.

Story choice and story alteration are necessary skills in the use of story for healing and understanding. *A word of caution here*: When altering stories that are not in the public domain but under copyright, one must first consult the story's author (and/or copyright holder) to obtain his or her permission for a literal retelling. It is helpful to understand that copyright does not protect an idea, only the fixed form of expression of an idea. A more in-depth discussion of copyright issues related to storytelling is found in *The Storyteller's Guide* (Mooney & Holt, 1996).

As already noted, storytelling is an interaction between the listener and the teller. When you are telling a story in a way that makes use of all aspects of the self (mind, body, spirit) to engage and convey the story, you, the storyteller, will be changed by the reception of the listener(s). This is often true even in writing.

For instance, as I interact here with the imagined ear of you, the listener, someone with whom I wish to connect in a meaningful way, I imagine the story in the context of this book. I think about what the story might mean to you, am challenged by how I can describe what it means to me, and am curious as to what it might mean to the editor of this book, whom I appreciate and admire. I am informed by my belief that effective storytellers do more than tell a tale, they embody it (Stotter, 1994). I ask myself, "What should I add or take from my story experience that will bring you, the reader, with me into the written story? How can I create an environment so that its words can transmit meaning and resonance? Something to help this story encourage you to discover and use story in your work with children?"

In my experience one thing rings true: Stories that heal offer kinesthetic and emotional memories and possibilities, as well as intellectual ones. Stories that have the greatest potential for healing are those that have openings, places that listeners can claim for their own. These stories can create shifts in awareness, understanding, and well-being, and their emotional resonance may replace or surpass cognitive understanding.

The Crucial Role of Imagination

Following a loss, the abilities to imagine new possibilities and to reformulate old experiences are essential components for finding our way or growing through grief. This imaginative capacity is needed by children and adults alike. It allows us to re-create or reconstruct meaning and hope for a life that may be new or altered but still holds value and promise. The imaginative capacity also serves as a foundation for building resilient, purposeful, and unique human beings.

RECOGNIZING THERAPEUTIC STORIES

In choosing and developing stories for therapeutic value, I rely heavily on two sources as guidelines: First, I count on my understanding of practices and attributes derived from the literature and research on resilience, heartiness, and transformation and growth through loss and trauma, some of which I listed previously. Second, I have gained greatly from workshops and study with various professional storytellers, especially Donald Davis (1993), Robin Moore (1991), David Holt and Bill Mooney (1994, 1996), Jim Mays (1989), and Kendall Haven (1999). I often return to their teachings when I search for stories, or when I write or tell my own. All of these storytellers have published works with August House Publishers in Little Rock, Arkansas.

Finding and Telling Stories That Resonate Wholeness

There is a *Family Circle* cartoon in which a little boy is distraught after hearing the nursery rhyme Humpty Dumpty. He looks up seriously at his father and says, "Maybe they didn't try hard enough."

Story is the natural language of children. At an early age children know what is and what is not a satisfying story (McAdams, 1993) and are able to manipulate story images to obtain more satisfactory outcomes. In the case of the Humpty Dumpty cartoon, the child hearing the story knows that something is wrong with its ending.

At a weeklong training I attended, storyteller Donald Davis presented a three-part formula for determining whether a story is whole or complete. Davis sees this formula as a means to measure a story's ability both to entertain and to be known by the listener as a wholesome life experience. From his point of view, a whole story begins as the listener feels at home and in place in the world of the story.

This is done first by providing in the story descriptions that locate the time, place, and people of the narrative in the normal routine of the characters' daily lives and allow the listener to experience them. This first phase of the telling, the story foundation, or story setting, often takes the most words and time to construct and to deliver.

Second, with the storyteller's world now known to the listener, a crisis or some trouble begins to surface in the narrative and is worked through. Davis defines a "crisis" as anything that takes a piece of the world we are comfortable with and turns it upside down, so that we have to make adjustments to go forward. The grievous losses of children certainly fit this criterion. The crisis may be sudden and dramatic or subtle and drawn out. A crisis can be chosen or involuntary, positive or negative. Davis describes this story phase by saying, "Trouble's coming . . . trouble's coming . . . trouble's coming . . . trouble comes." Davis points out that a whole story gives much more attention and time to setting the stage and to presenting the "trouble's coming" component than to the part of the story in which the trouble or crisis actually happens and is worked through. In a whole story, a healing story, a working through, some solution must be realized. The boy in the cartoon (discussed earlier) had a valid point. He knew that the problem of Humpty Dumpty was not resolved. As he saw the story, nothing was learned or discovered. So while Humpty Dumpty may be useful as a rhyme presenting the notion of loss as permanent and irreplaceable, it does little as a story to teach the concepts of resilience or connection, both of which are known to foster hope and well-being for children experiencing a loss (Klass, Silverman, & Nickman, 1996). For these purposes we look to whole stories containing the three elements suggested by Davis.

The third part of a whole story is its briefest component. This is the learning that is achieved and/or discovery that is made. Here Davis warns us not to get caught up in long prescriptive teachings. Children love to learn but, like adults, they rarely love to be taught. Let them discover. Therefore, while the discovery or learning from a story is an important component, it needs only a short amount of narrative time.

In *The Healing Power of Stories*, Daniel Taylor (1996, pp. 85–86) gives three parallel requirements of stories with the potential for healing losses and fostering resilience. Taylor says that first the story must explain the experience, externally or internally. Second, these stories must have explanations that are satisfactory. They need to create a world in which we find it possible—even desirable—to live. Third, like Davis, Taylor tells us that healing stories must assure us that life is worth the pain, that meaning is not an illusion, that others share and value our experience.

Here, then, is an example of a different ending for the Humpty Dumpty story, one that honors connection and memory:

So while all the King's horses and all the King's men couldn't put Humpty Dumpty together again, they could nonetheless care for him and remember him. And this they did. Some of the King's men carefully gathered up every last piece of Humpty Dumpty's shell; others called Humpty Dumpty's family and friends. Some gathered round in silence, listening, while others told stories about what he was like before he fell and cracked into so many pieces. Those who had loved Humpty still felt their love for him. That hadn't changed, although now their love had a great sadness as well. When all the work was done, they held hands and remembered Humpty Dumpty by singing this song: "Humpty Dumpty sat on a wall, Humpty Dumpty had a great fall. All the King's horses and all the King's men would always remember him as their special neighbor and friend."

REASONS FOR USING STORIES
WITH BEREAVED CHILDREN AND FAMILIES

Stories can be used in many ways with children who are bereaved. When choosing a story for a therapeutic use, keep in mind the particular need the story embodies, remembering that the most useful stories often describe rather than prescribe. These stories may suggest or describe change, but they do not demand it through pedantic persuasion.

Stories that assist healing have spiritual elements, as well as intellectual and emotional content. They allow the teller and the listener to enter into the mystery of what is known and what is not known. They present possibilities rather than dispense solutions.

Stories can provide information and distractions from the burden of sorrow, encourage curiosity and imagination, give validation, and present alternatives. Stories may give a sudden burst of insight or provide a gradual, indirect entry into awareness.

Stories can give new or additional information to correct faulty assumptions and be used to normalize the grief process. Through story, we can remember the past, validate what a child holds important, memorialize and honor what has been lost, and build bridges of hope for future development (Gersie, 1991). By diminishing isolation, quickening hope, and making a child's world more familiar and safe, stories also aid his or her spiritual development (Coles, 1991).

STORY FORMS AND PRACTICES

With the rising interest and current research into narrative as a therapeutic practice, many story forms have promise. These include poetry reading and writing, journal keeping, story circles, read-aloud story sharing, and collaboratively written poems, plays, and stories.

Enhanced stories—those that can be enacted through puppetry, play, music, video, and theater—are beyond the scope of this chapter but are worth mentioning. To help grieving children, Steve Dawson and Laura Harris (1997, 1999) have developed an intriguing process called grief dramatics. Their work offers a 9-week children's bereavement group curriculum, as well as scripts and activity pages. Grief dramatics can be used in individual or group settings, or in bereavement camps for school-age children.

The *Aarvy Aardvark Finds Hope* story I discussed earlier provides another look at enacted story. Because his family has been taken away, young Aarvy Aardvark is all alone. He feels so sad and devoid of hope that he even wishes he were dead. Thanks to a wise rabbit that befriends Aarvy through sharing his own experiences and witnessing Aarvy's pain, Aarvy gradually finds his own inner strength and begins to imagine a future. Through a slow and gradual awareness that culminates in a ritual of remembrance, Aarvy discovers the courage to grieve his losses. After the ritual, a time when Aarvy honors the memory of his mother, he can once again remember the beauty of rainbows of every color.

Aarvy's story, adapted as a live puppet show, is regularly performed by trained volunteers in two urban North Carolina school systems and by the Jewish Counseling Center of Norfolk, Virginia. By using Aarvy's story in this enhanced manner, hundreds of performances of the Aarvy story are given yearly to fourth-grade students and to adults and children in church, synagogue, and educational organizations.

The use of *Aarvy Aardvark Finds Hope* as a puppet show has helped teachers and school counselors identify and respond to many bereaved children. Other young students not currently suffering a loss learn to recognize the universality of loss, and the feelings and behaviors of grief as natural and normal. Students participating in the live puppet programs, who are assisted to interact with the puppets and do drawings and group activities, are thus able to change the story to show their personal needs and coping patterns.

Bereavement counselors can learn to use stories in several distinct ways: (1) spoken stories, (2) written stories and bookmaking, (3) storybooks—story readings, and (4) sharing personal stories and story listening.

Spoken Stories

For therapeutic value, storytelling in spoken form is perhaps the most compelling medium of all the story forms. I have had many opportunities to present stories about loss and grief, and death and dying, to individuals and to audiences large and small, young and old. These are stories I have either composed or have chosen and adapted from folk literature. During and after the storytelling I have witnessed the depth and breadth of learning as people respond, resonate, and extract what they need. People can and do enter into stories to create and discover their own meaning.

Telling Homemade, Individualized Stories

Doris Brett, an Australian psychologist and practitioner of therapeutic storytelling, has effectively constructed stories to help children deal with fear, pain, hospitalization, and death (Brett, 1988, 1992). She began her use of stories with her daughter Annie as together they faced various developmental hurdles and challenging life events. Later she fashioned her stories using materials and circumstances faced by troubled youngsters who were her clients. Brett gives the following outline for making up your own therapeutic stories:

1. *Model the story character after the child.* This assists the child in using the story through identifying with the character.
2. *Make the problems and conflicts echo those of the child.* The narrative tone of the story should match how the child sees the conflict, not how you see it. This assists identification with the story character. The idea is to have the child think, "Yes, that's exactly how I feel." After the child has identified with the character, you introduce the way the story character comes to shift its thinking as it struggles with and then resolves its concern.
3. *Keep things simple.* Use concepts and language the child can understand. Tailor the length of the story to the child's attention span.
4. *Have the story honestly portray real conflict, uncertainty, and struggle.* Children have internal experiences of these feelings that need to be matched by the story characters if the story is to be believable.
5. *Remember to identify the strengths of the child and weave them into the story.* This helps the child recognize these traits in him- or herself and to increase the individual sense of worth and potency.
6. *Use humor whenever possible.* It, too, allows for psychic shifts to take place and helps to release tension.
7. When the child is tense, use your voice as an instrument to encourage relaxation.

8. *As you tell the story, watch the child's body language for cues.* If the child is engaged, you are on target. If the child is disinterested, you might be on the wrong track, or the content may be something he or she is not ready to hear.
9. *If you are unsure of where to go next, ask the child.* "What do you think Tommy did then?" Encourage responses through such a guessing game, until you have enough direction to continue.
10. *Give the child hope by ending in a way that relieves the story character's distress.* Brett suggests that these positive endings be honest and possible, something the child can use.

Mutual Storytelling

Brett's guidelines apply when creating a story for a specific situation. Another method of creating stories for therapeutic use is the mutual storytelling technique developed by Richard Gardner (1993). His work is thorough and instructive, and provides considerable insight into ways the mutual storytelling technique can be effectively used in therapy situations. His work, based on the psychodynamic interpretation of the child's story themes, may seem challenging to persons who offer supportive rather than therapeutic bereavement counseling.

The work of Joyce Mills and Richard Crowley (1986) shifts the focus from psychodynamic analysis to the behavioral subtleties they observe and extrapolate in their work with children. Using metaphors and stories, Mills and Crowley parallel a child's situation with metaphors that the child has not overtly identified. Their clinical success with metaphors and simple stories is a tribute to the healing power of the interactive story, especially when the content is carefully and sensitively chosen, and is altered by a child's verbal and nonverbal responses. Their approach favors the story *process,* one in which the child cocreates the story, over the story content. Mills and Crowley believe a story can bring about positive internal shifts and gains even when the child is unable to articulate that change through cognitive recognition.

Written Stories and Bookmaking

There has been an increase in popularity of personal stories for adults, as well as for children. The *Chicken Soup for the Soul* (Canfield & Hansen, 1993) books that tell short, personal stories of inspiration have enjoyed many months on best-seller lists. National publishing houses publish hundreds of personal stories each year, and many authors— unable to negotiate contracts with publishers—have self-published their memoirs.

Bookmaking can be used by parents and professionals alike, as discussed earlier in the father–son publication, *When I Die, Will I Get Better?* (Breehaart & Breehaart, 1993). The technique of bookmaking as a therapeutic process is carefully outlined for parents and practitioners in *Homemade Books to Help Kids Cope*, by Robert Ziegler (1992).

Storybooks—Story Readings

Many of us remember a particular book, poem, song, or story that came to us at just the right time. We remember how we were given some glimpse of hope or some insight to face some challenge. The story *The Little Engine That Could* (Piper, 1990) evokes many such remembrances. A train faces a big hurdle in taking its load of toys across a great hill to waiting children. It seems an impossible task. But the Little Engine, empowered with resilient traits, turns boldly to the task. Although the going is steep and difficult, the Little Engine never loses hope: "I think I can, I think I can" is its constant refrain.

Many stories have been told of how *The Little Engine That Could* has been used by children and adults to help them complete tasks that appeared impossible. One of these stories reports how an elementary school child pulled his mother, who was injured and unable to walk, from a wrecked car and up an incline to safety. The mother remembers hearing her son's repetitive refrain, "I think I can, I think I can," as he cajoled her to move while he dragged and pulled her away from danger.

As the author of *Aarvy Aardvark Finds Hope*, I have experienced the power of a tale to heal. I have been privileged to receive many poignant phone calls and letters from adults and children whom I would otherwise not have known. They have told me how they used Aarvy's story and Ralphy's imaginary presence to hold onto hope during periods of despair and loneliness. One such woman was a single parent, whom I doubt I will ever meet but cannot imagine I will ever forget. On the phone she told me how her only child had been killed in a car crash. She told me how desperately she herself had wished to die. This, she said, was the only way she could imagine being reunited with her daughter. For months she had reached out to touch the copy of *Aarvy Aardvark Finds Hope* that a friend had given her. She kept the book on her bedside table, beside a night-light, which she kept on. She said that on the many nights when she could not sleep, she would reach out and touch the book cover. As she did so, she would hope that, like Aarvy, she, too, might find the will to live; that she might someday, like him, be able to imagine a rainbow of every color.

This woman told me how one day while she was walking from the grocery store to her car, she saw a brilliant rainbow that arched across the city. She immediately felt a momentary burst of hope and joy. She said that in that instant, she felt reconnected to her daughter, to everything, everywhere. For her it marked a turning point. She had a long way to go, she told me, but she knew now that she was not alone, that she belonged, and that somehow she would find her way.

I am convinced there is more at work here than the story itself. For me there is experience, cocreation, and no small amount of mystery. Through the stories we tell, especially those with which we resonate and retell ourselves, not only do we construct ourselves (Engel, 1995) but we are also held in the arms of the mystery we sometimes call love. Indeed, storytelling can diffuse isolation and help us find our way.

Sharing Personal Stories and Story Listening

As a person who has experienced healing and growth through many different story forms, I would be remiss if I did not speak of the inherent value of personal dialogue and listening in various settings. Whether in individual encounters, in dyads, in story-sharing circles, or in other group settings, story sharing enables us to see and reformulate our world. Through the transparency of self we can externalize beliefs, validate what gives meaning to our lives, and release internalized or repressed feelings. Sharing like this allows our own words to be mirrors in which we can see ourselves from the inside out.

Thus, in listening to our own words, we are better able to decide whether to appreciate and maintain the story as it stands or take steps to alter it through present experience, knowledge, desire, and awareness. Additionally, we, as cocreator helpmates, benefit from listening to the stories of others. Listening stimulates opportunities for new insights as we learn about the many and varied ways individuals experience similar circumstances. Benevolent listening with nonjudgmental awareness can greatly enrich our ability to understand ourselves and others.

OUR CHALLENGE: TO FOSTER NARRATIVE DEVELOPMENT IN CHILDREN

If we are to raise resilient children, we will do well to nurture children in the telling of stories. Susan Engel (1995) suggests that we can enhance the natural abilities of children to tell stories by listening attentively, responding substantively, and using collaboration to clarify and expand the tales. Engel also recommends a multiplicity of voices and genres for story expression, encouraging the use of a wide range of forms and permitting, even encouraging, stories about things that matter to the individual child.

As adults desiring to prepare children for the vicissitudes of life, we are called to encourage, reformulate, hold, and witness the stories of those we cherish. Together, as we make the transgenerational journey, we can find our way with the help of such stories. For healing stories are more than fiction—they can be our means of recognition, insight, and liberation. Stories are how we can connect with our children, how we can connect with ourselves. Stories can make us real.

DISCUSSION QUESTIONS AND ROLE-PLAY EXERCISES

1. Imagine that you are a school social worker who has been asked to provide a consultation to a third-grade classroom teacher regarding the death of one of her students in a car accident. The teacher has asked you to give her the names of some books she can read to the class. How would you prepare for this consultation? Discuss this in terms of both possible resources for the teacher and suggested activities to help the children grieve their loss.

2. Review three stories from folk literature or books mentioned in this chapter, such as *When I Die, Will I Get Better?* and *Aarvy Aardvark Finds Hope*, to identify factors that contributed to the resilience of the story characters. Write these factors down. Then find someone else to read the books and to identify what assisted their healing. Discuss and collaborate on your findings as to what factors and qualities enhanced healing.

3. Do you think that everyone can learn to use storytelling with bereaved children? What might interfere with a counselor's willingness or ability to use this modality, and how could he or she become more comfortable using this method?

4. Discuss some of the pros and cons of reading a story to a bereaved child compared to telling the story in your own words or creating one together with the child. What are some of the advantages of using a video such as *Aarvy Aardvark Finds Hope* in a bereavement group like those conducted by some hospice programs. How may the facilitator stimulate group discussion following the viewing of the video?

5. Role play: Using animal characters, create a story about the death of a parent. After selecting the age and abilities of the child with whom the story will be developed, indicate how you might help the child incorporate Donald Davis's three-part formula for an effective story. Role-play this process with someone who will play the part of the child.

REFERENCES

Breebaart, J., & Breebaart, P. (1993). *When I die, will I get better?* New York: Bedrick Books.

Brett, D. (1988). *Annie stories.* New York: Workman.

Brett, D. (1992). *More Annie stories.* Washington, DC: Magination Press/American Psychological Association.

Canfield, J., & Hansen, M. (1993). *Chicken soup for the soul.* Deerfield Beach, FL: Health Communications.

Coles, R. (1991). *The spiritual life of children.* New York: Houghton Mifflin.

Corr, C. A. (2000). Using books to help children and adolescents cope with death: Guidelines and bibliography. In K. Doka (Ed.), *Living with grief: Children, adolescents, and loss* (pp. 295–314). Washington, DC: Hospice Foundation of America.

Corr, C. A., Nabe, C. M., & Corr, D. M. (2000). *Death and dying, life and living* (3rd ed.). Belmont, CA: Wadsworth.

Davis, D. (1993). *Telling your own stories.* Little Rock, AR: August House.

Dawson, S., & Harris, L. (1997). *Adventures in the land of grief.* Wilmore, KY: Words on the Wind.

Dawson, S., & Harris, L. (1999). *Death of a forest queen.* Wilmore, KY: Words on the Wind.

Dwivedi, K. N. (1997). *The therapeutic use of stories.* New York: Routledge.

Engel, S. (1995). *The stories children tell.* New York: Freeman.

Flach, F. (1988). *Resilience: Discovering a new strength at times of stress.* New York: Ballantine Books.

Gardner, R. (1993). *Storytelling in psychotherapy with children.* Northvale, NJ: Aronson.

Gersie, A. (1991). *Storymaking in bereavement.* London: Jessica Kingsley.

Harvey, J. (1996). *Embracing their memory: Loss and the social psychology of storytelling.* Needham Heights, MA: Allyn & Bacon.

Haven, K. (1999). *Write right! Creative writing using storytelling techniques.* Little Rock, AR: August House.

Haven, K. (2007). *Story proof: The science behind the startling power of story.* Westport, CT: Libraries Unlimited.

Haven, K. (2008). *Reluctant heroes: True five-minute-read adventure stories for boys.* Westport, CT: Libraries Unlimited.

Holt, D., & Mooney, B. (Eds.). (1994). *Ready-to-tell tales.* Little Rock, AR: August House.

Holt, D., & Mooney, B. (1996). *The storyteller's guide.* Little Rock, AR: August House.

Jevne, R., & Miller, J. (1999). *Finding hope.* Fort Wayne, IN: Willowgreen.

Johnson, S. (2004). *Mind wide open: Your brain and the neuroscience of everyday life.* New York: Scribner.

Klass, D., Silverman, P., & Nickman, S. (1996). *Contuining bonds.* Washington, DC: Taylor & Francis.

Kobasa, S. (1985). Stressful life events, personality, and health: An inquiry into hardiness. In A. Monat & R. S. Lazarus (Eds.), *Stress and coping* (2nd ed.). New York: Columbia University Press.

Mays, J. (1989). *The farm on Nippersink Creek.* Little Rock, AR: August House.

McAdams, D. (1993). *Stories we live by.* New York: Morrow.

Mills, J., & Crowley, R. (Eds.). (1986). *Therapeutic metaphors for children and the child within.* New York: Brunner/Mazel.

Mooney, B., & Holt, D. (1996). *The storyteller's guide.* Little Rock, AR: August House.

Moore, R. (1991). *Awakening the hidden storyteller.* Boston: Shambhala.

Obama, B. (1995). *Dreams from my father.* New York: Three Rivers Press.

Obama, B. (2007). *The audacity of hope.* New York: Three Rivers Press.

O'Connell Higgins, G. (1994). *Resilient adults.* San Francisco: Jossey-Bass.

O'Toole, D. (1988). *Aarvy Aardvark finds hope.* Burnsville, NC: Compassion Press.

O'Toole, D. (1989). *Growing through grief: A K–12 curriculum to help young-people through all kinds of loss.* Burnsville, NC: Compassion Press.

O'Toole, D. (1995). Using story to help children cope with dying, death and bereavement issues: An annotated resource. In D. W. Adams & E. J. Deveau (Eds.), *Beyond the innocence of childhood* (Vol. 2, pp. 335–346). Amityville, NY: Baywood.

O'Toole, D. (1998). *Aarvy Aardvark finds hope* [Video]. Burnsville, NC: Compassion Press.

O'Toole, D. (2009). *The compassion books catalog.* Burnsville, NC: Compassion Press. Available online at *www.compassionbooks.com.*

O'Toole, D., with Wood, S. (2002). *Stories of lead, stories of gold* [storytelling CD]. Burnsville, NC: Compassion Press.

Piper, W. (1990). *The little engine that could.* New York: Platt & Munk.

Rando, T. (1993). *Treatment of complicated mourning.* Champaign, IL: Research Press.

Rowling, J. K. (1998). *Harry Potter and the sorcerer's stone.* New York: Scholastic.

Rowling, J. K. (1999). *Harry Potter and the prisoner of Azkaban.* New York: Scholastic.

Rowling, J. K. (2000a). *Harry Potter and the chamber of secrets.* New York: Scholastic.

Rowling, J. K. (2000b). *Harry Potter and the goblet of fire.* New York: Scholastic.

Rowling, J. K. (2004). *Harry Potter and the order of the phoenix.* New York: Scholastic.

Rowling, J. K. (2006). *Harry Potter and the half-blood prince.* New York: Scholastic.

Rowling, J. K. (2007). *Harry Potter and the deadly hallows.* New York: Scholastic.

Schmidt, M. (1981). *Super Cystic Fibrosis and Fabulous Fran Fibrosis.* West Orange, NJ: Organon Inc.

Schneider, J. (2000). *The overdiagnosis of depression: Recognizing grief and its transformative potential.* Traverse City, MI: Season's Press.

Schneider, J. (2006). *Transforming loss: A discovery process.* Traverse City, MI: Season's Press.

Stotter, R. (1994). *About story.* Stinson Beach, CA: Stotter Press.

Taylor, D. (1996). *The healing power of stories.* New York: Bantam–Doubleday–Dell.

Walsh, F. (2006). *Strengthening family resilience* (2nd ed.). New York: Guilford Press.

Williams, M. (1995). *The velveteen rabbit.* New York: Doubleday. (Original work published 1922)

Wood, S. (1998). *Mama mockingbird.* Omaha, NE: Centering Corporation.

Ziegler, R. (1992). *Homemade books to help kids cope.* New York: Brunner/Mazel.

PART V

HELP FOR COUNSELORS, PARENTS, AND TEACHERS

CHAPTER 17

Professional Self-Care and Prevention of Secondary Trauma

TINA MASCHI
DEREK BROWN

My father was dying of cancer. A social worker came over to the house to talk to the family. He was such a caring, kind person—I knew right then and there that this is what I wanted to do.

—ELLIE, practitioner

I always enjoyed helping others, listening to their problems, problem solving, and brainstorming. I thought I could make a difference—one-to-one, especially with children. I'm cynical about "mankind," but I think everyone has some goodness and neediness I could tap into.

—ISABELLE, practitioner

My father had died 8 months after I'd graduated from college with BA degrees in History/Political Science and Spanish. I felt like I was on a quest to learn more about human behavior, loss, and why bad things happen to good people.

—JOHN, practitioner

As illustrated throughout this book, practitioners represent a pillar of compassion and support for bereaved children and their families. As they share in the opening quotes, they also are often highly motivated to help others cope and solve complex problems, and often experience a high level of job satisfaction for doing so. However, this level of caring does not come without a price tag. As Jennifer Freyd (1996) so eloquently noted about humanity, "if we look at the world conscious of both of our eyes, we will see peace and violence, love and hate, joy and pain, and even beauty and the beast. There is a bittersweet taste to this human reality" (p. 3). That is, in addition to job satisfaction, practitioners who work with bereaved children often experience work-related stressors that impact them at the personal, interpersonal, and organizational levels.

On a personal level, working with bereaved children may trigger unresolved feelings of loss. On an interpersonal level, practitioners' use of empathy with bereaved children often reflects tragic circumstances that may embitter their positive worldview. On an organizational level, practitioners may experience additional stressors, such as high caseloads and working long hours, that impact their ability to function most effectively. All of these factors make it critical for practitioners to identify and manage work-related stress. This includes the use of self-care strategies to sustain and reinforce practitioners' personal well-being and practice effectiveness.

This chapter provides an overview of job-related risks for practitioners who work with bereaved children, with special attention to the prevention and management of compassion fatigue/secondary and vicarious trauma.

THE CONTINUUM OF LOSS

Practitioners working with bereaved children often help them to cope with loss. In addition to the death of a loved one, loss involves "any separation from someone or something whose significance is such that it impacts on our physical or emotional well-being, role, and status" (Weinstein, 2006, p. 5). Practitioners help children with the "bereavement process," which, specifically, is their response to varying types of loss. For example, a practitioner may work with children who experienced the anticipated death of a significant other (e.g., a grandmother diagnosed with cancer) or an unexpected or traumatic death (e.g., witnessing the murder of a parent) (Webb, 2002, 2004; Weinstein, 2006). It is particularly the unexpected and traumatic types of death, where loss and trauma intersect, that place practitioners at a heightened risk for experiencing indirect or secondary trauma (Cunningham, 2004; Figley, 1995; Jenkins & Baird, 2002).

THE BENEFITS OF CARING: COMPASSION SATISFACTION

Many practitioners are drawn to the field because of a desire to help those in need. The term "compassion satisfaction" refers to satisfaction from helping other people (Radey & Figley, 2007; Stamm, 2002).

The *Merriam Webster Dictionary* (2008) defines "compassion" as the "sympathetic consciousness of others' distress together with a desire to alleviate it" (p. 254). Daisy, a licensed clinical social worker, noted that compassion motivates her work. She said, "I love what I do—helping others to change their lives and possibly making an impact on their lives. It was a field that was the right fit for me as far as finding satisfaction in helping people who are disenfranchised and oppressed." It is the satisfaction with helping that often drives practitioners to help others in distress (Radey & Figley, 2007). It is also this drive for compassion, which does not easily succumb to stressors, that allows practitioners to remain resilient and to thrive throughout their professional careers. One veteran practitioner noted, "After 20 years of social work, I realized that I was always a clinician in the 'trenches.' I always worked with women and children [who were] victims in their homes and in group settings. I realized I was effective as a clinician."

Empathy as the Conduit

Empathy, like compassion, is a central aspect of practitioners' work with bereaved children. Carl Rogers (1980) eloquently describes the nature of "empathy":

> It means entering the private perceptual world of the other and becoming thoroughly at home in it. It involves being sensitive, moment by moment, to the changing felt meanings which flow in this other person, to the fear or rage or tenderness or confusion or whatever that he or she is experiencing. It means temporarily living in the other's life, moving about in it delicately without making judgments. (p. 251)

As Rogers suggests, empathy is both a cognitive skill and an affective skill that involves seeing the thought and feeling world of others from their perspectives. It does not mean the helper loses his or her own perspective, but that he or she temporarily suspends his or her frame of reference while looking at another's world through his or her own eyes (Pearlman, 1999). It is this empathetic openness that helps practitioners effectively connect with their clients. However, it also places them at risk for adverse emotional, psychological, social, and behavioral effects (Pearlman & Saakvitne, 1995a; 1995b).

THE PRICE TAG FOR CARING

The literature has documented occupational risks for practitioners who work with children and adults who have experienced loss (Cunningham,

2004; Figley, 1995; Hooyman & Kramer, 2006; Ryan & Cunningham, 2007). Practitioners who work with bereaved children, especially if it involves trauma, are at risk for work-related adverse effects, including chronic bereavement, psychological distress, countertransference, burnout, secondary trauma/compassion fatigue, and vicarious trauma.

Bereavement, Grief, Mourning, and Chronic Bereavement

Practitioners who work with bereaved children are exposed to children's responses to that loss. Bereavement is a core human experience that varies across cultures and historical periods. In the practitioner–client dyad, grief is the interpersonal or psychological expression of the bereavement process. Practitioners who work with a caseload of bereaved children may be exposed to chronic bereavement, that is, "multiple loss in which chronic anticipatory, unresolved grief, and the compounding effects of experiencing several episodes of grief concurrently" (Cho & Cassidy, 1994, p. 275). For example, practitioners who work in the juvenile justice system may consistently hear from youth on their caseloads about the loss of family members and friends due to drug overdoses or terminal illnesses. Practitioners' chronic exposure to grieving children may subsequently cause them to be adversely impacted physically, psychologically, socially, and spiritually (Cunningham, 2004; Gamble, 2002; Meyers & Cornille, 2002; Weinstein, 2006).

General Psychological Distress

General psychological distress is considered a minor occupational risk among practitioners that occurs in response to clients' material. "General psychological distress" refers to transitory feelings that arise after a practitioner has been exposed to a client's disturbing material and is a natural occurrence when the practitioner interacts with the client (Cunningham, 2004). For example, in a session in which a child details the deteriorating health of a parent, the practitioner may feel upset or helpless. However, for a particular practitioner, this feeling of distress is temporary and does not impact his or her ongoing practice effectiveness.

Countertransference

Countertransference is another occupational risk that occurs in the context of the relationship with a client. Related to psychodynamic therapy, "countertransference" generally refers to unresolved personal issues that account for the practitioner's reactions to the client and/or the situation

(Freud, 1959; Wilson & Lindy, 1994). That is, the content within the child's narratives evokes a personal reaction based on the practitioner's past history (Ryan & Cunningham, 2007). For example, a child grieving over the death of a parent may trigger unresolved feelings related to the death of the practitioner's own parents. This infusion of the practitioner's personal history may compromise his or her ability to be effective with the client.

Countertransference is relatively easy for practitioners to prevent or eliminate if they use strategies, such as self-insight and if they make it a routine to practice self-integration, empathic ability, anxiety management, and conceptualizing skills (Cunningham, 2004; Figley, 1999).

Burnout

Burnout is another occupational risk in which practitioners are considered at high risk. In contrast to countertransference, burnout is not contingent on the practitioner-client relationship, but rather the workplace. "Burnout" has been described as a psychological syndrome of emotional exhaustion, depersonalization, and reduced personal accomplishment that can occur in individuals who work with other people in some capacity (Maslach, 2003). An important feature is that it starts out slowly and becomes progressively worse if no intervention is in place. It may have an adverse impact on practitioners' sense of well-being and their level of effectiveness with clients and overall job performance (Maslach & Leiter, 1997).

A practitioner experiencing burnout has increased feelings of emotional exhaustion, and may feel that he or she is no longer psychologically or emotionally available for others. A practitioner may experience depersonalization, often in the form of negative, cynical attitudes and feelings about one's clients. Practitioners experiencing burnout syndrome also may feel a sense of reduced personal accomplishment and view themselves and their work negatively. Factors that may contribute to burnout include high caseloads, lack of supervision at work, and so forth (Maslach, Jackson, & Leiter, 1996, 1997; Rothschild, 2006).

It is well documented in the literature that burnout may have serious consequences for workers, their clients, and the larger organizations in which they are employed (Lloyd & King, 2002). Studies that use the Maslach Burnout Inventory (MBI) have shown that burnout (emotional exhaustion, depersonalization, and reduced personal accomplishment) among practitioners is the result of work-related problems, such as low morale, absenteeism, and staff turnover, as well as personal problems, such as physical exhaustion, insomnia, substance abuse, mental health problems, and marital and family conflict (Lloyd & King, 2002; Maslach, 2003).

Secondary Traumatic Stress and Compassion Fatigue

Secondary traumatic stress (STS), or its more user-friendly term, compassion fatigue (CF), is another occupational risk directly related to a practitioner's work with bereaved children. This is especially true when the child's loss is due to sudden traumatic circumstances, such as the loss of a parent in a terrorist attack or an unexpected natural disaster. In contrast to burnout, which is not necessarily linked to work with clients, STS *is* related. STS (or CF) is defined as the "natural consequent behaviors and emotions resulting from knowing about a traumatizing event experienced by a significant other—the stress resulting from helping or wanting to help a traumatized or suffering person" (Figley, 1995, p. 7). Similar to a person directly exposed to a traumatic event, through the context of the work relationships, practitioners are exposed secondarily.

Paralleling the DSM-IV-TR criteria for posttraumatic stress disorder (PTSD), practitioners may develop secondary traumatic stress disorder (STSD) in response to clients' trauma-related material (American Psychiatric Association, 2000; Figley, 1995). According to Figley's criteria and the DSM, the stressor to which the practitioner is exposed must be outside the range of usual human experiences, and would be markedly distressing to most people. Afterwards, the practitioner may continue reexperiencing the traumatic event, which may include having recollections (including dreams) of the client's traumatic experiences (Stamm, 1999, 2002).

Practitioners may have physiological and psychological reactions to their memories of clients' materials (Adams, Boscarino, & Figley, 2006). These reactions may include avoidance and numbing, and persistent arousal. Avoidance and numbing include practitioners' efforts to avoid thoughts or feelings, activities, and situations that remind them of the client or event. They also may experience adverse psychological and emotional changes as part of their avoidance and numbing strategies, such as psychogenic amnesia, diminished affect, negative thinking patterns, decreased interest in activities, and detachment from others. Practitioners may also experience persistent arousal. This may include somatic symptoms such as difficulty falling or staying asleep, irritability, anger outbursts, and trouble concentrating. They may also experience hypervigilance for the traumatized person, exaggerated startle response, and physiological reactivity to cues (Bride, 2007; Bride, Radey, & Figley, 2007; Figley, 1995, 1999; Valent, 2002).

CF/STS has been called "a disorder that affects those who do their work well" (Figley 1995, p. 5). Practitioners may experience emotional, cognitive, and physical effects from assisting others (Stamm, 1999, 2002). CF also is characterized by deep emotional and physical exhaustion, and by a shift in a helping professionals' sense of hope and optimism about the future and the value of their work. Additionally, the symptoms of CF/STS are usually sudden in onset and associated with a particular event. As a result of listening to a client's material, a practitioner may feel afraid, have trouble sleeping, or have disturbing images. The level of CF a practitioner experiences can ebb and flow from one day to the next and can even impact a very healthy helper with optimal life/work balance. However, practitioners may experience a higher than normal level of CF when working with a lot of traumatic content or when CF is coupled with burnout, in which they experience large case overloads and unsupportive work environments, and are generally overworked (Figley, 1995; Maslach, 2003; Stamm, 2002).

Recently, Radey and Figley (2007) have posited that CF should be viewed from a broader positive context as opposed to only its potential negative consequences; that is, practitioners' focus also should be on the positive fulfillment and satisfaction from work as opposed to primarily an avoidance of occupation-related stress. Based on the work of Frederickson (1998), Radey and Figley (2007) proposed a conceptual model based on positive affects, and internal and external resources as important in reducing symptoms of CF and increasing feelings of compassion satisfaction.

Vicarious Trauma

Vicarious trauma (VT) is another occupational risk of working with bereaved children, especially if children's losses are trauma related. Whereas STSD is based on clinical symptoms and diagnostic criteria, its related "cousin" VT is based on theoretical constructs and is important for practitioners to understand (Pearlman, 1999; Saakvitne & Pearlman, 1996; Saakvitne, Gamble, Pearlman, & Tabor Lev, 1999). Pearlman and Saakvitne (1995a) defined VT as

> the transformation that occurs within the trauma counselor as a result of empathic engagement with clients' trauma experiences and their sequelae. Such engagement includes listening to graphic descriptions of horrific events, bearing witness to people's cruelty to one another, and witnessing and participating in traumatic reenactments. It is an occupational hazard and reflects neither pathology in the therapist nor intentionality on the part of the traumatized client. (p. 31)

Another distinct difference between these constructs is that STS can have a sudden onset, whereas VT has a gradual onset in response to an accumulation of memories of clients' traumatic material and affects practitioners' perspective of themselves, others, and the world (Figley, 1995; Pearlman, 1999).

Constructivist Self-Development Theory

Constructivist self-development theory (CSDT) is the theoretical framework most commonly used to describe VT among practitioners (Saakvitne & Pearlman, 1996). According to CSDT, vicarious trauma causes "profound changes in the core aspects of the therapist's self" (Pearlman & Saakvitne, 1995b, p. 152). VT causes disruptions in practitioners' cognitive schemas that involve self-identity, beliefs, perceptions, and memories. Because VT is a natural consequence of trauma-related work, the ongoing challenge for practitioners is to identify, address, and transform it.

According to the theory, practitioners are at risk for VT because their open, empathetic engagement with clients involves both positive and negative material (Pearlman & Saakvitne, 1995b). VT is the result of persistent exposure to clients' traumatic material that causes cognitive disruptions in practitioners that adversely impact their perceptions of themselves, others, and the world (Figley, 1995; Pearlman, 1999). The shift to a negative worldview can have devastating effects on practitioners' personal and professional lives, if it remains unchecked.

According to CSDT, in the face of trauma, each person will adapt and cope (Pearlman, 1999). Therefore, adaption and coping are integral internal factors that influence what the theory refers to as the "developing self" (Saakvitne & Pearlman, 1996). Positive adaption and coping protect the health and well-being of the practitioner's self, whereas negative adaption and coping compromise that self. Internal and external factors that influence a practitioner's ability to adapt and cope include environmental, interpersonal, and intrapersonal factors, such as the current context; the practitioner's prior history of loss and trauma; and familial, social, and cultural factors (Saakvitne et al., 1999). Parts of the developing self that are at risk when exposed to traumatic material include the practitioner's frame of reference, self-capacities, ego resources, psychological needs, cognitive schemas, and memory and perception (Pearlman & Saakvitne, 1995a; Saakvitne et al., 1996, 1999; see Figure 17.1).

FRAME OF REFERENCE

CSDT argues that each self has a *frame of reference,* which consists of self-identify, worldview, and spirituality, influenced by personal and

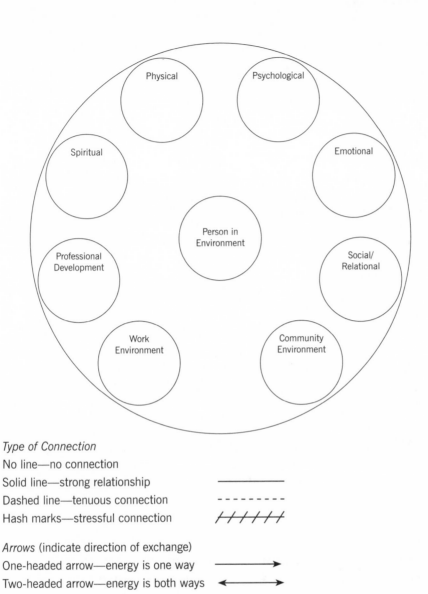

Type of Connection

No line—no connection

Solid line—strong relationship

Dashed line—tenuous connection

Hash marks—stressful connection

Arrows (indicate direction of exchange)

One-headed arrow—energy is one way

Two-headed arrow—energy is both ways

FIGURE 17.1. Self-care (inner and outer) ecomap: Maschi and Brown. This visual assessment tool that we developed can help practitioners identify strong and positive areas, area of neglect, and areas of conflict (see the key code). In the center circle, the practitioner should list his or her name. Each self-care circle should list the activities, relationships, and so forth, associated with the self-care area. This ecomap can also be used with clients.

professional experiences. An individual's frame of reference shapes his or her interpretation of the self, relationships, and experiences.

SELF-CAPACITIES

The concept of self-capacities represents a person's quest to maintain inner balance, which also includes the ability to self-soothe. On a practical level, it involves a practitioner's ability to (1) manage strong feelings, (2) feel entitled to be alive and deserving of love, and (3) have an inner awareness of others (Saakvitne et al., 1999). A practitioner's frame of reference may be disrupted when working with high levels of trauma material that impacts his or her ability to manage emotions, and personal and professional relationships.

EGO RESOURCES

An individual's ego resources also may be impacted by VT. The concept "ego resources" refers to the ability of the individual to negotiate interpersonal situations, as well as to exercise good decision making and judgment (Pearlman, 1999). It consists of self-awareness (insight), being able to take the perspective of another (empathy), use of willpower and initiative, and striving for personal growth. A practitioner's effective use of ego resources includes being able to foresee consequences, make self-protective judgments, and establish healthy boundaries between self and client (Pearlman & Saakvitne, 1995a; Saakvitne et al., 1999). When practitioners are adversely influenced by VT, these ego resources are compromised, if left unchecked.

PSYCHOLOGICAL NEEDS AND COGNITIVE SCHEMAS

Practitioners' psychological needs and cognitive schemas also may be influenced by VT. There are five basic psychological needs: safety, esteem, trust (or dependence), control, and intimacy. According to CSDT, these basic psychological needs are critical factors that protect practitioners from VT, or being unduly influenced by others' trauma content and placed in a vulnerable position (Pearlman & Saakvitne, 1995a).

MEMORY AND PERCEPTION

Practitioners' memory and perception also are susceptible to adverse changes when they have prolonged experiences with client material that involves loss and trauma (Pearlman, 1999). Because memory and perception are multimodal, they involve the different senses (i.e.,verbal, visual, emotional, somatic and sensory, and interpersonal). Any experience is processed, and recall modalities, including the cognitive (verbal), visual, affective (emotional), somatic and sensory, and interpersonal, can be affected (Pearlman & Saakvitne, 1995b; Saakvitne et al., 1996; 1999). Verbal memory and perception involve the narrative of what happened before, during, and after the traumatic event; imagery involves the mental picture of the event; affect involves the emotions related to the event; somatic sense involves the bodily experiences that represent the traumatic events, and interpersonal involves the relational patterns and behaviors that reflect the abusive traumatic relationship (Saakvitne et al., 1996). The challenge for practitioners in preventing or remediating VT effects is to maintain the integration and interconnectedness of the different parts of memory and perception, so that disconnection or dissociation does not occur.

Signs and Symptoms of VT

Practitioners who work with bereaved children are at risk for experiencing VT. Therefore, practitioners need to be aware of the signs and symptoms of VT. For example, the memory of a practitioner impacted by VT often becomes fragmented; that is, the practitioner may be unable to recall a client's trauma narrative without also recalling his or her feeling in reaction to it (e.g., panic or terror). The practitioner may also experience an image (e.g., flashback) without connecting it to the client's trauma narrative or associated feelings.

Because VT is the "transformation of the helper's inner experience resulting from empathic engagement with the client's trauma material" (Saakvitne et al., 1996, p. 40), Saakvitne and colleagues noted general and specific symptoms that may impact a practitioner's developing self. A practitioner who works with bereaved children may lack energy and feel disconnected from loved ones, socially withdrawn, and more sensitive to loss and trauma. He or she may have increased feelings of cynicism, despair, and ongoing nightmares, or experience specific intrapersonal changes, such as disruptions or impairment in frame of reference (i.e., self-identify, worldview) and spiritual beliefs; self-capacities, ego resources, psychological needs and cognitive schemas; and memory and perception (e.g., intrusive imagery, dissociation, and depersonalization) (Pearlman, 1999; Saakvitne et al., 1999). This shift may result in practitioners assuming negative attitudes about themselves and the world. This type of negative shift compromises their personal well-being and practice effectiveness (Pearlman, 1999). Figure 17.2 provides for practitioners a self-assessment checklist for VT.

Use this worksheet to assess for vicarious trauma. Rate how much you agree which each of these statements using the following scale: 1 = strongly disagree, 2 = disagree, 3 = neutral, 4 = agree; 5 = strongly agree. Put a plus sign next to those items that are a source of strength and a check mark next to those items that are of concern.

FRAME OF REFERENCE

____ I have a strong sense of self-identity.

____ Overall, the world is a good place.

____ I am a spiritual person.

____ I am connected to my faith.

____ My life has meaning.

____ I have a purpose to fulfill.

SELF-CAPACITIES

____ I can manage my strong feelings.

____ I keep my loved ones in mind.

____ My loved ones care about me.

____ I am worthwhile.

____ I am deserving of good things.

____ I am lovable.

EGO RESOURCES

____ I use resources on my own behalf.

____ I make good decisions in my personal life.

____ I make good decisions in my professional life.

____ I can protect myself.

____ I have strong personal boundaries.

____ I have strong professional boundaries.

____ I know how to use resources for self-growth.

____ I keep growing personally.

____ I have deep insight into myself.

____ I keep growing professionally.

BASIC PSYCHOLOGICAL NEEDS

Safety

____ I feel reasonably safe.

____ I feel my loved ones are reasonably safe.

Self-Esteem

____ I feel proud of who I am.

____ I trust my judgment.

Trust

____ I believe I can trust others.

____ I feel I can depend on others.

Control

____ I believe I have control over my life.

____ I have the power to influence others.

Intimacy

____ I am good company for myself.

____ I feel I am close to others.

PERCEPTION AND MEMORY

____ I sleep well at night.

____ I never experience nightmares.

____ I get triggered by clients' experiences.

____ I experience stress in my body.

____ I feel nervous.

____ I feel numb.

FIGURE 17.2. Self-assessment checklist for vicarious trauma.

Adapted from Saakvitne, Gamble, Pearlman, and Tabor Lev (1999), with permission from the Sidran Institute, in *Helping Bereaved Children: A Handbook for Practitioners* (3rd ed.), edited by Nancy Boyd Webb (The Guilford Press, 2010). Permission to photocopy this figure is granted to purchasers of this book for personal use only (see copyright page for details). Purchasers may download a larger version of this figure from the book's page on The Guilford Press website.

Factors Influencing VT

Despite the risk, VT is very amenable to self-prevention and intervention (Pearlman, 1999). The nature of social–environmental and individual-level factors may protect or place practitioners at risk for VT (Saakvitne et al., 1999). Environmental factors, such as the nature of the work, the clientele, cumulative exposure to trauma material, organizational context, and social and cultural context, can influence how VT impacts practitioners (Bell, Kulkarni, & Dalton, 2003; Catherall, 1995). Additionally, characteristics such as personal history, personality, coping style, current life context, training and professional history, and level of participation in supervision or personal therapy also may influence how much VT adversely impacts practitioners (Crestman, 1999; Saakvitne et al., 1996).

In general, the less practitioners are exposed to trauma content in their work and the more they receive support from their agencies and communities (i.e., the environment), and the more reinforcement they receive for personal characteristics of resilience and adaptive coping, the more likely they are to prevent or remediate trauma-related work symptoms (Adams & Riggs, 2008; Bell, 2003; Figley, 1995, 1999; Radey & Figley, 2007). These individual and social–environment characteristics apply to both VT and STSD. It is important that practitioners who work with bereaved children conduct regular self-assessments of the impact of trauma-related content. In the following section we discuss a number of assessment tools that can assist practitioners.

ASSESSMENT TOOLS

There are a number of user-friendly standardized assessment tools for identifying occupational risks such as burnout, STS/CF, and/or VT (Bride et al., 2007). These instruments include the Professional Quality of Life Scale (ProQOL; Stamm, 2005), the Secondary Traumatic Stress Scale (STSS; Bride, Robinson, Yegidis, & Figley, 2004), and the Trauma and Attachment Belief Scale (TABS; Pearlman, 2003).

The ProQOL (Stamm, 2005) is a 30-item scale that has three subscales: (1) Compassion Satisfaction, (2) Burnout, and (3) Compassion Fatigue/Secondary Traumatic Stress. The ProQOL can be self-administered and is known to have good psychometric properties (Bride et al., 2007; Stamm, 2005). It is available for download at *www.isu. edu/~bhstamm/tests.htm,* and can be completed and self-scored in about 10 minutes.

The STSS (Bride et al., 2004) is a 17-item summative scale that measures the frequency of intrusion, avoidance, and arousal symptoms associated with indirect exposure to traumatic events in practice over a 7-day period. The items on the scale are consistent with the DSM-IV-TR criteria for PTSD, with subscales for Intrusion, Avoidance, and Hyper-arousal (B, C, and D criteria) and takes about 5 minutes to complete. A copy of this measure is available online at *mailer.fsu.edu/~cfigley/cfas/stssweb.htm.*

The TABS (Pearlman, 2003) is a reliable and valid instrument based on CSDT. It consists of 84 items that assess practitioners' beliefs about self and others, and the five areas of psychological need (safety, trust, esteem, control, and intimacy) that may be impacted by VT. A sample of the TABS is available at *www.isu.edu/~bhstamm/tests/tsisample.htm.* The entire scale can be purchased from Western Psychological Services at *portal.wpspublish.com.* After an assessment for trauma-related work symptoms, practitioners may engage in number of self-care strategies to prevent or ameliorate their impact.

THE SELF-CARE TRIANGLE:
AWARENESS, BALANCE, AND CONNECTION

It is generally agreed that self-care prevention and intervention strategies should target the three realms of practitioners' lives: personal, professional, and organizational (Gamble, 2002; Ryan & Cunningham, 2007; Yassen, 1995). While the pathways to work-related burnout, STS, and VT may vary, practitioners often experience similar adverse physiological, psychological, emotional, social, and behavioral consequences. (See Figure 17.3 for a self-care activity checklist.

Thus, self-care represents a critical component of every practitioner's plan (Pearlman, 1999; Trippany, White Kress, & Wilcoxon, 2004). Saakvitne and colleagues (1996) identified the three interlocking legs of the practitioner's self-care triangle: (1) awareness, (2) balance, and (3) connection. "Awareness," the first leg of the self-care triangle is described by Saavkitne et al. (1996) as a practitioner being in touch with his or her own needs, limits, emotions, and resources; that is, if a practitioner can identify the problem, he or she can prepare the self-care solution. Self-care necessitates that a practitioner pay careful attention to his or her body, mind, and emotions. Allowing time for quiet and reflection, and the practice of "mindfulness" (which is acceptance of what is in the moment without modification or judgment) is considered an essential self-care strategy (Cunningham, 2004; Gamble, 2002). Allowing self-time can help to facilitate the personal grief process that a practitioner

Rate how frequently you do these self-care activities using the following scale: 0 = never, 1 = rarely, 2 = sometimes, 3 = frequently. Put a check mark next to those self-care activities you want to continue doing and a double check mark next to those activities you would like to do.

PHYSICAL SELF-CARE
____ Get enough sleep.
____ Eat three meals a day.
____ Eat healthy foods.
____ Exercise.
____ See a doctor if needed.
____ Get massages.
____ Be sexual.
____ Rest.
____ Other physical self-care activities.

PSYCHOLOGICAL SELF-CARE
____ Make time for reflection.
____ Practice self-awareness.
____ Use guided imagery.
____ Practice relaxation.
____ Attend counseling.
____ Write in a journal.
____ Read for entertainment.
____ Make efforts to minimize stress.

SOCIAL SELF-CARE
____ Spend quality time with family.
____ Spend quality time with friends.
____ Attend social events.
____ Participate in social action activities.
____ Ask for help when needed.

WORK SETTING
____ Take a lunch break.
____ Eat during my lunch break.
____ Participate in rewarding projects.
____ Attend work-related trainings.
____ Get regular supervision.
____ Negotiate for needs (pay raise, benefits).
____ Participate in a peer support group.
____ Do some nontrauma work.

EMOTIONAL SELF-CARE
____ Enjoy the company of others.
____ Love myself.
____ Allow myself to cry when needed.
____ Laugh.
____ Engage in creative activities.
____ Express anger with social action.
____ Other emotional self-care activities.

SPIRITUAL SELF-CARE
____ Make time for self-reflection.
____ Spend time in nature.
____ Belong to a spiritual community.
____ Practice positive thinking.
____ Meditate.
____ Pray or chant.
____ Do yoga.
____ Read spiritual teachings.
____ Practice mindfulness.
____ Embrace hope and optimism.
____ Other spiritual activities.

PROFESSIONAL SELF-CARE
____ Maintain professional boundaries.
____ Keep to a regular work schedule.
____ Attend training and workshops.
____ Review agency policies.

COMMUNITY ENVIRONMENT
____ Participate in community activities.
____ Attend community groups.
____ Participate in social activism.
____ Volunteer in the community.
____ Garden at home.
____ Participate in creating a community garden.
____ Give donations to charity.
____ Provide community leadership.

FIGURE 17.3. Self-care activities checklist.

Adapted from Saakvitne, Gamble, Pearlman, and Tabor Lev (1999), with permission from the Sidran Institute, in *Helping Bereaved Children: A Handbook for Practitioners* (3rd ed.), edited by Nancy Boyd Webb (The Guilford Press, 2010). Permission to photocopy this figure is granted to purchasers of this book for personal use only (see copyright page for details). Purchasers may download a larger version of this figure from the book's page on The Guilford Press website.

experiences when working with bereaved children, which the practitioner emerges from a symbolic type of psychological death into an inner world free of client-related trauma content (Figley, 1995).

In the second leg of the practitioner's self-care triangle, Saavkitne and Pearlman (1996) refer to "balance" in both inner and outer activities. Practitioners who lead balanced lives are able to balance work, play, and rest activities. Although they are active, they are also in touch with their inner resources and allow ample time for self-reflection and freedom of choice (Saavkitne et al., 1996).

Connection is the third leg of the practitioner's self-care triangle. Practitioners who foster connection with themselves, others, and something larger than themselves are practicing preventive self-care (Saakvitne et al., 1996). Being connected to oneself and others offers a powerful antidote to living under the shadow of despair and isolation that characterizes practitioners with untreated STS/VT. Practitioners in tune with their inner selves can more readily recognize and respond to their changing perceptions and needs (Pearlman, 1999). Studies have shown that practitioners who maintain their internal and external connections sustain hope, along with a positive outlook relative to themselves, others, and the world (Adams & Riggs, 2008). Connection also serve to distract practitioners from falling into a pattern of nihilistic attitudes, despair, and isolation.

After practitioners identify symptoms of STS/VT, they need to address and transform them. The literature emphasizes self-care as an essential strategy to address the ongoing positive development of the mind, body, emotions, and spirit of the practitioner. Additionally, since there are negative consequences of grief and trauma work, the practitioner must actively work to transform and to release negative beliefs, feelings of despair, helplessness and hopelessness, and a loss of meaning (Pearlman, 1999).

The literature suggests that the despair of STS/VT can be transformed when practitioners engage in meaning making that involves thought and action. Saakvitne et al. (1996) recommend that practitioners integrate their current activities with renewed meaning. It also is important for to practitioners constantly challenge negative beliefs and assumptions, such as nihilism, cynicism, and despair, with actions such as participating in community building activities (Yassen, 1995). Cunningham (2004) has recommended the use of mindfulness and relationship building. For example, working with other community members for a common good or goal, such as combating family and community violence, creates a community of personal and group connection and empowerment. According to Saakvitne and colleagues (1999), the processes of addressing and transforming STS/VT often go hand in hand.

ECOLOGICAL MODEL FOR PREVENTION

Another useful practitioner self-care model is Yassen's (1995) ecological prevention model (EPM; see Figure 17.4). EPM uses an ecological framework for preventing STS/VT. This multidimensional approach to reduction of stress and burnout, and prevention planning uses knowledge-building strategies and techniques. The model assumes that STS/VT is a normal reaction to abnormal (e.g., violence) or unusual events (e.g., natural disasters). EPM assumes that the enduring or negative effects of trauma can be prevented from developing into a psychological symptomatology, such as STSD, depression, or anxiety (Bride, 2007; Crestman, 1999). EPM consists of the following four steps: (1) prepare, (2) plan, (3) attend, and (4) transform. For example, practitioners can develop healthier lifestyle skills that give them a solid grounding for exposure to the ebb and flow of the trauma-related experiences inherent in working with bereaved children.

Similar to a public health model, EPM adapts three levels of prevention: primary, secondary, and tertiary. *Primary prevention* for STSD and VT targets underlying social causes. *Secondary prevention* addresses specific strategies that reduce risk or prepare for trauma should it occur. *Tertiary interventions* are part of the aftermath of traumatic events that engender loss, such as the 9/11 terrorist attacks, in which many children lost their parents and other relatives. An example of a tertiary intervention would be a practitioners' crisis hotline during an emergency that resulted in the sudden death and loss of community members (Yassen, 1995).

Since EPM adopts an ecological approach, it targets both the psychological and social impacts of diseases that occur at work or home, and in the community. According to this model, *primary prevention* efforts may consist of practitioners and other community members engaging in activities that target long-term social and societal change (e.g., educational and social service interventions that target the elimination of community violence in which family members' and friends' lives are lost; Yassen, 1995).

Secondary prevention efforts target practitioners' personal and environmental conditions through planning and practice; that is, practitioners applying secondary prevention have developed a self-care plan, and are monitoring their own progress. This strategy helps them cope with traumatic loss (e.g., social work and counseling programs that not only prepare students to help clients but also provide self-care strategies to cope with trauma and loss) (Cunningham, 2004).

Tertiary prevention is the level of crisis intervention for individuals and communities (e.g., in the wake of natural disasters in which many

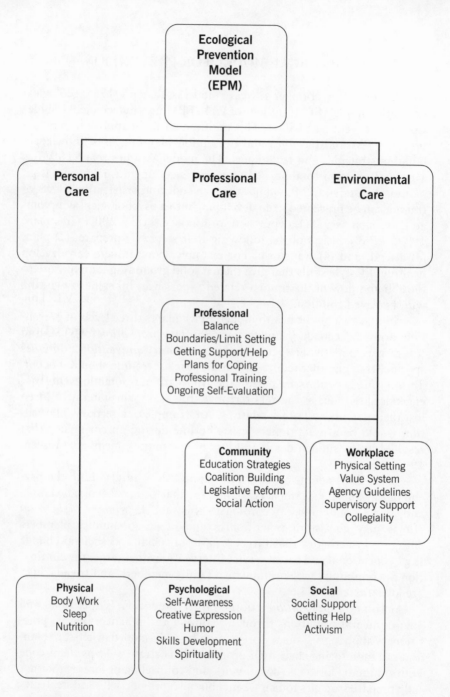

FIGURE 17.4. A visual depiction of Yassen's (1995) ecological prevention model (EPM) and the three levels of self-care: personal care, professional care, and environmental care.

children lose family members and friends). At this stage, a practitioner's self-care strategies focus on the reduction of long-term effects of STS/VT (Yassen, 1995).

Primary, secondary, and tertiary prevention target both individual and community–environment levels.

Personal Self-Care

Personal self-care is aimed at self-development activities, such as self-awareness and strategies in the physical, psychological, emotional, spiritual, and social domains.

Self-Awareness

Similar to other self-care models, EPM underscores the importance of self-awareness as a critical factor for prevention of STS and VT. This approach, corroborated by studies, has shown that the character and personality of individuals may influence the level of trauma-related symptoms when working with bereaved children. It is important for practitioners to assume a nonjudgmental and compassionate attitude toward themselves and others, and to have a good understanding of their current life situations. They also should be aware of power dynamics in their lives (i.e., what they do and do not have power over and control), especially when they need to ask for help. Good self-awareness skills are critical for recognizing adverse signs of somatic, psychological, emotional, and spiritual shifts in practitioners' belief systems.

Self-Care Strategies

At the individual level, practitioners should practice self-care strategies that target physical, psychological, cognitive, behavioral, interpersonal, and spiritual well-being (Saakvitne et al., 1999). It is vital for the practitioner to maintain physical health by receiving adequate sleep and to have a healthy diet. In addition, self-care strategies include physical activities that increase practitioners' strength, endurance, clarity of mind, and feelings of well-being. It is important for practitioners to adopt exercises that fit their specific lifestyles (Cunningham, 2004). Some common physical exercises of practitioners include jogging, aerobics, playing on competitive sport teams, dog walking, yoga, and tai chi. The use of yoga as a self-care activity is featured in Figure 17.5.

Psychological and emotional self-care strategies can also reduce practitioners' symptoms of physical arousal (Gamble, 2002; Jenkins & Baird, 2002). Practitioners should balance their work with outside inter-

Yoga is a preventive, personal self-care activity at the social and interpersonal levels. Yoga is a Hindu philosophy or way of life that integrates the mind, body, and spirit. It consists of eight dimensions or limbs of practice, such as building concentration, meditation, spirituality, and physical practice called *asanas*. The limbs build on one another and represent the practitioner's integration and progression to his or her highest spiritual attainment. The most common limb practiced at most yoga studios or homes in the United States is *asanas*. Studios and home practitioners also often incorporate higher order limbs of yoga, such as meditation, into their practice.

Yoga is an activity in which the practitioner positively develops the psychological, physical, and spiritual self. Evidence indicates that yoga builds strength, flexibility, endurance, and mental acuity. As yoga is practiced, the practitioner builds self-awareness and mindfulness.

Yoga is considered a preventive self-care activity, because it builds awareness, balance, and connection. Awareness is built when yogis participate in yogic meditation and mind–body movement, or *asanas*. For example, a yoga instructor guides a practitioner on how to adjust his or her body into the alignment of the posture, which requires mental processing of what body parts are necessary to adjust to create a posture. Yoga helps with life balance. When practitioners take time out for activities of play, such as yoga, they are creating a stronger work–play–rest balance. Yoga's primary purpose is to build a connection to the practitioner's self and something larger than him- or herself in order to build relationships with others, such as clients. Yoga is a holistic self-care activity that is preventive in nature.

The evidence base for yoga as a self-care regimen is growing and suggests that it would be a beneficial activity for practitioners to cope with STDS. Studies (e.g., de Silva, Ravindran, & Ravindran, 2009) demonstrate that yoga reduces stress and PTSD symptomatology, including avoidance, numbing, persistent arousal, dissociation, and reexperiencing a client's traumatic life event.

Basic yogic *asanas* and meditation can be practiced at the home or office during breaks, or in between sessions. Below are safe and easy yogic exercises that can help bereavement counselors and other practitioners cope with VT and alleviate symptoms of STDS.

1. Yogic *Asana*: Corpse Pose (aka *Savasana* or *Mrtasana*)

Step 1: Lie on the floor exactly as if you were standing erect, except relax your feet and let them fall to the sides of your body.

Step 2: Let your hands relax away from your body and onto the floor. Then, flip your palms, so that they are open and facing the ceiling.

2. Yogic Meditation

Step 1: Sit in a chair with your:
- Head facing forward and your chin at a 90-degree angle to the floor.
- Shoulders resting naturally against the chair.
- Back against the chair.
- Hands resting on your knees.

(cont.)

FIGURE 17.5. Yoga as a self-care activity.

1. Yogic *Asana*: Corpse Pose (aka *Savasana* or *Mrtasana*) *(cont.)*

Step 3: Ensure that the center of the back of your head rests on the ground. Your neck should be relaxed, so it should be neutral and not stretched forward or backward.

Step 4: Close your eyes and try to release any stress, tension and intruding thoughts by:

- First, telling yourself to relax your toes then your ankles, and continue up the body with different muscles and joints. Please don't forget to relax your tongue away from the roof of your mouth and your eyes in their sockets.
- Second, taking in the sounds of your external environment (not resisting them).
- Last, letting go of any concentration on the inhalations and exhalations of your breath.
- Take as much time as you can afford and need and just rest on the floor.
- For further guidance on this pose, see *www.yogajournal.com/poses/482*.
- Other, active poses should be done in consultation with a Yoga Alliance-certified and -registered instructor; see *www.yogaalliance.org*.

2. Yogic Meditation *(cont.)*

- Knees at a 90-degree angle to the floor.
- Feet planted on or close to the ground.
- Eyes closed.

Step 2: Try to calm your mind by concentrating on your breath.

- Start by breathing in.
- Mentally follow the flow of air in and out of your nose (and eventually in and out of your throat and lungs).
- For every inhale and exhale, count (1, 2, 3, etc.).
- As you count, try to release any intruding thoughts about the session you just had with your client, the argument with your significant other, or any other issues that may be bothering you. Take in the internal silence. Remember that yoga is not about winning or losing. It is more important to be aware of intruding thoughts than it is to win at this activity by forcing yourself not to have any intruding thoughts. Over time, the intruding thoughts will wither away, and you will be connected with yourself and relaxed.

FIGURE 17.5. *(cont.)*

ests that include a social life, personal time, and recreational activities. Daily relaxation, guided imagery, and breathing exercises or spending time in nature are consistently recommended in the literature as helpful strategies that are not time intensive (Cunningham, 2004; Gamble, 2002; Yassen, 1995). Creative activities also help in the processing of psychological and emotional materials that prevent and remediate STS/VT. Creative arts activities include writing, poetry, drama, photography, cooking, drawing, painting, dancing, humor, playing music, and journal writing. Additionally, humor has been shown to reduce stress, release tension, and increase physical, psychological, and emotional health (Moran, 2002). Self-care strategies should also address cognitive and behavioral skills development (Yassen, 1995). Some examples of skills development include assertiveness training, stress management, time management, and individual and group communication skills training.

Spiritual practices and meditation also have been shown to be helpful self-care strategies (Ryan & Cunningham, 2007). Practitioners generally report the positive impact of meditation and spiritual practices on feelings of well-being (Cunningham, 2004). Meditation and spiritual practices have been shown to offer benefits such as lowering blood pressure, improving breathing, relaxing muscles, and increasing feelings of hope and well-being among practitioners (Trippany et al., 2004).

Social and Interpersonal-Level Interventions

Prevention and reduction of stress in trauma-related work with bereaved children requires interventions at the social and interpersonal levels. Social support in the form of being connected to other people has been associated with prevention and reduction of trauma-related symptoms among survivors and practitioners (Cunningham, 2004). Social support has restorative powers for both clients' and practitioners' ability to cope with trauma and loss (Pearlman, 1999). Practitioners who participate in supportive social networks have access to others, such as family members, friends, and professional colleagues, who can provide vital feedback that can help to facilitate ongoing self-awareness. Having a supportive social network also provides a safety net for practitioners to access and receive help in a timely manner (Yassen, 1995). In EPM, social activism, especially activities that target violence, is another way to work with others to foster hope and a sense of purpose that can ward off the insidious effects of STS/VT. Even small acts of activism, such as participating in an autism awareness walk, can combat the feelings of helplessness and powerlessness that practitioners who work with bereaved children may be prone to feel.

Professional Self-Care

Practitioners also must attend to professional self-care to maintain their job performance, high morale, good citizenship, and responsible behaviors (Bell, 2003). Yassen (1995) identified professional care strategies that include maintaining balance and boundaries, limit setting, seeking assistance from peers and supervisors, self-care plans, and ongoing professional training.

Practitioners who practice self-care set consistent time boundaries, such as set appointment times and avoidance of overwork. Professional self-care also includes maintaining strong professional boundaries with clients and effectively managing dual or multiple roles. These practitioners also are open to consulting with coworkers, such as getting support and help, which includes talking honestly about their own experience. In fact, peer support is critical for both receiving and giving feedback. Receiving supervision and/or consultation from a seasoned professional or mentor can provide an outside perspective and the needed guidance and support to celebrate the triumphs and weather the difficulties that result from working with bereaved children (Saakvitne et al., 1999; Yassen, 1995).

EPM recommends that practitioners who work with loss and trauma should have a self-care plan. These plans include coping strategies for before, during, and after a meeting with a nonbereaved child clients, as well as emergency situations with bereaved children. Professional training, workshops and conferences, and membership in professional organizations are important for professional growth and preventing and combating STSD and VT. These additional learning opportunities enable practitioners to supplement their existing knowledge and skills and to continually evaluate their values and assumptions.

Components of Environmental Prevention: Work and Community Settings

In addition to the individual environment, components of EPM include both *work and community settings*. Assessment of the work setting includes attention to the physical surrounding, such as the overall look of the agency, including wall decorations, type of furniture, and use of lighting. Less tangible items include the agency's values, expectations, and culture. Additionally, subtle aspects of the work environment, such as management policies, should be clear to practitioners. To work most effectively, practitioners should be knowledgeable about the values, tasks (e.g., job descriptions, philosophy, realistic expectations, task variety, adequacy of supervision), in-service and career opportunities, training, and orientation.

Additionally, the work setting should promote a positive work climate. Agency guidelines and norms should foster respect for differences, social support and mutual aid, cooperation and trust among staff members, and sensitivity to the well-being of the workers (e.g., personal days, stress management training, lower caseloads) (Bell et al., 2003; Yassen, 1995).

Community setting prevention and intervention efforts target the society at large (Yassen, 1995). Practitioners can become involved in combating personal and community denial, misinformation, injustice, and prejudice. Educational interventions require activities aimed at changing attitudes or providing information, coalition building, building alliances with various groups to exert a greater influence, legislative reform (using the legal system to enforce rights), social activism (planning actions that include public activities to draw attention to a problem, usually, but not consistently, through the law), mass media education, and global communications. These activities engage practitioners in empowerment and community work that can combat feelings of hopelessness and powerlessness, and foster positive personal and social change (Bell, 2003; Herman, 1992; Lee, 2001).

Eight-Step Prevention and Intervention Plan

EPM uses an eight-step prevention or remediation plan for practitioners (Yassen, 1995, p. 204):

1. Review current self-care and prevention functioning.
2. Select one goal from each category (individual and environmental).
3. Analyze the resources for and resistance to achieving this goal.
4. Discuss goals and implementation plan with support person(s).
5. Activate the plan.
6. Evaluate the plan weekly, monthly, and yearly with support persons.
7. Notice and appreciate the changes.
8. Repeat steps 1 through 7.

ACCELERATED RECOVERY PROGRAM

Practitioners may prefer participating in a formal program, such as the Accelerated Recovery Program (ARP) to prevent or combat STS/ VT (Gentry, Baranowsky, & Dunning, 2002). The ARP model was developed to prevent or remediate CF or STS. It is a comprehensive, self-administered assessment and self-care program, a brief, five-session treatment program designed to assist professionals in reducing intensity, frequency, and duration of CF symptoms. It is a standard treatment, and its major objectives are symptom identification, recognition of CF triggers, identification and use of resources, review of personal and professional history to the current time, mastery of arousal reduction containment skills, creation of a contract for life enhancement, initiation of conflict resolution, implementation of a supportive aftercare plan using the Pathways Self-Care Program. Despite its promise as an intervention for practitioners, little is known about its efficacy (Gentry et al., 2002).

CASE EXAMPLE

Since the time she lost her father at the age of 5, Wanda wanted to grow up to be a counselor for children whose parents had died. At age 35, she is doing just that. Wanda is a clinical social worker at an inner-city agency that has a program for bereaved children between the ages of 5 and 17. Fifteen of the 25 children in Wanda's caseload have lost one or more family members due to community violence. After 3 years on the job, Wanda's enthusiasm for helping has given way to a feeling of emptiness. In a discussion with her supervisor, she cannot pinpoint any single child client's story that concerns her; rather, she experiences a general sense of malaise and hopelessness. She is surprised by her self-deprecating thoughts and has stopped going out with her friends on Friday nights. For the past 3 months Wanda has had trouble sleeping, and she regularly skips meals. She does not receive regular supervision at work because her supervisor is "too busy." She has just about given up hope that anything will change in her community, and she can no longer stand the pain and suffering of so many young people. When she talks about her clients in treatment team meetings, she discusses their issues in a monotone voice and flat affect. *Based on the chapter content reading, how would you describe what Wanda is experiencing? If you were helping Wanda develop an assessment and self-care plan, what might it look like?*

DISCUSSION QUESTIONS AND ROLE-PLAY EXERCISES

Discussion Questions

1. Thinking back to your decision to enter the profession, what reasons led you to choose your profession? What role, if any, did compassion satisfaction (e.g., the desire to help other people) have in your decision-making process? What roles does it play in your current professional life?

2. Which of the psychological needs and cognitive schemas (i.e., safety, esteem, trust, control, and, intimacy) are most challenged by the type of work you do?

3. Download and complete the ProQOL (available at *www.isu.edu/~bhstamm/ tests.htm*). What are your scores for satisfaction, CF/STS, and burnout? Based on the results, which areas have you identified as needing intervention? (This exercise can be completed individually or in a group.)

4. Using the self-care ecomap (Figure 17.1), what have you identified as areas of strength and vulnerabilities? What self-strategies do/can you use to develop or maintain your strength and reduce your vulnerabilities?

5. Using the self-care activities checklist (Figure 17.3), what activities do you already do? What additional activities are you willing to incorporate into your daily life routine?

6. Using the EPM eight-step model, develop an intervention plan for yourself.

Role-Play Exercises

Dyad role plays can be conducted in two parts by using the following vignette. For the first set of role plays, Person 1 (the supervisor) role-plays the client and reenacts the narrative of witnessing a family member's death. Person 2 (the practitioner) role-plays listening to the narrative. During the second part of the role play, Person 2 follows up as the same practitioner discussing with the supervisor (Person 1) his or her feelings related to the session material.

Peter, a 14-year-old incarcerated youth, describes his thoughts and feelings on watching the slow death of his father from drug-related complications:

"In a way I am mad, and in a way I'm sad, but in a way I am happy, because he ain't in misery anymore. A lot of people I tell I am happy that my dad is dead. It doesn't sound right, but you have to understand. He was suffering. He would just stare in front of a black TV screen for hours. Every time my mom would say, 'You are going to the hospital,' he would phase in and say, 'No, I'm not.' And she would let it go until he urinated in the bed. She said, 'That's it. You are going into the hospital.' He had blotches on his skin and they were turning dark green and light green, cause he shot up with a bad needle and the needle must have been dirty and it got into his blood. Now I am not going to be like that, because I know that I grown without a father around my teenage years. I know how it feels and I am not going to leave my kids like that."

REFERENCES

Adams, R. E., Boscarino, J. A., & Figley, C. R. (2006). Compassion fatigue and psychological distress among social workers: A validation study. *American Journal of Orthopsychiatry, 76*(1), 103–108.

Adams, S. A., & Riggs, S. A. (2008). An exploratory study of vicarious trauma among therapist trainees. *Training and Education in Professional Psychology, 2*(1), 26–34.

American Psychiatric Association. (2000). *Diagnostic and statistical manual of mental disorders* (4th ed.). Washington DC: Author.

Bell, H. (2003). Strengths and secondary trauma in family violence work. *Social Work, 48*(4), 513–522.

Bell, H., Kulkarni, S., & Dalton, L. (2003). Organizational prevention of vicarious trauma. *Organizational Prevention of Vicarious Trauma, 84*(4), 463–470.

Bride, B. E. (2007). Prevalence of secondary traumatic stress among social workers. *Social Work, 52,* 63–70.

Bride, B. E., Radey, M., & Figley, C. R. (2007). Measuring compassion fatigue. *Clinical Social Work Journal, 35,* 155–163.

Bride, B. E., Robinson, M. M., Yegidis, B., & Figley, C. (2004). Development and validation of the Secondary Traumatic Stress Scale. *Research on Social Work Practice, 13,* 1–16.

Catherall, D. (1995). Preventing institutional secondary traumatic stress disorder. In C. R. Figley (Ed.), *Compassion fatigue: Coping with secondary traumatic stress disorder in those who treat the traumatized* (pp. 232–248). New York: Routledge/Taylor & Francis.

Cho, C., & Cassidy, D. E. (1994). Parallel process for workers and their clients in chronic bereavement resulting from HIV. *Death Studies, 18,* 273–292.

Crestman, K. R. (1999). Secondary exposure to trauma and self-reported distress. In B. H. Stamm (Ed.), *Secondary traumatic stress: Self-care issues for clinicians, researchers, and educators* (pp. 29–36). Baltimore: Sidran Press.

Cunningham, M. (2004). Avoiding vicarious traumatization: Support, spirituality, and self-care. In N. B. Webb (Ed.), *Mass trauma and violence: Helping families and children cope* (pp. 327–346). New York: Guilford Press.

de Silva, T. L., Ravindran, L. N., & Ravindran, A. V. (2009). Yoga in the treatment of mood and anxiety disorders: A review. *Asian Journal of Psychiatry, 2*(1), 6–16.

Figley, C. R. (1995). Compassion fatigues as secondary traumatic stress disorder. In C. R. Figley (Ed.), *Compassion fatigue: Coping with secondary traumatic stress disorder in those who treat the traumatized* (pp. 1–20). New York: Routledge/Taylor & Francis.

Figley, C. R. (1999). Compassion fatigue: Toward a new understanding of the costs of caring. In B. H. Stamm (Ed.), *Secondary traumatic stress: Self-care issues for clinicians, researchers, and educators* (pp. 3–28). Baltimore: Sidran Press.

Fredrickson, B. L. (1998). What good are positive emotions? *Review of General Psychology, 2,* 300–319.

Freud, S. (1959). The dynamics of the transference. In E. Jones (Ed.) & J. Riviere (Trans.) *Collected papers* (Vol. 2, pp. 312–322). New York: Basic Books.

Freyd, J. J. (1996). *Betrayal trauma: The logic of forgetting childhood abuse.* Cambridge, MA: Harvard University Press.

Gamble, S. J. (2002). Self-care for bereavement counselors. In N. B. Webb (Ed.), *Helping bereaved children: A handbook for practitioners* (2nd ed., pp. 346–362). New York: Guilford Press.

Gentry, G. E., Baranowsky, A. B., & Dunning, K. (2002). The Accelerated Recovery Program (ARP) for compassion fatigue. In C. R. Figley (Ed.), *Treating compassion fatigue* (pp. 123–138). New York: Routledge/Taylor & Francis.

Herman, J. (1992). *Trauma and recovery.* New York: Basic Books.

Hooyman, N. R., & Kramer, B. J. (2006). *Living through loss: Interventions across the lifespan.* New York: Columbia University Press.

Jenkins, S. R., & Baird, S. (2002). Secondary traumatic stress and vicarious trauma: A validational study. *Journal of Traumatic Stress, 15,* 423–432.

Lee, J. (2001). *The empowerment approach to social work practice* (2nd ed.). New York: Free Press.

Lloyd, C., & King, R. (2002). Social work, stress and burnout: A review. *Journal of Mental Health, 11,* 255–265.

Maslach, C. (2003). *Burnout: The cost of caring.* Cambridge, MA: Malor Publishing.

Maslach, C., Jackson, S. E., & Leiter, M. P. (1996). *Maslach Burnout Inventory* (3rd ed.). Palo Alto, CA: Consulting Psychologists Press.

Maslach, C., Jackson, S. E., & Leiter, M. P. (1997). Maslach Burnout Inventory (3rd ed.). In C. P. Zalaquett & R. J. Wood (Eds.), *Evaluating stress: A book of resources* (pp. 191–218). Lanham, MD: Scarecrow Press.

Maslach, C., & Leiter, M. P. (1997). *The truth about burnout: How organizations cause personal stress and what to do about it.* San Francisco: Jossey-Bass.

Merriam Webster Dictionary. (2008). Compassion. Retrieved April 10, 2008, from *www.merriam-webster.com/dictionary/compassion.*

Meyers, T. W., & Cornille, T. A. (2002). The trauma of working with traumatized children. In C. R. Figley (Ed.), *Treating compassion fatigue* (pp. 39–56). New York: Routledge/Taylor & Francis.

Moran, C. C. (2002). Humor as a moderator of compassion fatigue. In C. R. Figley (Ed.), *Treating compassion fatigue* (pp. 139–154). New York: Routledge/Taylor & Francis.

Pearlman, L. A. (1999). Self care for trauma therapists: Ameliorating vicarious traumatization. In B. H. Stamm (Ed.), *Secondary traumatic stress: Self-care issues for clinicians, researchers, and educators* (pp. 51–64). Baltimore: Sidran Press.

Pearlman, L. A. (2003). *Trauma and Attachment Belief Scale (TABS) manual.* Los Angeles: Western Psychological Services.

Pearlman, L. A., & Saakvitne, K. W. (1995a). *Trauma and the therapist.* New York: Norton.

Pearlman, L. A., & Saakvitne, K. W. (1995b). Treating therapists with vicarious traumatization and secondary traumatic stress disorders. In C. R. Figley (Ed.), *Compassion fatigue: Coping with secondary traumatic stress disorder in those who treat the traumatized* (pp. 150–177). New York: Routledge/Taylor & Francis.

Radey, M., & Figley, C. R. (2007). The social psychology of compassion. *Clinical Social Work Journal, 35,* 207–214.

Rogers, C. R. (1980). *A way of being.* Boston: Houghton Mifflin.

Rothschild, B. (2006). *Help for the helper: Self-care strategies for managing burnout and stress.* New York: Norton.

Ryan, K., & Cunningham, M. (2007). Helping the helpers: Guidelines to prevent vicarious traumatization of play therapists working with traumatized children. In N. B. Webb (Ed.), *Play therapy with children in crisis: Individual, group and family treatment* (3rd ed., pp. 443–460). New York: Guilford Press.

Saakvitne, K. W., Gamble, S., Pearlman, L. A., & Tabor Lev, B. (1999). *Risking connection: A training curriculum for working with survivors of childhood abuse.* Baltimore: Sidran Press.

Saakvitne, K. W., & Pearlman, L. A. (1996). *Transforming the pain: A workbook on vicarious traumatization.* New York: Norton.

Stamm, B. H. (Ed.). (1999). *Secondary traumatic stress: Self-care issues for clinicians, researchers, and educators.* Lutherville, MD: Sidran Press.

Stamm, B. H. (2002). Measuring compassion satisfaction as well as fatigue: Developmental history of the Compassion Satisfaction and Fatigue Test. In C. R. Figley (Ed.), *Treating compassion fatigue* (pp. 107–122). New York: Routledge/Taylor & Francis.

Stamm, B. H. (2005) Professional Quality of Life Scale. Retrieved March 19, 2007, from *www.isu.edu/~bhstamm/tests.htm.*

Trippany, R. L., White Kress, V. E., & Wilcoxon, S. A. (2004). Preventing vicarious trauma: What counselors should know when working with trauma survivors. *Journal of Counseling Development, 82,* 31–37.

Valent, P. (2002). Diagnosis and treatment of helper stresses, trauma, and illnesses. In C. R. Figley (Ed.), *Treating compassion fatigue* (pp. 17–38). New York: Routledge/Taylor & Francis.

Webb, N. B. (Ed.). (2002). *Helping bereaved children: A handbook for practitioners* (2nd ed.). New York: Guilford Press.

Webb, N. B. (2004). The impact of traumatic stress and loss on children and families. In N. B. Webb (Ed.), *Mass trauma and violence: Helping families and children cope* (pp. 3–22). New York: Guilford Press.

Weinstein, J. (2006). *Working with loss, death and bereavement: A guide for social workers.* Thousand Oaks, CA: Sage.

Wilson, J. P., & Lindy, J. (Eds.). (1994). *Countertransference in the treatment of PTSD.* New York: Guilford Press.

Yassen, J. (1995). Preventing secondary traumatic stress disorder. In C. R. Figley (Ed.), *Compassion fatigue: Coping with secondary traumatic stress disorder in those who treat the traumatized* (pp. 178–208). New York: Routledge/Taylor & Francis.

CHAPTER 18

Guidelines to Help Parents and Teachers of Bereaved Children

NANCY BOYD WEBB

The purpose of this book is to help practitioners and students who are working with bereaved children and adolescents. There are many facets to this work, and it is not always focused on the child. Any young person's world inevitably involves numerous adults who serve as supports in his or her daily life. No matter how compassionate these adults are, however, they may not know how to help and comfort children who are bereaved, and they may be quite uncomfortable at the prospect. Often it becomes the role of practitioners to help such parents and teachers involved with bereaved children on a daily basis, who are eager for very specific suggestions about what to say and do. This chapter offers such practitioners concrete suggestions about how they can assist parents and teachers when children have suffered the death of someone important to them. Some guidelines apply for *both* parents and teachers, whereas others are specific to the particular role of each. The chapter begins with principles that can be used by both groups and later addresses topics specific to either the home or school.

ISSUES AND GUIDELINES
FOR *BOTH* PARENTS AND TEACHERS

Death is a difficult reality of life that may and does confront people of any age at any time. The reactions of those who learn about a death vary depending on many factors, such as their relationship with the person who died, the circumstances of the death, and also their own unique past history with other deaths. I refer to these three groups of factors as the "tripartite assessment" and discussed this in some detail in Chapter 2.

Regardless of the specific circumstances, *anyone seeking to help bereaved children must keep in mind the following principles:*

1. Adults must pay attention to their own need to mourn, and admit their own sad feelings to the child. (It is never appropriate to try to cover up one's feelings of grief, since the child will notice and get the message that these feelings cannot be discussed.) Because some children become concerned when they see adults crying, it may be appropriate to say, "I'm crying because I am so sad, but I can still take care of you and do most of the things that I have to do." (Children worry about who will take care of them, especially when they see their caregiver in a very upset condition.)

2. Keep in mind that the child's ability to comprehend the reality of death varies with his or her age. Try to use simple language that will not be confusing. The word *"dead"* is preferable to terms such as "passed on," "eternal rest," or other euphemisms. Young children (preschool through first or second grade) may not understand the *finality* of death, and they may expect the dead person to return for special occasions, such as birthdays. Adults must be patient and be prepared to repeat the fact that "when people die, they cannot come back, no matter what." Older children have a more mature understanding, but they may think that something they did or did not do caused the death. It may help to say, "The doctors did everything possible, and *it was nobody's fault.*"

3. Be honest with the child regarding the cause of death, without going into excessive detail.

4. Inform the child that it is still OK for him or her to go to school and to play. Children should not be expected to spend long periods of time sitting and talking about the dead person during a wake or a shiva, because children typically have a "short sadness span" (Webb, 2002) and become restless.

5. Understand that cultural/religious practices dictate how much the child will be included in rituals following death. We must be open to learning about and accepting diverse practices.

6. Emphasize to the bereaved child that his or her friends will still be friends. Sometimes children feel painfully "different" because someone in their family has died. Most children want their families to be like everyone else's, and they feel conspicuous and uncomfortable about the absent/dead family member. They need reassurance that their friends

will still want to spend time with them despite the fact that a member of their family has died.

7. Help the child recall and preserve happy memories of the person who died, and encourage him or her to talk about these memories.

8. Be prepared for possible regressive behavior related to the child's expressed or unexpressed anxiety about the death. This can include an array of sleep problems, clinging and withdrawal behaviors, difficulty concentrating, and deterioration in school grades. These may be related to the youth's ongoing fears and anxieties about the death, and should be responded to with sensitivity. If the behavior continues beyond a couple of weeks, a child therapist who specializes in bereavement should be consulted.

ISSUES AND GUIDELINES FOR PARENTS

When parents of bereaved children are themselves coping with their own grief, this reality must come first, prior to dealing with their young children, who look to them for clues and guidance after a significant death has occurred. The parent's own mourning may compromise his or her ability to attend to the child's special needs. This is especially true when the death is that of a family member, in comparison with the death of a teacher or a peer.

As previously mentioned, the parent should not attempt to hide or minimize his or her own grief and should explain to the child that "all of our family is sad because Grampa died. We will all go to the funeral together, and the minister will say some prayers and some people will talk about Gramps, and many of the adults will be crying. It is OK for adults to cry after someone dies, and it's OK for you to cry also, if you feel like it; everyone understands that." *The principle is to prepare the child for what to expect at the funeral service.*

Depending on the child's age and the anticipated length of the funeral service, it may be wise to arrange to have a relative, or someone the child knows, sit with him or her during the service, and if the child gets restless, this person can escort the child outside. Again, children's short sadness span may preclude their ability to pay attention during a long funeral service even though they loved their deceased relative very much.

If there will be a wake with an open casket, the child also needs an explanation about what to expect. A parent can say, for example, "Some people want to see Grampa even though he is dead, and the wake lets them do that. Grampa will be lying very still in a special box called a casket, and because he is not alive or breathing, he will look different.

Sometimes people like to kneel and say a prayer in front of the dead person's body. Usually people sit around the room and talk about things they remember about Grampa."

It is very important to emphasize to the child that when a person is dead, his or her body does not have any more feelings. The body does not feel cold or hot, and it does not get hungry or have to go to the bathroom! *When a person is dead, his or her body stops working and it doesn't feel anything.*

The child's attendance at the burial service also needs to be considered. If it is a Jewish burial, for example, it is important to explain to the child that after the rabbi says some prayers, the family and friends may take turns shoveling dirt onto the casket. Children usually are fascinated by the fact that the casket will be lowered into the ground and buried. Emphasize once again that the body inside the casket is dead and cannot feel anything.

Any other family rituals related to death should be similarly explained to the child. *The principle is that if the child knows what to expect, he or she will be more able to participate appropriately.* The fact that many visitors whom the child may not know come to the house can be somewhat confusing. This, of course, can be explained as family friends, coworkers, neighbors, and other people who knew the dead person wanting to come and speak to the family and say they are sorry. Sometimes they bring food and flowers.

ISSUES AND GUIDELINES FOR TEACHERS

The Death of a Student's Family Member

The role of the teacher differs, depending on the age of the child and the degree of daily contact between the teacher and the bereaved youth. For example, a first-grade teacher sees her students every day for several hours and often has a close relationship with her students. The parent could serve as an important resource for them in a situation of the death of a classmate. This might be less true of teachers in the upper grades, who see students only for a few hours in the week.

Regardless of the age of the child or the grade, *teachers must first contact the family to express condolences and to ask for permission to inform the child's classmates about the death.* Sometimes school policy specifies drafting a memo that states the facts of the death, with instructions to teachers about when to read the memo. This memo would be read by the teacher in any class in which the deceased child was a student. In some schools, the policy following the death of a student requires that the principal send home a letter to all parents advising them of the death.

In discussion with the bereaved student's parent the teacher might inquire about whether the child will be absent for several days, and whether it would be acceptable to arrange for classmates to send their condolence messages to the child. Sometimes classmates want to attend the service to offer support to the bereaved child. I remember one such situation in my own private practice, when a 9-year-old's mother died of cancer and several of her classmates, plus her teacher, attended the funeral.

Often students do not know what to say to a classmate who is bereaved. The teacher can bring this up with the pupils and suggest that it helps the person when friends and fellow students simply say that they know about the death, and that they are sorry. The classmate also might mention attending a future event to which he or she would like to accompany the bereaved student (thereby emphasizing that the usual school activities will still take place).

The teacher should be mindful that some children may become upset when they hear that the mother or father of one of their classmates has died. This may be because a child is particularly sensitive, or because his or her own parent has been sickly, and the child now is worried that his or her own parent might die. In a situation like this, the teacher should refer the child to the school social worker or guidance counselor, who in turn would establish contact with the worried child's family and determine whether the child needs some counseling.

When the bereaved child returns to class the teacher should speak to the student privately, acknowledging the death and expressing condolences. The teacher also may tell the student that his or her classmates know about the death, and that some of them may choose to speak privately to him or her, but that no general announcement will be made, except to say that everyone is glad to welcome the student back to class.

Counseling should be available for all students and teachers, and an announcement/memo should indicate where and when this can be obtained.

The Death of a Student or a Teacher

Each school should have in place policies about how to handle the death of a student or teacher. Many schools have a crisis team whose responsibility is to deal with such situations. Doka (2008) points out that it is important that the same information be shared with different classes and members of the school community to reduce the likelihood of rumors. A memo (as described earlier) would facilitate this. See Chapter 9, this volume for more discussion.

In a situation of terminal illness, it is appropriate that someone known to the pupils communicate with them as a group about the reason for their classmate's or teacher's absence. When students have some advanced knowledge about a medical condition, they are in a better psychological state to deal with it. When this information is conveyed in a group format, the students can voice their questions or concerns. It is not uncommon for a student to ask whether the terminally ill person is going to die, and the response should be that "everything possible is being done," and that the ill person might very much appreciate a card/message or drawing from his or her pupils/classmates.

When a student or teacher dies unexpectedly, it is more difficult for everyone, but the students must be informed nonetheless, and it is likely that some of them will become quite anxious. Depending on the circumstances of the death, the person informing the student body can mention that knowing someone can die so suddenly makes us all concerned. If the death is from an unexpected heart attack, the person giving the news can stress how unlikely this is to happen to anyone, especially to a young person. If the death is from a car or other accident, the unexpected shock of this should be recognized. Often the crisis team or the school social workers/guidance counselors are expected to be present during the announcements of deaths of this type, since they are specially trained to help in situations of traumatic loss.

REFERENCES

Selected Resources for Parents and Teachers*

The books listed below are just a small fraction of available titles. It is recommended that teachers and parents make these books available at *all* times, not just following a death. Children who have read about death prior to experiencing it personally are generally better prepared to deal with their own losses.

Books

General

Cassini, K., & Rogers, J. (1990). *Death and the classroom.* Cincinnati, OH: Griefwork of Cincinnati.

Doka, K. J. (2008). *Living with grief: Children and adolescents.* Washington, DC: Hospice Foundation of America.

Fitzgerald, H. (1992). *The grieving child.* New York: Simon & Schuster.

---

* Children's librarians can help to locate many sources.

Goldman, L. (1994). *Life and loss. A guide to help grieving children*. Muncie, IN: Accelerated Development.

Grollman, E. (1967). *Explaining death to children*. Boston: Beacon Press.

Huntley, T. (1991). *Helping children grieve: When someone they love dies*. Minneapolis, MN: Augsburg Fortress.

Webb, N. B. (Ed.). (2002). *Helping bereaved children: A handbook for practitioners* (2nd ed.). New York: Guilford Press.

For Preschoolers

Brown, M. W. (1955). *The dead bird*. Reading, MA: Addison-Wesley.

De Paola, T. (1998). *Nana upstairs and Nana downstairs*. New York: Putnam.

Fox, M. (1994). *Tough Boris*. New York: Harcourt Brace.

Gryte, M. (1988). *No new baby*. Omaha, NE: Centering Corporation. [Also available in Spanish]

Heegaard, M. E. (1988). *When someone very special dies*. Minneapolis, MN: Woodland Press.

Hodge, J. (1999). *Finding Grampa everywhere: A young child discovers memories of a grandparent*. Omaha, NE: Centering Corporation.

Krasny Brown, L., & Brown, M. (1998). *When dinosaurs die: A guide to understanding death*. Boston: Little, Brown.

O'Toole, D. (1988). *Ardy Aardvark finds hope*. Burnsville, NC: Compassion Books.

Woodson, J. (2000). *Sweet, sweet memory*. New York: Hyperion Books.

For Elementary School Children

Alexander-Greene, A. (1999). *Sunflowers and rainbows for Tia: Saying goodbye to Daddy*. Omaha, NE: Centering Corporation.

Barron, T. A. (2000). *Where is Grandpa?* New York: Philomel Books.

Bunting, E. (1999). *Rud's pond*. New York: Clarion.

Buscsglia, L. (1982). *The fall of Freddie the leaf*. Thorofare, NJ: Charles B. Slack.

Coerr, E. (1977). *Sadako and the thousand paper cranes*. New York: Putnam.

Copland, K. M. (2005). *Mama's going to heaven soon*. Minneapolis, MN: Augsburg Fortress.

Fassler, J. (1983). *My Grandpa died today*. Springfield, IL: Human Sciences Press.

Grollman, E., & Johnson, J. (2006). *A complete book about death for kids*. Omaha, NE: Centering Corporation.

Johnson, J., & Johnson, M. (1982). *Where's Jess?* Omaha, NE: Centering Corporation.

Old, W. (2001). *Stacy had a baby sister*. Morton Grove, IL: Albert Whitman.

Smith, H. I., & Johnson, J. (2006). *What does that mean?: A dictionary of death, dying, and grief terms for grieving children and those who love them*. Omaha, NE: Centering Corporation.

For Middle School Students

Dragonwagon, C. (1990). *Winter holding spring.* New York: Atheneum/Simon & Schuster.

Gignoux, J. H. (1998). *Some folk say: Stories of life, death, and beyond.* New York: Foulketale.

Krementz, J. (1983). *How it feels when a parent dies.* New York: Knopf.

Little, J. (1984). *Mama's going to buy you a mockingbird.* New York: Viking.

Paterson, K. (1977). *Bridge to Terabithia.* New York: Cromwell.

Smith, D. B. (1973). *A taste of blackberries.* New York: HarperCollins.

Techner, D., & Hirt-Manheimer, J. (1993). *A candle for Grandpa: A guide to the Jewish funeral for children and parents.* New York: UAHC Press.

Traisman, E. S. (1992). *Fire in my heart, ice in my veins: A journal for teenagers experiencing a loss.* Omaha, NE: Centering Corporation.

White, E. B. (1952). *Charlotte's web.* New York: Harper.

For High School Students

Craven, M. (1973). *I heard the owl call my name.* New York: Dell.

Grollman, E., & Malikow, M. (1999). *Living when a young friend commits suicide.* Boston: Beacon Press.

Guest, J. (1976). *Ordinary people.* New York: Viking.

O'Toole, D. (1995). *Facing change: Falling apart and coming together again in the teen years.* Burnsville, NC: Compassion Books.

Scrivani, M. (1991). *When death walks in.* Omaha, NE: Centering Corporation.

Videos

For Adults Who Are Helping Grieving Children

Dougy Center. (1992). *Dougy's place: A 20-20 video.* Portland, OR: Author.

Ebeling, C., & Ebeling, D. (1991). *When grief comes to school.* Bloomington, IN: Bloomington Educational Enterprises.

Wolfelt, A. (1991). *A child's view of grief.* Fort Collins, CO: Center for Loss and Life Transition.

For Children

O'Toole, D. (1988). *Aarvy Aardvark finds hope.* Burnsville, NC: Compassion Press.

Rogers, F. (1993). *Mr. Rogers talks about living and dying.* Pittsburgh: Family Communications.

RESOURCES

Selected Training Programs and Certifications

PLAY THERAPY

Boston University School of Social
  Work
Postgraduate Certificate Program in
  Advanced Child and Adolescent
  Psychotherapy
264 Bay State Road
Boston, MA 02215
Phone: 617-353-3756
Fax: 617-353-5612
Website: *www.bu.edu/ssw/continue.*
  html

California School of Professional
  Psychology
Alliant University
5130 East Clinton Way
Fresno, CA 93727
Phone: 559-456-2777, ext. 2273
Fax: 559-253-267
Website: *www.cspp.edu/www.*
  alliant.edu

Center for Play Therapy
University of North Texas
P.O. Box 311337
Denton, TX 76203-1337
Phone: 940-565-3864
Website: *www.coe.unt.edu/cpt*

Chesapeake Beach Professional
  Seminars
3555 Ponds Wood Drive
Chesapeake Beach, MD 20732-3916
Phone: 410-535-4942
E-mail: *cbps@sbpsseminars.com*
Website: *www.cbpseminars.com*

New England Center for Sandplay
  Studies
31 Boston Avenue
Medford, MA 12155
Phone: 978-342-6070
E-mail: *JKneen@bu.edu*

International Society for Child
  and Play Therapy/Play Therapy
  International
Fern Hill Centre, Fern Hill
Fairwarp, Uckfield
Sussex TN22 3BU, United Kingdom
Phone: 44-1825-712360
Website: *www.playtherapy.org*

Theraplay Institute
1137 Central Avenue
Wilmette, IL 60091
Phone: 847-256-7334
E-mail: *theraplay@aol.com*
Website: *www.theraplay.org*

Play Therapy Training Institute
P.O. Box 1435
Hightstown, NJ 08520
Phone: 609-448-2145
Website: *www.ptti.org*

Post-Master's Certificate Program in
Child and Family Therapy
New York University
Rockland Branch Campus
Sparkill, NY 10976-1050
Phone: 845-398-4120
Website: *www.socialwork.nyu.edu/cft*

Vista Del Mar Child and Family
Services
3200 Motor Avenue
Los Angeles, CA 90034
Phone: 310-836-1223; Toll-Free:
888-22-VISTA
Website: *www.vistadelmar.org*

Vision Quest into Symbolic Reality
1946 Clemens Road
Oakland CA 94602
Phone: 510-530-1383
E-mail: *gisela@vision-quest.us*
Website: *vision-quest.us/vqisr/
trainings.htm*

GRIEF COUNSELING

Association for Death Education
Headquarters
60 Revere Drive, Suite 500
Northbrook, IL 60062
Phone: 847-509-0403
Website: *www.adec.org*

Certificate Program in Thanatology
College of New Rochelle
29 Castle Place
New Rochelle, NY 10805-2339
Phone: 914-654-5561; 914-654-5418
E-mail: *gs@cnr.edu*

Children's Hospice International
1101 King Street, Suite 131
Alexandria, VA 22314
Toll-Free: 800-242-CHILD

Dougy Center for Bereaved Children
P.O. Box 86582
Portland, OR 97286
Phone: 503-775-5683
Website: *www.doughy.org*

Hospice Foundation of America
2001 S Street, NE
Washington, DC 20002
Phone: 202-638-5419
Website: *www.hospicefoundation.
org*

Make-A-Wish Foundation of America
100 West Clarendon, Suite 2200
Phoenix, AZ 85013
Phone: 800-722-9474

National Center for Death Education
Mount Ida College
777 Dedham Street
Newton Centre, MA 02459
Phone: 617-928-4649
Website: *www.mountida.edu*

TRAUMA/CRISIS MENTAL HEALTH COUNSELING

American Academy of Experts in
   Traumatic Stress
368 Veterans Memorial Highway
Commack, NY 11725
Phone: 631-543-2217
Website: *www.aaets.org*

American Association of Suicidology
5221 Wisconsin Avenue, NW
Washington, DC 20008
Phone: 202-237-2280
Website: *www.suicidology.org*

Child Trauma Academy
5161 San Felipe, Suite 320
Houston, TX 77056
Phone: 281-932-1375
Website: *www.childtrauma.org*

Child Trauma Institute
P.O. Box 544
Greenfield, MA 01302-0544
Phone: 413-774-2340
Website: *www.childtrauma.com*

EMDR International Association
P.O. Box 141925
Austin, TX 78714-1925
Phone: 512-451-5200
Website: *www.emdria.org*

National Institute for Trauma and
   Loss in Children
900 Crook Road
Grosse Pointe Woods, MI 48236
Phone: 313-885-0390; Toll-Free:
   877-306-5256
Website: *www.tlcinst.org*

Suppliers of Play Materials

Sunburst Visual Media
(Childswork/Childsplay)
45 Executive Drive, Suite 201
P.O. Box 9120
Plainview, NY 11803-0760
Toll-Free: 800-962-1141
E-mail: *info@guidancechannel.com*
Website: *www.sunburstvm.com*

Childcraft Education Corporation
P.O. Box 3239
Lancaster, PA 17604
Toll-Free: 800-631-5652
Website: *www.childcrafteducation. com*

Creative Therapeutics
155 County Road
Cresskill, NJ 07626-0317
E-mail: *ct39@erols.com*;
    drgardnersrescources@yahoo.com
Website: *www.rgardner.com*

Magic Cabin
3700 Wyse Road
Dayton, OH 45414
Phone: 800-247-6106
Website: *www.magiccabin.com*

Rose Play Therapy
3670 Travelers Court
Snellville, GA 30039
Toll-Free: 800-713-2252
Website: *www.roseplay.com*

School Specialty
W6316 Design Drive
Greenville, WI 54942
Toll-Free: 888-388-3224
Website: *www.schoolspecialty.com*

Self-Esteem Shop
32839 Woodward Avenue
Royal Oak, MI 48073
Toll-Free: 800-251-8336
E-mail: *deanne@selfesteemshop.com*
Website: *www.selfesteemshop.com*

Toys to Grow On
2695 East Dominguez Street
P.O. Box 17
Carson, CA 90895
Toll-Free: 800-874-4242
E-mail: *toyinfo@toystogrowon.com*
Website: *www.lakeshorelearning. com/www.toystogrowon.com*

U.S. Toy Co., Inc.
Constructive Playthings
13201 Arrington Road
Grandview, MO 64030
Phone: 816-761-5900 (Kansas City
    area only); Toll-Free: 800-832-
    0572 or 800-448-4115
E-mail: *ustoy@ustoyco.com*
Website: *www.constplay.com*

Western Psychological Services
12031 Wilshire Boulevard
Los Angeles, CA 90025-1251
Toll-Free: 800-648-8857
Website: *www.wpspublish.com*

Bereavement Resources

American Hospice Foundation
2120 L Street, NW, Suite 200
Washington, DC 20037
Toll-Free: 800-447-1413
Website: *www.americanhospice.org*

Trains school professionals who work with grieving students. Supports programs for terminally ill and grieving individuals of all ages.

Association of Death Education and Counseling
60 Revere Drive, Suite 500
Northbrook, IL 60062
Phone: 847-509-0403
Website: *www.adec.org*

A multidisciplinary professional organization that provides information, support, and resources related to care of the dying, grief counseling, and research in thanatology.

Children's Hospice International
1101 King Street, Suite 360
Alexandria, VA 22314
Toll-Free: 800-24-CHILD
E-mail: *info@chionline.org*

Encourages the inclusion of children in existing hospice and home care programs, including pediatric care and training for those who care for children with life-threatening conditions and their families.

Compassion Books and The Compassion Books Catalog (formerly the
    Rainbow Collection)
7036 Highway 80 South
Burnsville, NC 28714

Toll-Free: 800-970-4220
Website: *www.compassionbooks.com*

Compassion Books is a mail-order catalog and Internet resource center of professional books, videos, and CDs related to loss and grief for children and adults across the lifespan.

National Alliance for Grieving Children
P.O. Box 1025
Northbrook, IL 60062
Phone: 866-432-1542
Website: *www.nationalallianceforgrievingchildren.org*

Provides resources and education to those supporting children and teens grieving a death. Has a searchable, state-by-state database of children's grief centers and programs.

National Center for Death Education Library
Mount Ida College
777 Dedham Street
Newton Center, MA 02159
Phone: 617-969-7000, ext. 249

Maintains a collection of print and audiovisual materials on all aspects of dying, death, and bereavement. Some may be borrowed on interlibrary loan. For information, contact Coordinator of Resources.

References on Religious/ Cultural/Ethnic Practices Related to Death

Berger, A., Badham, P., Kutscher, A. H., Berger, J., Perry, M., & Beloff, J. (1989). (Eds.). *Perspectives on death and dying: Cross cultural and multidisciplinary view*. Philadelphia: Charles Press.

Coles, R. (1990). *The spiritual life of children* [Christian salvation, pp. 202–224; Islamic surrender, pp. 225–248; Jewish righteousness, pp. 249–276]. Boston: Houghton Mifflin.

Corr, C. A., Nabe, C. M., & Corr, D. M. (2000). *Death and dying: Life and living* (3rd ed.). Belmont, CA: Wadsworth. [See pp. 119–120, 508–519, and 521–523 for discussion about different religious perspectives on death.]

Grollman, E. A. (Ed.). (1967). *Explaining death to children*. Boston: Beacon Press.

Johnson, C. J., & McGee, M. G. (Eds.). (1991). *How different religions view death and afterlife*. Philadelphia: Charles Press.

Kastenbaum, R. J. (2008). *Death, society, and human experience* (10th ed.). Boston: Pearson. [See pp. 438–442 for a discussion about how different religions view the topic of survival after death.]

McGoldrick, M., Almeida, R., Hines, P. M., Garcia-Preto, N., Rosen, E., & Lee, E. (1991). Mourning in different cultures. In F. Walsh & M. McGoldrick (Eds.), *Living beyond loss: Death in the family* (pp. 176–206). New York: Norton. [A list of references at the end of this chapter cites additional sources related to the following cultural/religious groups: Irish, Indian, African American, Jewish, and Puerto Rican.]

Ryan, J. A. (1986). *Ethnic, cultural and religious observances at the time of death and dying*. Boston: Good Grief Program.

Index

Violent death *(cont.)*
  crisis response teams for, 196,
    199–200
  disenfranchised grief, 100–104
  disenfranchised grief and, 95–96
  education about and prevention of,
    194–195
  resources on, 200, 201
  of siblings, 77
Volunteers
  for bereavement camps, 307–309
  in crisis teams, 204
VT. *See* Vicarious trauma

W

Wakes, attendance at, 18, 376–377
Walsh, F., 41, 326
War
  media exposure to, 215–216,
    220–228
  PTSD and exposure to, 228–234
War-related death
  case example, 152–154, 158–160
  cycles of deployment and, 149
  financial support after, 156
  intervention issues in, 154–158
  notification of, 156–157
  overview of, 147–148, 150
  resources for, 157–158
  statistics on, 151–152
  unexpected, 150
Webb, N. B., 3, 12, 22, 29, 32, 55,
71, 109, 114, 115, 116, 117, 119,
121, 122, 129, 160, 168, 170,
173, 181, 192, 220, 243, 256,
263, 272, 281, 284, 297, 298,
300, 301, 305, 306, 346, 374,
375
Websites
  on bereavement, 390–391
  chat lines, 138
  grief counseling, 386
  play material suppliers, 388–389
  play therapy, 385–386
  trauma and crisis mental health
    counseling, 387
  www.remembered-forever.org,
    207
When I Die, Will I get Better?
  (Breebaart and Breebaart), 323,
  325–326, 337
Wholeness, stories that resonate,
  331–333
Wolfelt, A., 7, 9, 16, 18, 22, 36–37,
  40, 129, 141
Wolfenstein, M., 11, 12, 16
Wood, S. K., 321–322
Worden, J. W., 9, 45, 156, 296, 297,
  298, 309, 310, 312
Work settings, and ecological
  prevention model, 367–368

Y

Yoga, as self-care activity, 364–36